Nutrition and Safety for Preschoolers

MW00979180

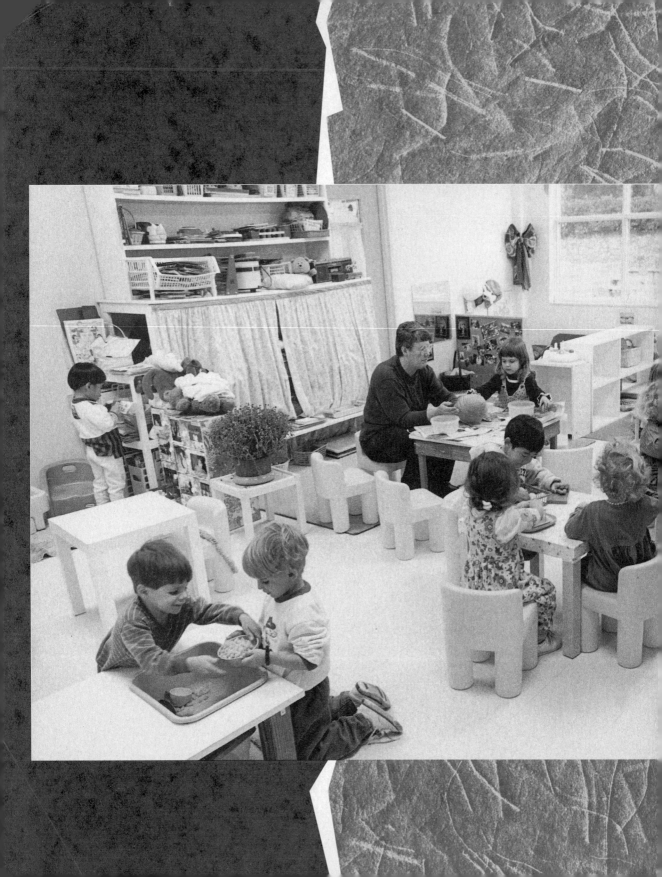

Nutrition, Health, and Safety for Preschool Children

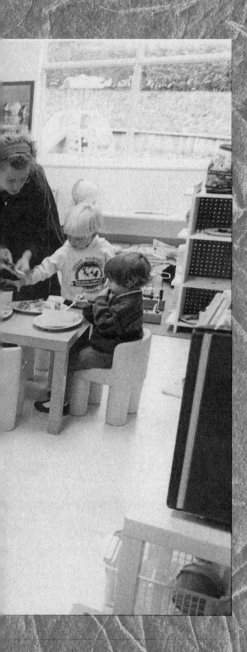

Roberta L. Duyff
Food and Nutrition Consultant
President, Duyff Associates
St. Louis, Missouri

Susan C. Giarratano
Professor, Health Science Department
California State University, Long Beach

Mary F. Zuzich
Project Director, Open Horizons
Tempe, Arizona
Visiting Faculty, Early Childhood Development
Scottsdale Community College

GLENCOE

McGraw-Hill

New York, New York
Columbus, Ohio
Mission Hills, California
Peoria, Illinois

Copyright © 1995 by Glencoe/McGraw-Hill. All rights reserved. Except as permitted under the United States Copyright Act, no part of this publication may be reproduced or distributed in any form or by any means, or stored in a database or retrieval system, without prior written permission of the publisher.

Send all inquiries to:
Glencoe/McGraw-Hill
936 Eastwind Drive
Westerville, OH 43081

ISBN 0-02-802089-8 (Student Edition)
ISBN 0-02-802091-X (Instructor's Guide)
ISBN 0-02-802092-8 (Study Guide)
ISBN 0-02-802093-6 (Test Bank)

Printed in the United States of America

1 2 3 4 5 6 7 8 9 10   POH   00 99 98 97 96 95 94

Library of Congress Cataloging-in-Publication Data

Duyff, Roberta Larson.
    Nutrition, health, and safety for preschool children / Roberta L. Duyff,
Susan C. Giarratano, Mary F. Zuzich.
        p.   cm.
    Includes bibliographical references and index.
    ISBN 0-02-802089-8 (Student ed.) — ISBN 0-02-802091-X (Instructor's guide) —
    ISBN 0-02-802092-8 (Study guide)
    1. Preschool children — Health and hygiene.   2. Preschool children — Care.
    3. Preschool children — Nutrition.   I. Giarratano, Susan.
    II. Zuzich, Mary F.   III. Title.
    RJ101.D89   1995
    613.2 ' 083 ' 3 — dc20
                                                                    94-4626
                                                                    CIP

Co-developed by
Glencoe/McGraw-Hill
and Visual Education Corporation
Princeton, NJ

Consultants and Reviewers

Consultants

Roseanne Dlugosz
Program Coordinator, Early Childhood Development
Scottsdale Community College
Scottsdale, California

Gail C. Frank
Professor of Nutrition
California State University, Long Beach
Adjunct Professor of Medicine and Pediatrics
University of California, Irvine

Reviewers

Ginny A. Buckner
Assistant Professor and Program Coordinator
Early Childhood Education
Cuyahoga Community College
Cleveland, Ohio

Margaret S. Budz
Program Coordinator, Early Childhood Education
Triton College
River Grove, Illinois

Robyn Flipse
Nutrition Consultant
Ocean, New Jersey

Harriet S. Nagel
Director and Head Teacher
Nutritional Sciences Preschool, Rutgers University
New Brunswick, New Jersey

Credits and Acknowledgments

Special thanks to:

Carnegie Family Center, Princeton, NJ

The Harmony Schools, Princeton, NJ

Janssen Child Development Center, A Quality
    Program of Resources for Child Care
    Management, Titusville, NJ

Princeton University League Nursery School,
    Princeton, NJ

Mercer Children's Center, Mercer Medical Center,
    Trenton, NJ

Photo Credits:

Denise Applewhite: 287

Dwight Cendrowski: 171, 181, 227, 362

Kent and Donna Dannen: 116

H. Armstrong Roberts: 143, 240, 313
    J. Nettis: 64

Cliff Moore: Title page, 2–3, 5, 15, 24–25, 26, 29, 31, 48,
    53, 55, 56, 67, 68, 69, 74, 77, 85, 87, 88, 91, 93, 95,
    100–101, 102, 106, 113, 126, 139, 145, 150, 165, 167,
    176, 179, 191, 193, 200, 203, 211, 213, 222–223, 224,
    229, 231, 242, 244, 250, 253, 256, 264, 280, 285, 290,
    299, 308, 319, 328, 333, 340–341, 342, 346, 349, 357,
    366, 376, 381, 383, 385

PhotoEdit:
    Cleo: 119, 129
    Robert Brenner: 41
    Mary Kate Denny: 6
    Myrleen Ferguson: 39
    Tony Freeman: 216
    W. Rosin Malecki: 110
    Tom McCarthy: 235
    Elena Rooraid: 316
    Wolfgang Spunbarg: 9
    David Young-Wolff: 295, 347

Kathy Sloane: 272

Terry Wild Studio: 43, 60, 140, 168, 351

Shirley Zeiberg: 20, 154, 206, 373

Preface

Nutrition, health, and safety are primary concerns in the care and teaching of young children. Understanding nutritional needs, principal health issues, and safety considerations helps early childhood professionals provide an environment in which children can grow and develop to their full potential. Teaching young children about nutrition, health, and safety helps them become self-caring individuals as time goes on.

This book focuses on those aspects of nutrition, health, and safety that are most important to those who work with young children as professional caregivers and teachers.

Content

The book begins with an overview of nutrition, health, and safety that emphasizes their interrelationship and the influences of heredity and the environment on each. These themes and their practical implications are interwoven throughout the book.

Part 1 presents basic information that forms a foundation for discussion of the nutritional needs of young children. It contains chapters on food patterns and how they form, basic facts about nutrients, and guidelines for healthful eating.

Part 2 is devoted to the nutritional needs of the growing child. It begins with a chapter on growth and development and nutritional influences on this process. This is followed by chapters on the nutritional needs of infants, toddlers, and preschoolers. A chapter on children with special nutritional needs completes this section of the book.

Part 3 addresses issues of health and safety in the child care setting. Of two chapters on health, one considers general health policies and procedures in the child care setting; the other covers infectious diseases affecting children. Safety

concerns that are discussed include providing safe environments for young children and teaching and practicing behaviors that promote children's safety.

The final part of the book provides general guidance on teaching children about nutrition, health, and safety. It consists of a chapter on curriculum with practical advice on lesson planning and a chapter on ways to involve parents in the nutrition, health, and safety program.

Throughout the text, the term used for early childhood professionals who work with children from birth to 3 years is *caregiver*; from 3 to 5 years the term used is *teacher*. For children, the following terms apply: infants—from birth to 1 year; toddlers—from 1 to 3 years; preschoolers—from 3 to 5 years; and school-age children—from 6 to 8 years. The term *parent* is intended to include guardian, thus the latter term will rarely be found. *Health care professional* or *health care provider* is used in preference to doctor or physician in recognition of alternative systems of health care. The text uses either female or male examples in order to avoid awkward he/she and him/her constructions. Where weights and measures are discussed, the system in common usage appears first and the metric conversion follows. The exception to this rule is the nutritional guidance on particular nutrients for which metric measurements such as gram and milligram have become well accepted.

Each chapter of the book begins with learning objectives and a list of important terms. Within the chapter, these terms are highlighted in *italics*; they are defined again in the Glossary at the back of the book. Author or title and publication date of each source are cited in the text (Pillitteri, 1992); full bibliographic information is provided in the References section at the back of the book.

Special Features

The book's practical emphasis is reinforced with a series of special features on topics of immediate concern to caregivers and teachers of preschool children. At least three of these appear in each chapter.

Focus on Cultural Diversity discusses a variety of topics designed to illustrate differences in customs and values among various groups of people. The theme of multiculturalism runs throughout the text as well.

Focus on Promoting Healthful Habits covers situations in which a child care professional can help children develop healthful attitudes and habits or must act on behalf of a child to protect his health. Students are asked to consider their own approaches to such a matter and how it might differ from the approach described.

Focus on Communicating presents discussions of both everyday problems and extremely sensitive topics. Written in dialogue format, the feature illustrates one way—not necessarily the best—that a caregiver or teacher might communicate with parents or children. It invites students to consider other ways of handling the communication.

One of three short pieces may complete a particular chapter's complement of special features. *Wholesome Snacks* are simple recipes for nutritious snack foods. *Health Tips* are short presentations of practical guidance on health concerns. *Safety Tips* provide quick guidelines on issues of safety.

End of Chapter Materials

Each chapter ends with a comprehensive review. This includes a *Summary* of important points covered; *Acquiring Knowledge*, a section that can be used to review chapter content; and *Thinking Critically*, a section that raises questions caregivers and teachers need to consider. *Observations and Applications* propose various situations in which students can practice observational skills and apply their knowledge of nutrition, health, and safety. *For Further Information* lists relevant publications and, where appropriate, organizations.

Supplementary Materials

The *Instructor's Guide* is a useful teaching support tool. It includes *Teaching Strategies* for each chapter in the text, *Chapter Tests,* and a list of sources for teaching nutrition, health, and safety.

The *Study Guide* is a workbook that provides students with a means of checking their mastery of the material covered in the text. *Study Questions* review the content, concepts, and vocabulary of each chapter. *Observation Activities* direct students to observe in the field firsthand the kinds of activities and behavior they are studying in the text. *Application Activities* require students to apply their knowledge to case studies and current issues in nutrition, health, and safety at the preschool level.

Test Bank. The computerized *Test Bank* provides a variety of questions that can be used to build a customized test for students. The software leaves room for instructors to add their own questions. Answers are included.

Contents

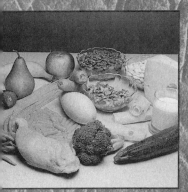

Part 1
Nutrition:
The Science of Food   24

Chapter 3:
Nutrition Basics   48

Chapter 4:
Overall Planning for Healthful Eating   74

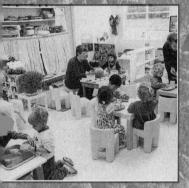

Part 2
Different Needs
at Different Ages 100

Chapter 5:
Growth and Development 102

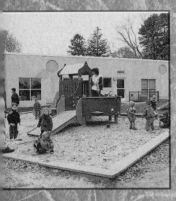

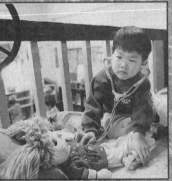

Part 4
Teaching Nutrition, Health, and Safety   340

Chapter 14:
Curriculum Design and Lesson Planning   342

Chapter 15:
Approaches to Parent Involvement 366

Introducing Nutrition, Health, and Safety

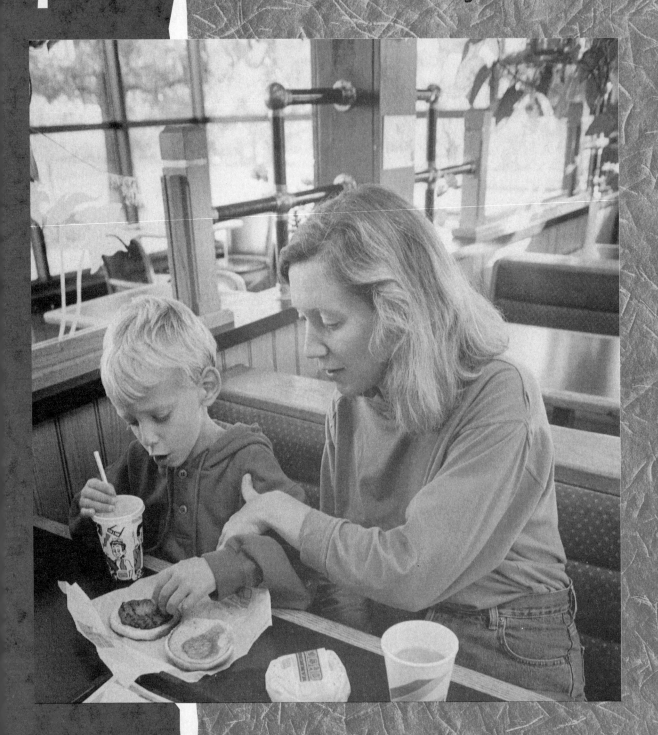

OBJECTIVES

Studying this chapter
will enable you to

- Describe the importance of
nutrition in the lives of young
children and the caregiver's role in
providing sound nutrition
- Discuss the variety of influences on
health and the caregiver's role in
protecting the health of children
- List and explain ways caregivers
can protect the safety of children
in their care
- Discuss the ways that nutrition,
health, and safety are interrelated
and describe the hereditary and
environmental influences that
affect the well-being of children

CHAPTER TERMS

health
heredity
malnutrition
nutrients
nutrition
overnutrition
safety
undernutrition

AT five o'clock, Lorraine left her office and drove over to the Busy Bee Child Care Center to pick up four-year-old Alexander. When she got there, Alexander was intensely involved in building a fort with one of his playmates. While Alexander played, Lorraine talked with Alexander's teacher, Bev.

"What a day!" Lorraine exclaimed. "One crisis after another. I only had time for an apple at lunch."

"I bet you'll be glad to get home," Bev answered. "You must be really hungry by now."

"I am," Lorraine said. "But that reminds me. I don't have a thing in the house for dinner! By the time I stop at the store, make dinner, and get it on the table it will be seven o'clock." She shook her head. "I think we'll just go out for dinner tonight."

Alexander, who had been engrossed in his game, suddenly paid attention to his mother's conversation. "Yippee!" he said. "Let's go for hamburgers and french fries! And root beer, Mommy, root beer!"

Lorraine shrugged her shoulders and gave Bev a guilty grin. "I feel a little bad about going to a fast-food restaurant for dinner. I know neither of us is going to get a balanced meal."

Bev glanced over at Alexander and back to Lorraine. "Well, you'll have a tough time getting him to go anywhere else, now. Fast food isn't bad now and then. But next time you feel too tired to cook, you might try the new place on Oak Lane. It has a great salad bar. My kids love it!"

"Sounds good to me," said Lorraine. "He likes being able to pick out his own vegetables." She turned to her son. "Come on Alexander, let's go eat."

Nutrition

Lorraine's story is worth telling—not because it is so unusual, but because millions of parents go through a similar experience every day. While the occasional fast-food meal is not cause for concern, the choices people routinely make, wherever they eat, are. Children need a balanced diet for their growth and development as well as their health. Understanding why a balanced diet is so important to health, growth, and development requires an understanding of nutrition.

Nutrition is the study and science of the foods people consume as well as the physical processes that are involved in taking in and using food. Nutrition is just one of the three major factors that contribute to a child's overall well-being. The other two factors—health and safety—are equally important. These three factors cannot be isolated from one another; any change in one affects the others.

Importance of Sound Nutrition

Substances in food that provide nourishment and help the body to function are called *nutrients*. The major nutrients are proteins, carbohydrates (sugars, starches, and fiber), fats, vitamins, minerals, and water. (You will learn more about individual nutrients in Chapter 3.) Each food contains a different combination of types and quantities of nutrients. People need different amounts of nutrients at different stages in their lives. The needs of an infant, for example, are quite different from those of a one- to three-year-old toddler. And the toddler's needs are different from those of a three- to five-year-old preschooler. (The different nutritional needs of infants, toddlers, and preschoolers are discussed in chapters 6, 7, and 8, respectively.) Child care professionals need a good working knowledge of the nutritional needs of the children in their care.

Nutrition is a very important factor in determining whether a particular individual will reach his full potential over time. Unlike some other health-related factors, nutrition is something over which people have direct control. Each time people put food into their mouths—or provide food for the children in their care—they make a choice. A number of factors influence those choices and play a part in determining the foods people eat.

A family's socioeconomic status will have a strong influence on the food they eat. People with low incomes may not be able to afford the variety of

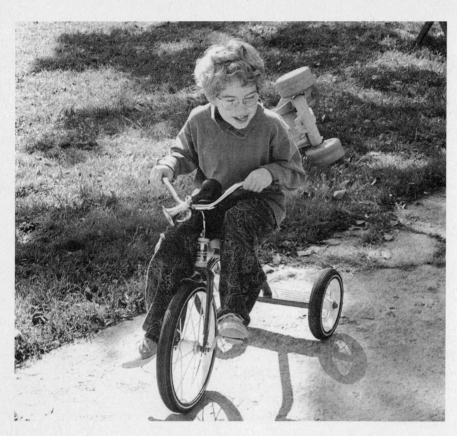

Active children need nutrients to help their bodies function.

foods they need. Their access to healthful food may also be limited by the stores they can get to. Many low-income families shop in small neighborhood groceries with limited selections of fresh fruits and vegetables.

A family's cultural background also influences the foods its members eat. Different ethnic groups tend to emphasize certain foods and food preparation styles. For example, the Chinese make extensive use of vegetables and rice in their diet; Italians often start their meals with pasta and make robust sauces with tomatoes, olive oil, garlic, and herbs. Children develop food likes and dislikes that are heavily influenced by the ethnic customs in their backgrounds. They generally carry these food preferences with them into adulthood. The social activities that families engage in also have an effect on what family members eat. Imagine a ball game without hot dogs or a movie without popcorn.

Yet another factor that affects what people eat is their emotional state. Emotions such as depression, excitement, anger, or stress may cause people to eat more than usual or to lose interest in food altogether.

Education also plays an important role. The more information people have about sound nutrition, the more likely it is that they will make wise food choices. Fortunately, making wise food choices is easier today than it used to be, thanks to the greater availability of year-round fresh fruits and vegetables and to the labeling information on most prepared foods.

Nutrition and learning go hand in hand. Well-nourished children are more alert and have longer attention spans.

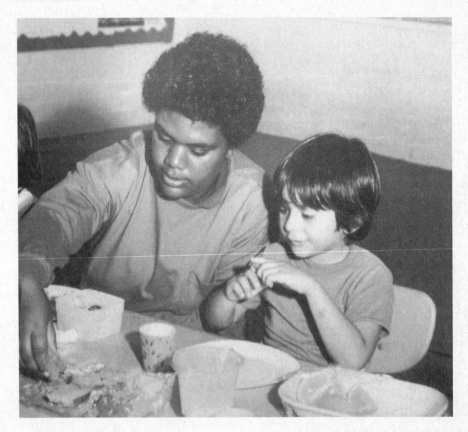

There are, then, many influences on people's food choices, and there are many foods from which they can choose. This is fortunate, because eating a variety of foods is the best way for people to be sure they are getting the nutrients they need. This is particularly important for young children. Studies have shown that nutritional deficiencies, or severe shortages of essential nutrients, during specific stages of infancy and early childhood can have an irreversible impact on physical development (Alford & Bogle, 1982). A prolonged severe episode of malnutrition in early childhood may also cause permanent mental retardation.

Malnutrition results when a person is poorly nourished for an extended period of time. Malnutrition can be caused either by undernutrition or by overnutrition. In *undernutrition,* people do not eat enough foods containing essential nutrients. When people do not take in the necessary nutrients, various disorders develop. For example, a diet lacking in iron can lead to anemia. (The most common deficiency disorders are discussed in detail in Chapter 9).

Overnutrition is caused by consuming too much of one or more nutrients and can be as damaging as undernutrition. Overnutrition can occur when a person frequently makes unwise food selections. If Lorraine and Alexander chose to eat hamburgers, french fries, and soft drinks every day, they would run the risk of being overnourished for some nutrients and undernourished for others. Eating habits that involve an excessive intake of sugars and fats at the expense of other important nutrients can lead to excessive weight gain and to the health problems associated with being overweight. They can also result in undernutrition with regard to particular vitamins or minerals that would be obtained from fresh fruits, vegetables, and milk. On a diet of hamburgers, fries, and soda, for example, Alexander would not get the calcium he needs for developing strong bones and teeth.

Nutrition also has an influence on learning. Children who are well nourished are more observant and alert and have longer attention spans. As a result, they are more likely to benefit from their educational experiences. Children who are undernourished or overnourished tend to have a more difficult time concentrating on the work at hand. These children are often withdrawn or hyperactive. Either type of behavior makes learning more difficult (Galler, 1984).

Nutrition and Child Care

Depending on the facility in which they work, caregivers will have either a direct or an indirect influence on the nutrition of the children in their care. Child care centers that provide meals can make sure that they supply a variety of foods and nutrients. Many prepare weekly menus that are distributed to parents, and parents are invited to comment.

Such comments from parents can be helpful in a number of ways. For example, parents can inform caregivers of strong family food preferences. Then parents and caregivers can discuss how to incorporate family favorites into the menu. Some parents might suggest that the center include certain ethnic foods on the menu from time to time. Other parents might get ideas from the menus for improving the nutritional variety in their own homes.

Not all child care facilities provide food for the children. In some cases, the children bring their own lunches and snacks from home. In such cases, caregivers maintain an interest in children's nutrition. Observing what children bring to eat can help caregivers spot potential nutritional problems and discuss them with parents in tactful ways. Most parents welcome information that benefits their children. In the story that opened this chapter, Bev was able to offer a helpful suggestion about the new restaurant without making Lorraine feel bad about her dinner plans for that evening. Familiarity with the child and the family is crucial, since a family's circumstances may place limits on their nutritional choices.

Health

The foods that people eat have an important influence on their health. *Health* is the state of a person's overall physical, mental, and emotional well-being. Two other factors that directly affect a person's health are heredity and the environment. The characteristics and conditions a person inherits from her parents and the surroundings in which the person lives play key roles in determining the level of health she experiences.

WHOLESOME SNACKS

Peanut Butter Raisin Snowballs

Ingredients:

1 cup creamy or smooth peanut butter
1 cup raisins
½ cup flaked coconut

Directions:

1. Mix peanut butter and raisins in a small bowl.
2. Spread coconut on a plate and roll ½ to 1 teaspoon of peanut butter mixture in the coconut until loosely covered.
3. Set aside on a sheet of waxed paper and continue until mixture is used.

You may substitute chopped dates or another chopped dried fruit for the raisins.

This recipe is intended for children over the age of four.

Yield: 15 servings

Each serving contains:

Calories: 140
Protein: 6 g
Fat: 9.5 g
Carbohydrates: 11 g

Role of Heredity

Heredity refers to the sum of the traits, characteristics, and defects that are passed from parents to their children through genetic mechanisms. At conception, a set of genes is produced; half come from the sperm cell of the father and half from the egg cell of the mother. The interaction of maternal and paternal genes at conception determines the blueprint, potential, and limits for various traits and disorders.

Eye color, blood type, and skin color are examples of traits that are inherited. Other traits such as height and build are thought to be controlled by both genes and the environment. Complex traits such as intelligence and personality also seem to be influenced by a combination of heredity and environmental factors.

Certain disorders, including sickle cell disease and cystic fibrosis, have been found to be hereditary. Heredity also plays a role in a person's resistance or susceptibility to certain disorders. The level of cholesterol in the blood, for example, is influenced by heredity. People who inherit a tendency to have high blood cholesterol levels run an increased risk of developing diseases of the heart and blood vessels.

While scientists have not yet been able to develop ways to correct defective genes, many genetic disorders can be treated. Treatment may involve special diets, as with phenylketonuria (PKU). Some mental disorders that involve an inherited chemical imbalance in the brain can be kept in check through drug therapy.

There is some hope for correcting defective genes through genetic engineering. Scientists have been able to identify and locate several missing or abnormal genes. The challenge now is to find a way to replace these defective genes with healthy ones.

Role of the Environment

Heredity is an important influence on health over which people have little control. Environment, another important influence, is more controllable. A child's environment—his physical, economic, social, and cultural setting—plays a significant role in determining his level of physical, mental, and emotional health.

The Physical Setting. A child's physical surroundings have an enormous impact on her health. A clean, comfortable, and stimulating environment allows a child to reach optimum levels of health and well-being.

However, the opposite is also true. The health of children who live in crowded and unsanitary conditions will be jeopardized. Such living conditions promote the spread of disease. So, too, do environments that have poor ventilation and temperatures that cannot be adequately controlled. And environments that are excessively noisy can pose a threat to children's hearing. Homelessness poses a particular threat to children's health. Studies of homeless children have shown that they suffer more physical and mental disorders than poor children who live in a permanent home (Bassuk & Rosenberg, 1990).

Any home, however, no matter how affluent, can pose a threat to children's health. Indoor air pollution—caused by smoke and other substances—can cause serious health problems. Recent research strongly links secondhand smoke from tobacco to asthma in children ("Stronger Data Link Smoking," June 15, 1993). Radon, a colorless, odorless radioactive gas that is released from natural materials in the ground, can reach dangerous concentrations inside buildings. Exposure to high levels of radon is linked to lung cancer.

The Economic Setting. Family economic circumstances can affect children's health in a number of ways. As already discussed, family income plays a significant role in the kind of physical environment provided for the child. It also affects the amount, the quality, and the variety of foods, particularly fresh foods, that the family can afford—and thus the supply of nutrients to the growing child.

Economic factors affect children's health in other ways as well. For example, the level of medical and dental care children receive is often influenced by family income. People with low incomes (or with no incomes) often do

Children from low-income families are at a higher risk of having health and developmental problems.

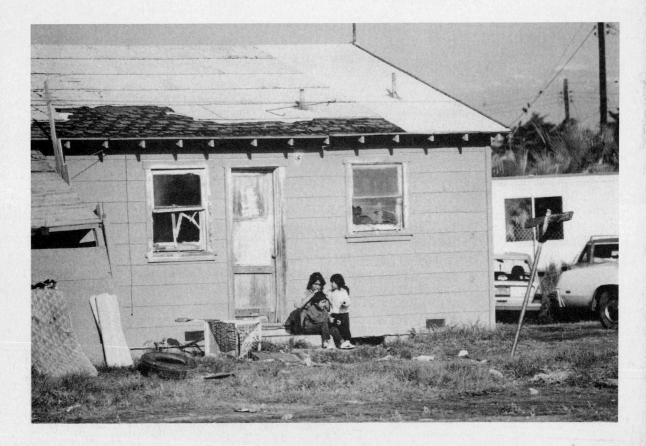

Limiting the Spread of Colds

It is the end of the day at the Bloomfield Avenue Kinderschool. Mrs. Finney, three-year-old Tamara's mother, has come to pick Tamara up. Mrs. Finney stops to talk to Joanne, one of the caregivers, about a health issue that has been bothering her.

MRS. FINNEY: Hello, Joanne. Is Tamara ready?

JOANNE: Hi, Mrs. Finney. Tamara is just putting away a puzzle. She'll be ready to go in a minute.

MRS. FINNEY: Has she been coughing much today?

JOANNE: Not that I've noticed. Has she had a cold?

MRS. FINNEY: It seems like she's had a cold since the beginning of the school year. She was never sick before she started here, and now she has a runny nose all the time.

JOANNE: A lot of the younger children's parents say the same thing.

MRS. FINNEY: There must be something the school can do to keep these kids from getting sick all the time.

JOANNE: Well, we send children home if Mrs. Owens, the director, thinks they're too sick to be here. We tell them to cover their mouths when they cough or sneeze, and to use tissues to wipe their noses. We also make sure they wash their hands after sneezing or wiping their noses and before meals and snacks.

MRS. FINNEY: What about the toys? The children cough and sneeze on them all the time.

JOANNE: Sometimes they do sneeze on the toys. If one of us sees that happen, we disinfect the toy right away.

MRS. FINNEY: How often do you clean all the toys?

JOANNE: All the rubber and plastic toys are washed and disinfected with a bleach solution at the end of each day. At least once a week, the wooden toys—the blocks and trucks—are wiped off and disinfected, too.

MRS. FINNEY: Aren't there some toys you can't wash?

JOANNE: I can't think of any toy here that can't be wiped off. It's school policy to buy toys that are easy to clean.

MRS. FINNEY: Well, I guess you clean as much as you can. And you can't keep the children from playing with the toys just because they have runny noses.

JOANNE: It would be pretty hard.

MRS. FINNEY: I still wish there was some way to keep Tamara from getting sick so often.

JOANNE: All I can tell you is that the older children—the ones who were here last year—don't get sick nearly as often as the younger ones. They seem to develop immunities after the first year.

MRS. FINNEY: I certainly hope so!

Do you think the information Joanne gave to Mrs. Finney was helpful? What else would you have said to reassure her?

not have health insurance, and they may be unable to afford to take their children to a doctor when the children are sick. They may also be unable to afford preventive medicine, such as immunizations for their children or pre-natal medical care. According to a 1992 U. S. government report, "The conse-quences of child poverty are well documented. From the womb to adulthood, poor children are at higher risk of health, developmental, and educational setbacks—problems that are likely to follow them through life" (Children's Defense Fund, 1992, p. 26).

The Social Setting.   A child's relationship with his parents, with mem-bers of his extended family, and with caregivers in a child care setting all af-fect his overall state of health. Warm, supportive relationships enhance physical, mental, and emotional health. In a classic study, one-year-old ba-bies were separated from their mothers for a few minutes. Some babies ex-hibited only mild distress, then sought their mothers out and were readily comforted by them upon the mothers' return. The pattern of attachment for these babies was defined as secure. Other babies exhibited great distress on their mothers' leaving and refused to be comforted on their return. Still oth-ers showed no reaction to the mother's departure or return. The pattern for both of these groups was defined as insecure (Ainsworth & Wittig, 1969). In a later study, when children who had been identified at the age of 18 months as securely attached to their mothers were observed 6 months later, they were found to be more enthusiastic, persistent, and cooperative than their insecurely attached counterparts (Matas, Arend, & Sroufe, 1978).

Traumas to a primary relationship, whether from death, separation, or in-adequate affection, can affect a child in many ways, ranging from a de-pressed or overactive appetite to a loss of achievement motivation or other serious emotional disturbances. It is important that caregivers be caring and competent and work with the same children consistently.

Other social relationships that affect health include extended familial re-lations and relations with peers. Strained relations among extended family members can place children in stressful situations they may not be equipped to handle. Children may have difficulty forming healthy peer relationships if they have poor role models for friendly behavior at home. Other children, such as those who are obese or extremely shy, may become targets for teas-ing. If children are taught or perceive that they are not valued by others, their self-esteem will be eroded.

The Cultural Setting.   The beliefs, customs, and social behaviors of a group can have a major impact on children's health. Just as parents tend to pass on the nutritional habits of their cultural groups, so they tend to follow other aspects of their culture's life-style that affect the health of their chil-dren. The Chinese, for example, regard a healthy body as a gift from ances-tors and believe that it must be cared for. This belief reinforces the importance of good nutrition. On the other hand, the Chinese also believe that, out of respect for the body, the body should be intact at death. This be-lief may prompt some Chinese to refuse surgery (Whaley & Wong, 1991).

Vietnamese people tend to regard certain illnesses as temporary and may do nothing about them. Because they feel the family is responsible for health, many Vietnamese people will not go to an outside agency for a health problem until they have exhausted all possible home remedies (Whaley & Wong, 1991). Meanwhile, a serious condition may worsen. In just about every culture, beliefs and behaviors such as these can be resources for or barriers to good health.

Developmental expectations are also different among cultures. The Japanese, for example, tend to be permissive about the behavior and emotional expression of children under five or six years of age. Older children, however, are encouraged to restrain their emotions and exhibit self-control. This emphasis on control can make it difficult for a health care professional to determine how much discomfort an older child is experiencing (Whaley & Wong, 1991).

Health and Child Care

Child care workers need to be aware of factors (hereditary, economic, social, and cultural) that affect the health of the children in their care. This knowledge will allow them to promote health most effectively and deal adequately with health problems that occur.

Caregivers also have a direct responsibility for protecting and promoting the health of the children in their care. This includes encouraging healthful patterns of exercise, rest, and quiet activities. Caregivers should also take action to prevent the spread of disease within the child care setting. Keeping the environment clean and free from germs is an important component of health. A child care setting that is not clean can contribute to the spread of infectious diseases, which threaten the health of children, their families, and their caregivers. Most of the communicable diseases that children contract in group settings are transmitted by coughing and sneezing, inadequate sanitation in diapering or toileting, direct contact, or contact with blood or other body fluids.

For each age group, specific sanitary concerns apply. The primary source of infection among infants is in the diaper-changing area. Inadequate disinfection of hands and surfaces can lead to a number of infectious diseases. Additional areas of concern for older infants and toddlers are the surfaces they play on and the toys they play with. Older infants frequently mouth their toys and pass them back and forth. Viruses and other sources of infection can go from the mouth to a toy or from the hands to a toy—and then to another child. With older children, the primary target of concern is the bathroom. Bathroom floors and surfaces should be washed and sanitized daily. Children should be given frequent instruction and careful supervision when washing their hands.

Child care workers can also learn to recognize the signs and symptoms of various childhood diseases and know what actions to take when a child is sick, both to protect the child and to protect those around him. Finally, caregivers can develop good communication with parents so that important

FOCUS ON — Promoting Healthful Habits

Picnic in the Park

It is the first day of spring. The four-year-old class from the Walker Child Care Center is about to leave for a picnic at a neighborhood park. "Hat check!" calls Annette, one of the caregivers. The Walker staff is always careful that the children wear brimmed hats to protect their faces from the sun, especially at midday.

Out the door they head, walking two by two and holding hands. There is one major intersection on the way. When the children reach it, Annette stops the group. She points to the traffic light and asks the children what color the light should be before they cross. "Green, green!" the children call out. This morning's traffic safety play is fresh in their minds.

"And let's not forget to look both ways before we step into the crosswalk," says Annette.

When they reach the park, Emilio, the other caregiver, finds a picnic table under a tree. The children help set out paper plates, napkins, and cups. Apple juice, kept cold in an insulated container, is a big hit with the thirsty four-year-olds. A lunch of peanut butter and jelly sandwich quarters, cheese cubes, carrot sticks, and banana chunks is also a treat. "Picnics have the best food!" pronounces Jeremy, enjoying a crisp carrot stick.

After everyone has finished, Emilio helps the children gather their plates, cups, and napkins and deposit them in the trash can. "Good job, everyone," says Emilio.

Meanwhile, Annette checks the nearby playground for pieces of broken glass, trash, and unsafe equipment. After she has made sure that the playground is safe, she and Emilio supervise while the children play on the swings and climber and in the sandbox.

Finally, the children line up for the walk back to the center. As they approach the intersection, Carey speaks up "Don't forget to look both ways!"

Could the caregivers have done anything else to keep the children safe on the trip to the park? What else would you have told the children?

health information can be freely exchanged. Chapters 10 and 11 in this book discuss these and other important health topics for caregivers.

Safety

The well-being of a child goes beyond nutrition and health. Where children are concerned, safety must be included as an integral part of the picture. *Safety* is freedom from risk, harm, and injury. Each year, more children die of injuries than of all diseases combined. Each year, one out of every five children requires medical attention for an injury (University of California at Berkeley Wellness Newsletter, April 1993). Clearly, a strong emphasis on safety is essential for anyone who works with children. The safety of the children in her care is, in fact, the first responsibility of any child care professional.

When it comes to safety, caregivers need to focus on three main aspects: creating a safe environment, teaching and modeling safe behaviors, and knowing what to do if there is an accident.

A Safe Environment

A safe environment is one that takes children's needs and abilities into account. To provide a safe setting for young children, caregivers need to understand children's developmental abilities. An environment that is perfectly safe for infants could prove treacherous for toddlers or completely inadequate for the needs of preschoolers.

Knowing the most likely sources of danger is the first step toward providing a safe environment. Caregivers should be aware of the most common hazards for young children. These include:

- Mechanical suffocation
- Aspiration and choking
- Burns
- Electrical shock
- Poisoning
- Falls
- Drowning
- Motor vehicle injuries

Chapter 12 provides detailed information for caregivers on how to prevent these types of injuries.

The Indoor Environment.   Indoor spaces for children should be appropriate for their ages and abilities. Most experts recommend separate play areas for infants, toddlers, and older children. This arrangement allows younger children to explore their area freely without fear of being knocked down by an older child. Furthermore, preschoolers need more room than younger children to roam and move about.

Furniture, equipment, and fixtures need to be checked regularly to make sure they are safe. The National Association for the Education of Young Children (NAEYC) recommends that early childhood caregivers get down on their hands and knees to see the space as the children do. Hazards that were not noticeable from a higher vantage point may become apparent (Kendrick, Kaufmann, & Messenger, 1991).

For infants and toddlers, it is important that cribs, high chairs, and other equipment meet recognized safety standards. Preschoolers need chairs and tables that are scaled to their size. Bathroom fixtures, such as toilets and sinks, should be low enough for preschoolers to use, but activity in the bathroom must be carefully supervised. (Water in any container can pose a drowning hazard for very young children.) The materials children play with also need to be carefully chosen to fit the children's developmental abilities, and they should be regularly examined to make sure they are in good condition.

The Outdoor Environment.   Children in child care settings will usually spend some part of their day outdoors. Outdoor playground equipment should be checked regularly to make sure that it is safe and sound. Any

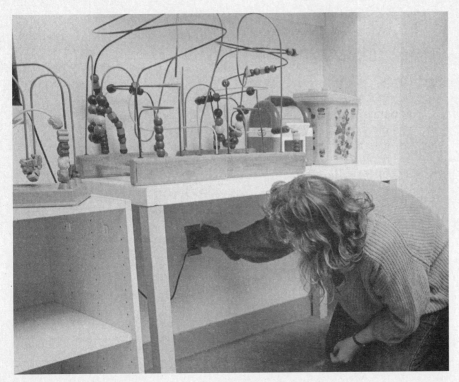

Early childhood professionals are encouraged to get down on their hands and knees to search for safety hazards from a child's point of view. This caregiver has discovered an unprotected outlet.

sharp edges or rough surfaces should be repaired or removed. Above all, playgrounds need to have impact-absorbent surfaces, since falls are the leading cause of playground injuries to children.

When infants, toddlers, and preschoolers are sharing the same playground, a fence should separate their play areas. Toddler play areas should have low climbers and emphasize sensorimotor activities. Preschooler play areas need to have climbers and swings at appropriate heights. Climbing equipment should take different ability levels into account, and it should allow the safe play of more than one child at a time. Chapter 12 discusses how caregivers can help to create and maintain safe indoor and outdoor environments.

Safe Behavior

Creating safe environments is only half the battle. If caregivers and children do not exhibit safe behavior, a large number of injuries may occur. Caregivers must know how to act safely themselves and how to set and enforce rules that help children to behave safely. Caregivers also have a responsibility to teach children about safe behaviors.

An extremely important factor related to child safety is the level and quality of adult supervision. Careful attention is needed to keep young children safe from injury. The appropriate ratio of adults to children varies with the ages and abilities of the children. NAEYC recommendations also vary with

TABLE 1.1
National Association for the Education of Young Children:
Recommended Child-Staff Ratios and Group Sizes

Age of child	Group Size							
	6	8	10	12	14	16	18	20
Birth to 12 mos.	3:1	4:1						
12 to 24 mos.	3:1	4:1	5:1	4:1				
24 to 30 mos.		4:1	5:1	6:1				
30 to 36 mos.			5:1	6:1	7:1			
Three-year-olds					7:1	8:1	9:1	10:1
Four-year-olds						8:1	9:1	10:1
Five-year-olds						8:1	9:1	10:1

Source: "Research Into Action. The Effects of Group Size, Ratios, and Staff Training on Child Care Quality," *Young Children*, 48(2), 65. © Copyright 1993 by the National Association for the Education of Young Children. Used by permission.

the size of the group. See Table 1.1 for specific child-staff ratios, but keep in mind that some children will not be at the expected developmental level for their age and may require more supervision than the table suggests.

Planning ahead can eliminate many safety hazards, especially when the children are away from the familiar child care environment—on a field trip, for example. By understanding when accidents are most likely to occur, caregivers can take extra measures to ensure everyone's safety. Chapter 13 discusses the many ways that caregivers can practice safe behaviors.

Safety for child care professionals involves more than inspecting the environment for potential hazards and supervising the children. Child care providers must also teach the children in their care ways to keep themselves safe. Caregivers can do this through rules about safe play and the use of equipment. They can also provide encouragement to children when they act and play in safe ways.

Caregivers have an additional responsibility to protect children's safety. They need to be alert to the signs of child abuse and neglect. By understanding the circumstances that lead to abuse and neglect and reporting suspected cases, caregivers can help children to be safe outside the facility as well as within it.

Emergency Preparedness

Of course, accidents can occur even under the best of conditions. That is why caregivers should be prepared for emergencies at all times. Fire drills and other periodic evacuations are an important way to prepare both caregivers and children to act quickly and calmly in an emergency. When there is an injury or sudden illness, caregivers must know whom to contact and how to communicate with them effectively. Advance planning and up-to-date record keeping will allow caregivers to contact both emergency personnel and parents as quickly as possible.

All caregivers should know basic first-aid procedures for dealing with the most common childhood injuries—from cuts and insect stings to falls and poisonings. In an emergency, quick action can mean the difference between life and death. Chapter 13 provides some information on responding to the most common child care emergencies. However, most child care professionals are required to take comprehensive first-aid training.

The Great Web

The well-being of an individual child is the product of many factors (see Figure 1.1). Nutrition, health, and safety all contribute in various ways to well-being. Each of these factors also affects the others so that overall well-being

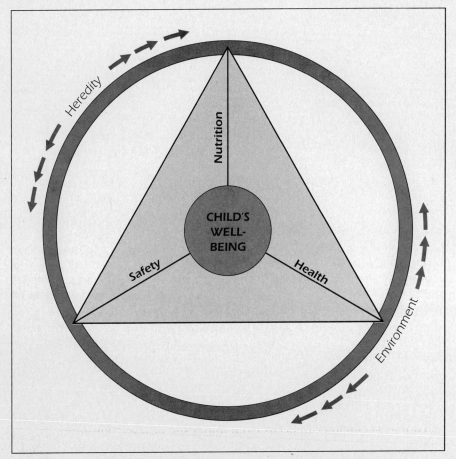

FIGURE 1.1   The Great Web of Well-being. Child care workers should be aware that the interrelated factors of nutrition, health, and safety, along with the influences of heredity and environment, all affect the well-being of each child.

FOCUS ON / Cultural Diversity

Attitudes About Touching

Touch is the most basic of the five senses. From their earliest years, children learn about things by touching them. And when it comes to touching other people, children learn the difference between touching that is "okay," and touching that is "not okay" by watching and listening to the people around them.

However, what is okay and not okay tends to vary from culture to culture. In Japan and China, for example, touching another person in public is unusual. Children whose parents or grandparents emigrated from those areas may be taught that emotions should not be expressed through physical contact. A child from such a cultural background may be less likely to hit another child but he may also be less inclined to give a warm hug.

In other parts of the world, physical contact between unrelated people is much more acceptable. Southern Europeans and people from Central and South America are among those who often embrace one another in public. Their children may hug teachers, friends, and friends' parents. This can sometimes cause problems in child care or playgroup situations when one child repeatedly tries to hug or hold hands with an unwilling playmate.

Religion also plays a role in determining touching behavior. Some religious groups, such as Hasidic Jews, prohibit touching between unrelated males and females, even in childhood. This ban on touching people of the opposite sex may also extend to social activities like dancing.

Knowing a child's ethnic and religious background can make a difference when it comes to understanding the physical gestures he makes toward others and how he responds to gestures himself.

can be maintained only when all three aspects are supported and preserved. In addition, hereditary and environmental influences on nutrition, health, and safety must be recognized and taken into account in order to promote the well-being of each child.

Interrelatedness

How does nutrition affect health and safety? A well-nourished child has better resistance to disease than a malnourished one and recovers more quickly from illness and injury. A healthful diet makes a child more alert, stronger, and better coordinated than an inadequate diet. The well-nourished child tends to be less accident-prone as a result. An overnourished child, on the other hand, may be slowed down by excess weight, be less alert, and be more likely to have accidents.

How does a person's state of health affect nutrition and safety? A healthy child generally has a better appetite than a child who is ill or who has a serious disorder. A healthy child is also more likely to digest and use food effectively. Illness places extra stress on the body. To recover, the body often has an increased need for certain nutrients.

Children who have access to the needed nutrients will recover more quickly than those who do not. Healthful habits like regular exercise promote proper bone growth by improving the bone's resistance to pressure, tension, and breakage. Regular exercise also improves muscle tone and coordination, and it is important to healthy development. Such effects make a healthy child less susceptible to accidental injury.

Completing the web of interrelatedness, safety affects nutrition and health. An injured child is less likely to have a good appetite; an injury may physically prevent the child from eating normally. An injured child may be more susceptible to illness, particularly if the injury is severe and interferes with good nutrition and other health-promoting activities.

Nature-Nurture Components of the Web

In addition to the effects that nutrition, health, and safety have on one another, each of these three areas is influenced by both heredity and the environment.

Some inherited disorders affect the body's ability to maintain good nutrition. For example, a child born with PKU cannot use protein normally and a child with cystic fibrosis cannot digest and use fats efficiently. Children need access to a variety of healthful foods as well as the support of the people who care for them to develop healthful food habits.

In terms of health, each person inherits a unique potential for a host of characteristics such as body structure, height, or a susceptibility to certain diseases. The environment provides the resources for meeting or moderating that potential. For example, children who are malnourished may never reach their maximum height potential. On the other hand, children who live in a healthful environment where sanitary procedures are carefully followed may never be exposed to diseases to which they would be susceptible.

Heredity and the environment can also affect safety. Genetic disorders such as cystic fibrosis can delay a child's physical development and make the child more accident-prone. Certain genetic disorders, such as Down's syndrome, can render a child unable to deal safely with otherwise age-appropriate tasks or materials. It is easy to see how environmental factors affect safety too. Very high water temperatures, unguarded open windows, or poisonous plants increase the chances that children will be injured.

The interrelatedness of nutrition, health, and safety makes it almost impossible to determine how each of these factors is affecting the well-being of a particular child. Child care providers need to recognize that the three areas are closely linked and that all are vitally important. Caregivers have a demanding and essential role to play in young children's lives.

Caring For and Teaching Young Children

Children, like adults, are complex individuals with a wide variety of needs. Their nutrition, health, and safety needs are part of the closely interdependent web described above. This interdependence has obvious relevance to

Careful attention to this child's nutrition, health, and safety will establish a firm foundation for his future attitudes and behavior.

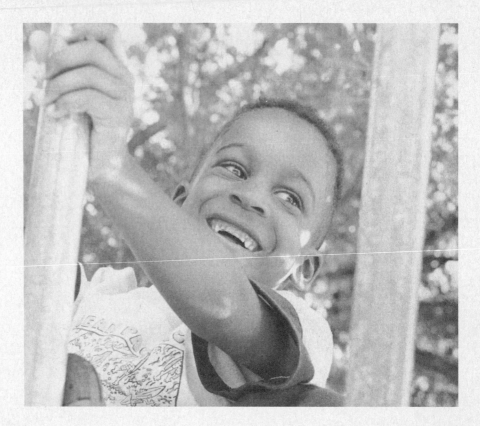

the care of young children. It is also an important consideration in teaching young children to care about and care for themselves.

Young children learn at an amazing rate from everything that goes on around them. Careful, caring attention to the many details affecting young children's nutrition, health, and safety can help set a firm, positive foundation for children's attitudes and behavior for a lifetime. Teaching children about nutritious foods, growing bodies, personal hygiene, exercise, and simple safety rules flows naturally from this kind of sound care of young children as they grow and develop. On the other hand, a poor selection of snack foods for a toddler, failure to teach proper handwashing to preschoolers, or skipping the use of a child safety seat for short automobile trips contributes to poor attitudes and behavior patterns in children.

Programs dedicated to improving the well-being of children must take all three areas—nutrition, health, and safety—into consideration. And the programs must combine them in a smoothly working framework for daily decisions and activities. Many programs work to build healthful habits in the areas of nutrition, fitness, sanitation, social relations, and safety. Such programs can help provide children with the resources and knowledge to become self-caring, responsible, healthy adults. By passing along these principles of healthful living, child care professionals can make a substantial difference in children's lives and in society for a long time to come.

SUMMARY

- Nutrition is the study of what people eat and how the body uses food.
- Nutrients are substances in food that nourish the body and help it to function. The choices people make about nutrition affect their total well-being.
- An individual's socioeconomic status, cultural background, emotional state, and education all have an effect on nutrition.
- Malnutrition occurs when a person is poorly nourished for a long time.
- Undernutrition happens when people do not consume enough foods with essential nutrients. Overnutrition is caused by eating too much of one or more nutrients and it can lead to undernutrition for other nutrients.
- Caregivers have an influence on the nutrition of children by providing healthful food choices and helping families make healthful food choices.
- Health is the state of a person's overall physical, mental, and emotional well-being.
- Heredity—the traits, characteristics, and defects passed from parents to children—has an influence on health. Some disorders are inherited. ✗
- A person's environment also has an influence on health.
- A child's physical, economic, social, and cultural setting can enhance or compromise her health.
- Caregivers should keep the child care environment clean to prevent the spread of disease. They should also recognize the symptoms of disease.
- Safety is the first responsibility of all child care providers.
- To maintain a safe environment, caregivers should be aware of children's developmental abilities and of potential hazards.
- Caregivers must also behave safely and teach children safe behaviors.
- Caregivers need to be prepared for emergencies. They should know how to obtain help as well as how to perform basic first-aid procedures.
- Nutrition, health, and safety are interrelated factors that affect children's lives. Changes in any one of the three factors affect both of the others.

ACQUIRING KNOWLEDGE

1. What is nutrition?
2. List the three factors that contribute to a child's overall well-being.
3. Define *nutrients* and name three major nutrients.
4. List four factors that influence the food choices people make.
5. What are some physical effects of nutritional deficiencies in young children?
6. What causes malnutrition?
7. Explain the difference between undernutrition and overnutrition.
8. Describe the way nutrition may affect learning.

9. Define health and list two factors that may influence health.
10. What is heredity?
11. List two hereditary disorders or susceptibilities that affect health.
12. Describe the effects of indoor pollutants on a child's health.
13. Why are poor children at a higher risk of health problems?
14. Describe how poor social relationships may affect a child's health.
15. Give an example of how a cultural belief can promote or hinder good health.
16. Name some ways communicable diseases are transmitted to children in group settings.
17. What is safety?
18. What are the three main aspects of safety for caregivers?
19. List five common hazards for young children.
20. How can caregivers make indoor spaces appropriate for children's ages and abilities?
21. Why are impact-absorbent surfaces crucial for children's playgrounds?
22. What factors are taken into account when child-staff ratios are recommended?
23. List two ways caregivers can be prepared for emergencies.
24. What does it mean to say that nutrition, health, and safety are interrelated? Provide an example.
25. What two factors also affect nutrition, safety, and health?

THINKING CRITICALLY

1. Make a list of the main factors that influence people's food choices. Which of these influences are strongest in the community where you live? If you were a caregiver in this community, how would this knowledge help you?
2. Explain how your own ethnic group influences your food choices and food preparation style. Do you believe that recognizing these influences on your eating practices can help you understand eating practices unlike your own?
3. Why is it important to look at both hereditary and environmental factors for an understanding of children's health?
4. Why do you think that safety experts recommend that caregivers examine a room from a child's point of view? What kinds of things might caregivers see there that they might not see from an adult height?
5. What is meant by the term *The Great Web* as it is used in this chapter? Why do you think this term is used?

OBSERVATIONS AND APPLICATIONS

1. Go to a local mall and observe what infants, toddlers, and preschoolers are eating and drinking. Are they drinking juices? Soda? Are they eating fruit? Ice cream? Are they consuming food they brought with them or food they bought at the mall? Does it seem that most of the children you

observe are consuming food? Be sure to observe children in areas where food is sold and in areas where it is not.

2. Suppose you work in a preschool. You notice that most children bring lunches that are filled with sweets. There are some children who eat only items that contain sugar—from the presweetened drink to the jelly on the peanut butter sandwich to the sweetened applesauce and the cupcake. What suggestions would you give to parents for improving the food choices they pack in their children's lunches?

3. Visit a child care center and observe measures that are taken to protect children's safety. Are the corners of the furniture rounded? Do rugs and mats have nonslip backings or pads beneath them? Are there safety gates at doorways and stairways? Are infants and toddlers separated? Observe the caregivers' actions. What do they do to protect children's safety? Do they keep children from running inside? Are spills quickly mopped up? On the playground, do they keep children from walking or running behind moving swings? Note any other safety promoting behaviors on the part of caregivers.

4. Suppose you work in a child care setting. You are planning an all-day field trip for preschoolers to a farm. Explain how you would prepare in advance for the nutritional, health, and safety needs of the children while they are on the trip.

FOR FURTHER INFORMATION

American Medical Association, Department of Adolescent Health. (1990). *Healthy youth 2000: National health promotion and disease prevention objectives for adolescents*. Chicago: Author.

Anspaugh, D. J., & Ezell, G. O. (1990). *Teaching today's health* (3rd ed.). New York: Macmillan.

Christian, J., & Greger, J. (1991). *Nutrition for living*. Redwood City, CA: Benjamin/Cummings.

Cook-Fuller, C. (Ed.). (1992). *Annual editions: Nutrition 92/93*. Guilford, CT: Dushkin.

Cresswell, W. H., & Newman, I. M. (1993). *School health practice* (10th ed.). St. Louis: C. V. Mosby.

Hamilton, E., Whitney, E., & Sizer, F. (1991). *Nutrition: Concepts and controversies*. St. Paul, MN: West.

Page, R. M., & Page, T. S. (1993). *Fostering emotional well-being in the classroom*. Boston: Jones and Bartlett.

U. S. Department of Health and Human Services. (1990). *Healthy people 2000: National health promotion and disease prevention objectives*. Washington, DC: U. S. Government Printing Office.

Whitney, E., & Rolfes, S. (1993). *Understanding nutrition*. St. Paul, MN: West.

PART 1

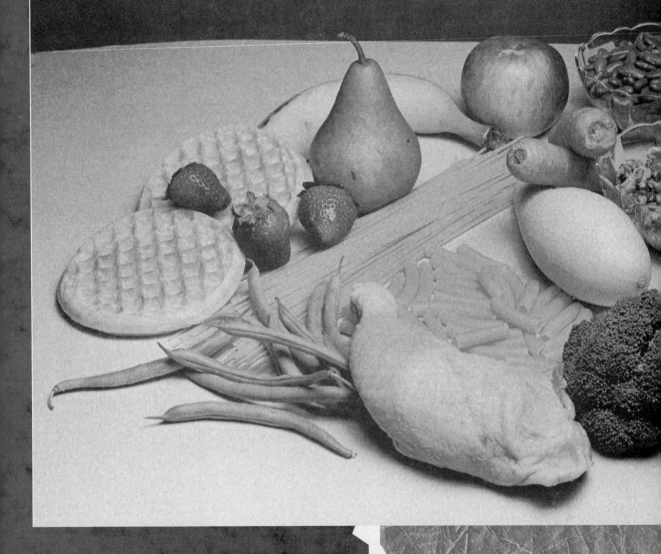

Nutrition: The Science of Food

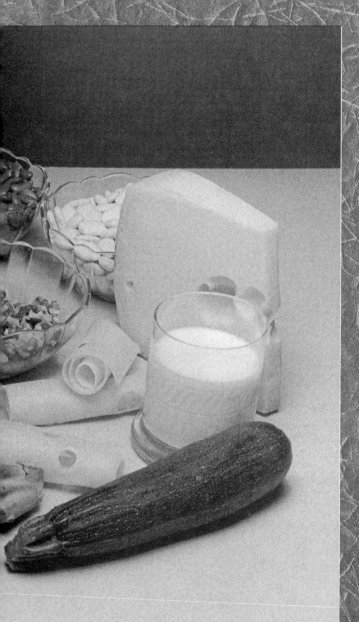

2

Food Patterns for Healthy Development

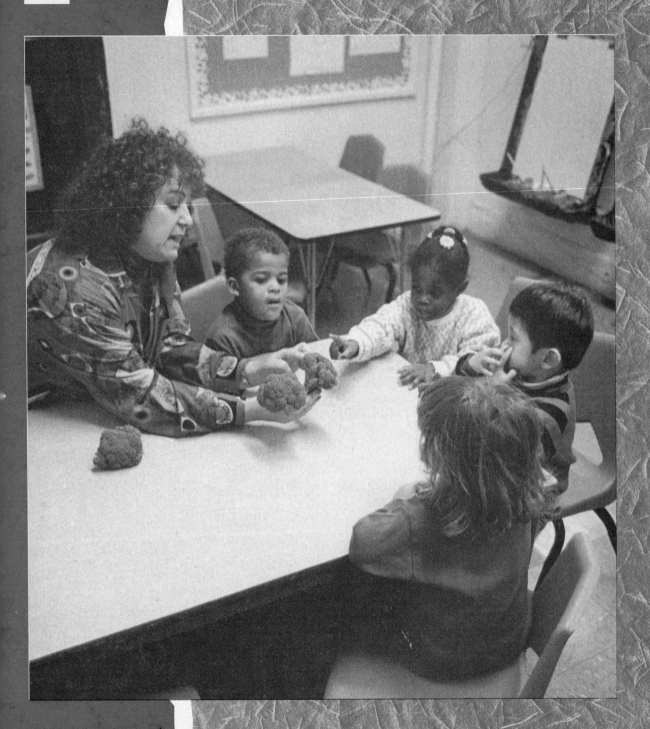

AFTER reading a favorite book with the children, Stacey took her seat at the small table. Four preschoolers—Michael, Janelle, Angela, and Luis—seated themselves in their child-sized chairs. Relaxed, washed, and hungry, they were ready to share an important part of their day together—a tasting party just before lunch.

Stacey knew that mealtimes and snack times at the center were important to the children's overall development. After all, they ate lunch and two snacks with her, which added up to more than half of their nutrient and caloric intake each day. And for Angela, whose family was homeless, meals at the center contained the most nutritious foods of the day. Stacey also knew that her role in helping children develop healthful food patterns was equally important.

"I brought in some broccoli today for you to see," she said to the children. "Let's talk about how it looks."

"It's green." "It looks like a tree with a bushy top!" several children responded.

"My Aunt Margie served that at her house for dinner, but no trunk," contributed Stacey.

"Do you think it comes from a plant or an animal?"

"A plant," Janelle exclaimed then paused.

"Then is it a vegetable, or is it a fruit?" Stacey guided the discussion as children came up with the answer.

Stacey cut the broccoli into small florets and ate the first bite saying, "Now, who will be the next food taster?"

Luis—always adventuresome—took one bite, then another. So did Angela, but she just took a little bite. Janelle picked up the broccoli, examined it for a while, then nibbled on the stalk. Stacey smiled approvingly to them. Michael just looked at the broccoli. "Maybe next time," Stacey thought as she winked at Michael.

"Now that you have had the chance to taste something different, let's have lunch," Stacey said. "If you'd like, you can have another bite of broccoli."

"Next week," thought Stacey, "the children will have another chance to try broccoli, and then again a week later. Each time, that food would become more familiar to them." Then she poured a glass of milk and sat down and enjoyed her meal with them.

Food Patterns in the Child Care Center

Healthful food patterns, formed during the early years of life, help ensure that children are adequately nourished. *Food patterns* refer to how, when, where, and how much food people eat. Early food patterns not only affect growth and development in the childhood years but also influence adult food behavior. The child who develops healthful eating habits is more likely to become an adult who eats wisely.

Parents and child care professionals like Stacey control which foods a child can choose from. They play a very important role in establishing healthful eating patterns.

The basic responsibility of a child care facility is to provide nutritious meals and snacks. However, child care professionals have the opportunity and responsibility to do far more than that. They can motivate and interest children in healthful eating and help them become successful in their eating skills. Healthful eating is, after all, a set of life skills that can be developed and reinforced through early childhood education.

The Food Environment in the Child Care Center

A positive food environment is safe, clean, pleasant, and physically comfortable. It promotes good eating habits and a child's overall enjoyment of food. The *food environment* takes the whole child into consideration and includes such elements as furniture and eating utensils, cleanliness, and all of the child's encounters with food and situations involving food.

Furniture and Eating Utensils.   Furniture and eating utensils should be developmentally appropriate, offering comfort, safety, and success to

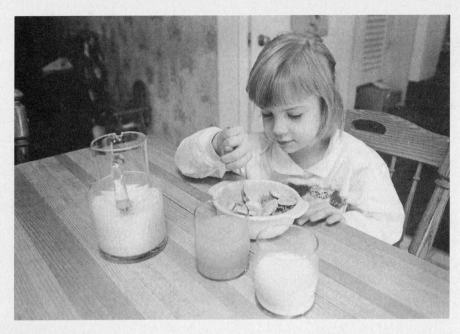

Ensuring that a child eats a nutritious breakfast helps to encourage healthful food patterns for years to come.

children as they strive to master self-feeding skills. Furniture and utensils need to be suited to the child's body size and level of physical dexterity.

Child care providers should serve meals and snacks at small tables (four to six people per table) with sturdy, child-sized chairs. Infants and young toddlers should be seated in high chairs or secured seats.

Small dishes, bowls, and glasses that are stable and nonbreakable are best for children. Choose dishes that have a slight lip to help children push food onto their forks or spoons. Glasses should have a broad flat base so they will not tip over easily. Avoid heavy mugs and cups with handles—most preschool children do not have the motor skills to hold them easily.

Broad spoons and forks with short, easily grasped handles work well for young children. Caregivers should make sure that all eating utensils are blunt to avoid injury. Chopsticks should be offered to youngsters who are accustomed to using them at home.

It is important to provide enough dishes, bowls, glasses, and utensils to allow for adequate cleaning and sanitizing between uses. Children should never share eating utensils.

Cleanliness. To protect against the spread of infectious disease, personal hygiene and cleanliness must be a priority in the food environment. Young children are especially vulnerable to colds, the flu, and other infectious illnesses because their immune systems are not fully developed. A clean, safe food environment also offers pleasant surroundings, which promote good eating habits.

Handwashing often signals mealtime. Proper handwashing before and after handling food and eating should be a routine habit for every child, staff member, and child care volunteer. Washing facilities need to be accessible,

FOCUS ON — Communicating with Parents

Encouraging Parent Participation

It is Friday at Willowdale Preschool. Karen, one of the teachers, is passing out next week's menus to the parents as they arrive to collect their children. Joyce Chang, a Chinese American parent, skims the menu and smiles. Ed Bukowski, of Polish ancestry, looks less happy.

JOYCE: I see you're serving rice on Thursday. Rosey likes that; we eat it at home almost every day.

KAREN: We try to accommodate the children's different backgrounds by including a number of ethnic foods each week.

ED: I notice that you have a lot of Mexican and Asian dishes on here, but not many traditional European foods like goulash, pirogi, sauerbraten, or spätzle. Is there a reason for that?

KAREN: I'm not sure. Our director, who plans the menus, might not be aware of the dishes you're suggesting. We also try to keep the dishes pretty simple, because we find that the children like them better.

ED: Pirogi are pretty simple. They're just a mashed potato and cheese filling wrapped in a macaroni dumpling. I make them for Toby all the time at home. How about if I send some in with him for the class to eat?

KAREN: That sounds delicious! I'm sure the children would love to try them, but there's one problem. Because of state regulations, we can't serve food prepared at home in the center.

ED: I see. That *is* a bit of a problem.

KAREN: But I have an idea. Would you be interested in visiting the center and showing the children how to *make* pirogi? I bet the children would even help you mash the potatoes and fold the dumplings.

ED: That's a good idea. I could bring in copies of my mother's recipe for the children to take home to their parents. I'll have to see if I can arrange to have a morning or an afternoon off.

KAREN: And I'll talk to the center's director so we can arrange to have the ingredients on hand for you. It sounds like fun—let me know when you're available so we can set up a time.

ED: Okay. We'll show these kids how to cook up a storm.

Did Karen address Ed's concerns well? What might you have done differently?

with sinks and liquid soap at a height that allows young children to use them independently.

Cleaning up adds another important dimension to the food experience. Most children like the "grown-up" feeling of helping with food cleanup. Keep covered refuse containers and a small, short-handled broom handy to encourage children to share this responsibility. And praise them for helping.

For sanitary and aesthetic considerations, food handling and eating areas need to be located well away from toilet and diaper-changing areas. Used tissues, wipes, and diapers should be stored in closed containers away from food, and they should be discarded daily.

Meal and Snack Schedules

Children need to eat when they are hungry. *Hunger* is a physical sensation that signals that it is time to eat. An empty stomach contracts, giving brief hunger pangs. Headaches and fatigue, often caused by low blood sugar, may be signs of hunger, too. Eating is pleasant because it eases sensations of hunger.

Appetite, on the other hand, is a psychological desire to eat. It usually involves a pleasant association with food, conditioned by experiences with food and by one's food habits. Appetite is stimulated by the body's senses—the way foods look, taste, and smell. An appetite stimulates the flow of digestive juices and aids the digestive process, thus promoting health.

While hunger helps regulate food intake, so do feelings of *satiety*. Satiety is a feeling of fullness or satisfaction that comes with eating. As adults, we often eat even after we are full. However, most children respond more readily to satiety; physical sensations naturally regulate their food intake.

Most young children need regular meal and snack schedules. While adults can often compensate for missed or late meals, children cannot usually do this. A meal or snack every two to three hours matches the need of most two- to five-year-old children to eat. The interval may be shorter for infants and young toddlers. Meals and snacks served at the same time each day tend to promote a healthful appetite.

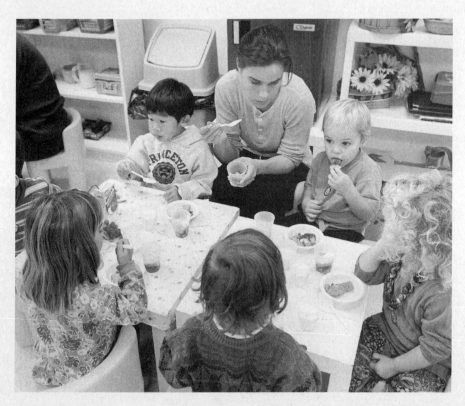

Children need a balanced and varied diet. Caregivers should offer a choice of foods at meals so that children can express their food preferences and not go hungry.

FOCUS ON Promoting Healthful Habits

Adjusting the Schedule to the Child

When three-year-old Ruth Ann arrives at the Twin Brooks Center, she seems to be in fairly good spirits. But her mother does mention to Peter, the caregiver, that the family was out quite late at a birthday party the night before. The little girl seems attentive during circle time and participates in the other early morning activities.

Later in the morning, though, Ruth Ann becomes unusually demanding about holding onto a few of the toys she especially likes.

At snack time, she picks up a wedge of apple, one of her favorite fruits, and throws it on the floor. As the other children look on, Ruth Ann bursts into tears.

Remembering her mother's comment about the late night, Peter takes Ruth Ann's hand and walks her over to one of the rocking chairs. He sits down and opens his arms to her. She climbs onto his lap, still sobbing, and drifts off to sleep after a few minutes of gentle rocking. Peter settles her on her cot in the sleeping nook.

Two hours later, Ruth Ann is awake and cheerful and hungry for the lunch that's about to be served. Peter remembered that, although schedules are important, sometimes a child's greater need should come first.

Do you think Peter did the right thing? Would you have tried something else first? What would you try next if the child didn't calm down and drift off to sleep?

Snacks should be planned events and not a series of sporadic nibbling episodes. Snacks should be spaced at least two hours before meals so they don't interfere with the meals. And they should be planned as part of the total food and nutrient intake for the day.

Meal and Snack Preparation

In order to thrive, children need the nutrients and energy supplied by a balanced, varied, and moderate diet. Caregivers can provide these by carefully following meal and snack patterns set by the child care facility where they work. For homeless children like Angela or children whose parents are unable to provide adequate food at home, the center's lunch or breakfast may be the only healthful meal of the day. (Chapter 4 discusses meal and snack planning and the differing nutrient and food needs of children at each age.)

Choice of Foods. At every meal, it's best to offer variety rather than just one food. In that way, children can express their food likes and dislikes without going hungry. Variety, along with balance and moderation, is the foundation of the healthful diet. The greater the variety of foods that children eat and enjoy, the more likely it is that they will choose a lifelong diet with an adequate amount of essential nutrients.

Most young children enjoy simple, unmixed foods. For example, children may put mixed peas and carrots into separate piles before eating them. In fact, it is common for young children to reject foods that touch each other. You might also avoid serving combination foods, such as casseroles or mixed fruit salads, until children are a little older.

Children generally prefer mild-tasting foods. Strong-flavored vegetables, such as spinach, onions, and brussels sprouts, often have less appeal than carrots and peas, for example. In general, it's best to avoid highly seasoned foods too; however, children who eat spicy foods at home may readily accept them.

Preparation of Foods.   A child's mouth is more sensitive to temperature than an adult's so serve cooked foods at warm, rather than hot, temperatures. Offer fruit, such as apples and pears, at room temperature. Some children stir ice cream until it is soft and not so cold.

Meals with a variety of textures develop different eating skills. Crisp food allows easy chewing and enjoyment of sounds in the mouth, and soft food is easy to eat. Chewy food develops emerging chewing skills, but it should be served in small quantities so children do not have too much to chew at one time. Chunks of meat are hard for two- and three-year-olds to chew; ground meat or poultry is easier for them to eat.

It's a good idea to avoid the excessive use of sugars, salt, and fats in food preparation; eating too much of these ingredients is linked to health problems later in life. Instead encourage children to enjoy and appreciate the natural flavor of fresh food.

Caregivers do well to offer food in small servings of bite-sized pieces that fit into small mouths. While young children may refuse a whole apple or banana, they usually enjoy apple or banana slices. Too much food can overwhelm a young child. If children are still hungry, they will ask for more.

Most children enjoy eating finger foods, such as quartered, hard-boiled eggs, string cheese, and orange sections. Finger foods are good choices for children of all ages because they are easy to pick up. This encourages independence, especially in toddlers and three-year-olds who may still find it hard to feed themselves using utensils. However, menus should still include foods that are best eaten with forks and spoons, so that children in these ages will have the opportunity to practice handling utensils.

Until children are about age four, avoid offering hard and small pieces of food that may cause choking. These include grapes, nuts, small pieces of raw vegetables, hot dog pieces, tough meat, popcorn, and snack chips. Regardless of the menu, be alert to the signs of choking. Observe children while they eat because they may not make choking sounds. Chapter 13 discusses first-aid procedures for infants and children who are choking.

Mealtime Management

The way child care professionals plan meals and snacks and their attitude toward children's developing eating skills and preferences can create an atmosphere conducive to positive eating behavior. It's better to plan quiet activities, such as reading, before meals to promote healthful appetites. Some children cannot settle down to a meal when they are still excited from play. Many also get fussy about eating when they feel tired.

Young children become bored and fidgety when they have to sit and wait for food. Food should be prepared and ready to serve when the children sit down to eat. Keep the atmosphere relaxed, never rushed. If children like to serve themselves, encourage them to do so. During meals and snacks, focus only on eating. Without distractions from stories, toys, or television, children can learn that eating in itself is an important, worthwhile event.

Respect a child's individual food preferences. Like adults, children have their personal food likes and dislikes. If a child repeatedly refuses a food, substitute another food with a similar nutrient content—for example, carrots instead of sweet potatoes or peaches instead of apricots (all good sources of vitamin A). Grapefruit or cantaloupe might appeal to a child who dislikes oranges, and all of these are rich in vitamin C. Child care providers should

FOCUS ON   Cultural Diversity

Table Manners

Table manners vary from culture to culture and in different places around the world. It's important for caregivers to realize that children from different cultures will bring different behaviors and expectations to the preschool lunch table. For example, for people in Japan and parts of China, it is customary for people to use a wet towel to wash their faces and hands at the table before the meal is served. In other places, diners wash their hands before coming to the table.

The dining table also takes various forms and heights in different cultures. In Japan and India, people often sit or kneel while eating at low tables. In some Middle Eastern countries, diners eat while seated on cushions on the floor.

Around the world, people use one hand or both hands to manipulate knives, spoons, forks, or chopsticks. In the Muslim tradition, the left hand is considered unclean and is kept out of sight during meals. The left hand is indispensable in the British Isles, Australia, and New Zealand, where it is used to hold the fork.

Most right-handed Americans hold the fork in the right hand to spear food, then switch it to the left hand while cutting large pieces.

Chopsticks are widely used in Asia, where foods are cooked and served in small pieces. Asians often drink soup directly from the bowl and eat noodles by holding the bowl close to their faces and scooping the food into their mouths with chopsticks. Slurping is perfectly acceptable. The same slurping would be frowned upon in the West.

Americans eat all kinds of foods, including whole fruits, with their fingers. This is also true in India. Mexicans fill tortillas with various foods and eat them with their fingers—even in fancy restaurants. Europeans are more likely to use knives and forks when eating fruits and even some sandwiches.

Children from different cultural backgrounds may eat the same foods in very different ways. The caregiver's role is to incorporate all the children's understanding of "good table manners" in a positive atmosphere of cultural diversity.

ask parents about food allergies or intolerances, but not about food dislikes. Allow children to explore and develop their individual tastes without the influence of adult expectations.

Avoid forcing children to finish everything on their plates. Besides creating unnecessary conflict, children need to regulate their own food intake and quit when they feel full. A "clean plate" policy, which encourages children to eat even after they are satisfied, reinforces a habit that often leads to obesity. Caregivers are responsible for what the child is offered to eat; the child is responsible for how much food is eaten and even whether to eat (Satter, 1986).

Spills and other messes are common as children develop self-feeding skills. Accept them without scolding as a normal part of development. Children can assist in wiping up spills, so they are part of the solution.

Establish realistic expectations with children about eating so they can feel successful. Reinforce positive food behavior with a smile, a kind word, and a caring look. Ignore undesirable behavior. Most children do want to learn adult food behavior. Like other skills, learning to eat in a healthful, appropriate way takes time, encouragement, patience, and practice.

As children move from the toddler to the preschool stage, they become more independent with their food behavior—what they eat, when they eat, and how much they eat. Child care professionals should give children the opportunity to make choices about the food they eat. Decision making is, after all, part of a lifelong process of making healthful food choices that match individual needs.

New Foods

Planning ahead and preparing young children for each new food experience lays the groundwork for getting them to try and accept new foods. Children learn from sensory experiences. Approach new food the way Stacey did in her introduction of broccoli. Have the children talk about and experience the food's qualities—color, size, texture, smell, where it comes from, perhaps even how it grows—before tasting it. Avoid asking them if the food tastes good or bad.

Consider timing. Offer new foods when children are not tired, excited, or already full from lunch or snacks. In a child care facility, snack time or before lunch—when children are hungry—is often a good time for tasting and learning about new foods. Trying a new food when hungry leaves a pleasant sensation, which translates to the next experience with that food (Pipes & Trahms, 1993).

Offer food tastings—one new food at a time. Plan to introduce a new food more than once. Over time, most children will try and even accept the food if they are not forced. Serve new foods with familiar favorites and offer tiny tastes at first. The first time, a child may try one green bean but not a full serving. Part of learning to be "grown up" about food is tasting a little more each time.

The Caregiver as Role Model

Caregivers—including parents and child care providers—may be the most important influence on children's food behavior. Because children imitate the behavior of adults and older siblings, setting a good example is essential for developing healthful food patterns. When adults enjoy nutritious foods, children usually accept those same foods.

By eating with children, child care providers can model positive eating behavior—for example, the proper use of utensils, trying all foods on the plate, talking without food in the mouth, saying "please" and "thank you" at the table, and eating mainly nutritious foods (rather than high-calorie, low-nutrient foods). Stacey, for example, drank milk rather than a soft drink as she ate with the children. When children and adults eat together, caregivers can also show children how to serve themselves and how to clean up when they are finished.

Influences on Children's Food Patterns

Why do children eat what they do? A child's food patterns are shaped by many interrelated influences (see Table 2.1). Life-style factors include the child's family resources, family structure, ethnic identity, religious beliefs, education, knowledge of nutrition and health, and geographic residence—either rural or urban (Kittler & Sucher, 1989). Emotional factors also affect what, how, and when a child eats. Other factors, such as the media, economy, politics, and food production and distribution, influence food availability as a whole. The child care professional should be sensitive to all the influences on what and how a child eats.

Family Resources, Structure, and Life-Style

The family is the main influence on a child's early food behavior. The child's food patterns are learned, not inherited; the family passes culture, including food culture, to the children. *Culture* includes the beliefs, customs, knowledge, and habits that people share (Kittler & Sucher, 1989).

Traditionally, the mother has been in control of the child's foods. However, because there are more families in which both parents work and more men who are single parents, fathers and older siblings may control food purchasing and preparation as well as the feeding of young children. Many children now take responsibility at an earlier age for feeding themselves.

Today's highly mobile nuclear family eats differently from the extended family of the past. Busy family schedules have spawned eat-and-run meals, microwaveable frozen foods, small breakfasts, fast foods, and grazing (or constant nibbling). Frequent reliance on fast foods may limit the variety of foods a child eats; some fast-food choices may accentuate a child's preference for foods higher in fat or added sugars. When nutritionally balanced home-cooked foods are replaced by quick meals and frequent snacking, children may not get the nutrients their bodies need.

TABLE 2.1
Influences on Children's Food Patterns

Factors	Influences
Family life-style	Fast foods, microwave dinners, and busy schedules may limit variety of foods. Some life-styles may expose children to a wider selection of foods.
Family structure	Food preparation may be done differently in one- or two-parent families, small or large families, or extended families.
Family income resources	Types of foods, places they are bought or eaten, and quantity and quality of food are all influenced by size of income.
Ethnic identity	Traditional food preferences are passed on for generations; food choices may be different at home from those at the center.
Religious beliefs	Some foods may be prohibited or not eaten with certain other foods. Some religions require fasting during certain times of the year.
Regional geographic differences	Climate, geography, and early settlers influenced regional foods; also, rural and urban dwellers may eat different foods.
Parent(s) knowledge of food and nutrition	Depending on the parents' food and nutrition knowledge, children may or may not benefit from basic principles needed for family meal planning.
Emotions	Stress, anger, boredom, excitement, depression, and pleasure all affect eating patterns.
The media	Television food ads are a major influence on food patterns and preferences.

   Food also plays a role in a family's social events. For example, children and their families may eat at parties, birthday celebrations, movie theaters, and sports events. Because these events tend to be pleasant, children associate foods eaten there—perhaps sweets, snack chips, soft drinks, and other less nutritious foods—with positive feelings that reinforce a preference for these foods.

   Family income influences which foods are purchased, the quantities available, and the places where they are eaten. Two-income families, for example, usually have enough money to provide an adequate variety of healthful foods for their families. A higher income, however, does not always mean a diet that is highly nutritious. Some families may spend more food dollars on eating out or on more costly but not necessarily more nutritious foods.

Low-income families may be limited in their ability to buy nutritious foods for their children. They may also lack transportation to stores offering a wide variety of nutritious foods. However, many families with limited incomes are skilled in buying foods that provide the best nutritional value for their food dollars.

Other family circumstances can adversely affect a child's food intake and nutritional status. These problems include substance abuse, homelessness, and child neglect and abuse.

As children get older and more independent, people other than family members can influence their food choices too. These people may include child care providers, teachers, other children, and perhaps the parents of children's friends.

Ethnic Identity

Ethnicity defines many food patterns. Some researchers would go so far as to say you eat what you are (Barer-Stein, 1991). Ethnicity means belonging to a group of people with common cultural characteristics; it is not defined strictly by race, country of origin, language, or minority affiliation. Everyone belongs to an ethnic group, even those who consider themselves stereotypically American.

Foods common to a specific ethnic group are often referred to as *ethnic foods*. Families usually pass these food preferences on to their children generation after generation. The basic diet for most ethnic groups is, to at least some degree, nutritionally sound. Otherwise that group would not have survived (Lowenberg, Todhunter, Wilson, Savage, & Lubawski, 1979). Child care professionals need to have an informed awareness, respect for, and understanding of ethnic foods in children's food patterns. Integrating ethnic and regional foods into the center's program is one way to show respect for children's diversity.

Each ethnic group has its own food traditions. Here are just three examples:

- **Chinese**. The Chinese diet comes mainly from plant sources of food— grains, vegetables, and legumes. Because of regional agricultural differences in China, rice is common in foods of southern China and noodles, made of wheat, are common in the north. Many of the dishes are stir-fried, steamed, or barbecued because traditionally these cooking methods required less fuel.
- **Mexican**. Beans, tortillas made from corn, chilies, and tomatoes are staples of the Mexican diet; these foods, which Native Americans ate before Columbus' time, are eaten at most meals. Fresh fruit is a common snack. Both adults and children drink hot chocolate and coffee made with a lot of milk. Besides beans, typical protein sources include chicken, fish, and other seafood. The Mexican diet is not typical of all Hispanic diets. The foods eaten by Puerto Ricans, Cubans, Colombians, and Argentineans are quite different.

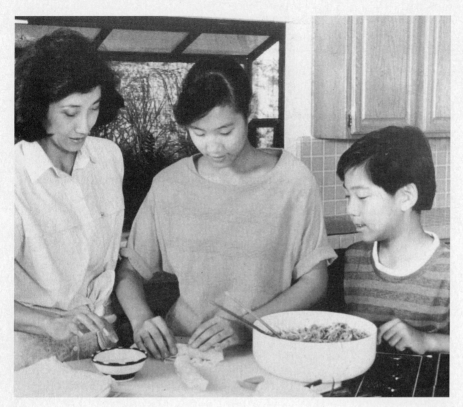

The food preferences of an ethnic group are often passed from generation to generation. Here, a Chinese American mother teaches her children how to prepare egg rolls.

- **Polish**. Whole grains, beets, potatoes, cabbage, and smoked meats are staples in the Polish diet and in many other Eastern European diets. These foods became popular because they could be stored over cold, harsh winters. Added flavor often comes from sour cream and mushrooms. This diet tends to be very hearty, with few fresh vegetables.

Subgroups within each ethnic group also have their unique food traditions. Italian food, for example, is not limited to the popular cuisine emphasizing pasta and red tomato sauces. While these foods are common in southern Italy, people from the north also eat cornmeal or rice dishes and sauces made with butter and cream.

Religious Beliefs

Food is central to many religious beliefs, often as a symbol of sacred rituals or as part of the celebration of religious holidays (Kittler & Sucher, 1989; Lowenberg et al., 1979). A family's religious practices influence a child's daily food choices and eating patterns. Child care providers need to be aware of any religious requirements that affect food practices of children and their families, and adjust menus accordingly.

Followers of Judaism, especially Orthodox Jews and some Conservative Jews, may follow dietary laws set down in religious writings. Many of these laws apply to the use of meat, dairy products, and other foods from animals. For example, meat and dairy products may not be eaten together. Pork and shellfish are considered unclean and unfit to eat. Children from homes that keep a kosher kitchen have very strict dietary restrictions. The term *kosher* or its symbol on food packaging indicates that the food has been prepared under the supervision of a rabbi.

Many Seventh Day Adventists are vegetarians. They avoid meat but not milk or eggs. They drink water before and after meals instead of with them, and in preference to coffee or tea. Highly seasoned foods, including some condiments, are avoided. And snacking is discouraged.

For Muslims, eating habits are part of religious practice. One of the five pillars of Islam is to fast from sunrise to sunset during the month-long religious period called Ramadan. Muslims are urged to share food and are expected to eat strictly for their health and to avoid both overeating and food waste. The Koran, or sacred writings, prohibits certain foods, including pork. Handwashing and mouthwashing before and after meals is required.

Regional Differences

In almost every country, there are regional differences in diet and cuisine. This is because climate and geography have influenced the agriculture and foods of each region. Many regional cuisines of the United States developed when areas of the nation were more isolated. The people who settled an area brought their foods with them and, over the centuries, adapted them to local agriculture.

Today food distribution systems make most foods available throughout the United States. Child care professionals are wise to consider regional foods that children enjoy, especially for children whose families have moved from another region of the country. Some examples of regional foods include:

- **The South**. The cuisines of the southern United States are heavily influenced by the Europeans who settled there, by African slaves, and by Native Americans who were important in its history. Chicken, pork, pecans, peanuts, okra, greens, and sweet potatoes are common ingredients in southern dishes. Soul foods, originally the fare of poor black and white populations, use inexpensive ingredients—such as chitterlings, ham hocks, and wild greens—in tasty, nutritious ways.
- **The Southwest**. Native American and Mexican peoples contributed many of the foods now characteristic of the Southwest. Tex-Mex foods such as enchiladas, tacos, and salsa are popular. Native Americans added cactus, squash blossoms, pine nuts, fried bread, chilies, corn, and beans to the Southwest menu.
- **The Northwest**. With its fertile valleys, mild climate, and rivers, the Northwest has abundant sources of foods, including freshwater fish, seafood, berries, apples, and other fruits.

Food patterns differ not only by region of the country. Urban, suburban, farm, and nonfarm families often eat differently too. They have access to different types of stores and restaurants, more or less opportunity to grow some of their own foods, and life-style differences that affect food patterns.

Knowledge of Food and Nutrition

Understanding simple nutrition principles helps people to develop healthful food patterns. And because people usually pass their food patterns on from generation to generation, the understanding that parents have of food and nutrition can have a lasting impact on their children.

The knowledge that caregivers have of food and nutrition also plays an important role in helping children develop healthful food patterns. To promote the children's health and the development of healthful eating habits, child care professionals can apply their understanding of nutrition principles to meal planning in the child care setting. Caregivers can also share nutrition information with parents.

Emotions

Emotions influence what, when, and how people of all ages eat. Feelings of stress, anger, boredom, excitement, or depression can either reduce appetite or trigger episodes of overeating.

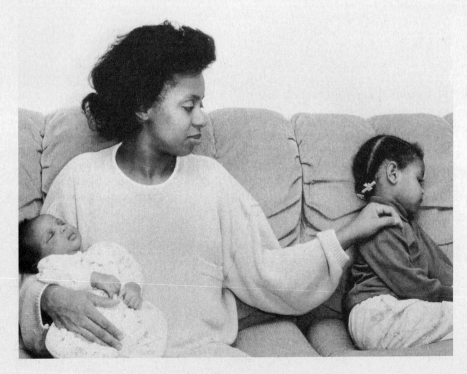

The arrival of a new baby can create stress in young children. Such emotions sometimes affect eating patterns.

WHOLESOME SNACKS

Banana Tropicana Sherbet

Ingredients:

1 cup sugar
⅛ teaspoon salt
2 cups water
1 cup nonfat dry milk powder
¼ cup lemon juice
⅓ cup orange juice
1 banana, mashed

Directions:

1. Dissolve sugar and salt in 1 cup water.
2. Add remaining water and milk powder and chill 1 hour.
3. Add juices and banana.
4. Pour into freezer tray and freeze until firm.
5. Turn into bowl and beat until fluffy.
6. Return to freezer tray and refreeze.

Yield: 8 servings

Each serving contains:

Calories: 146
Protein: 3 g
Fat: 0.1 g
Carbohydrates: 34 g

Source: DeBakey, M. (1984). *The living heart diet.* COPYRIGHT © 1984 by Raven Press Books, Inc. Reprinted by permission of Simon & Schuster, Inc.

If caregivers can deal immediately with disruptions in children's eating patterns caused by emotional upsets, such responses are usually short lived. However, if emotions repeatedly become cues for eating disruptions, these behaviors may be reinforced as lifelong habits.

Some emotions cannot be dealt with quickly. Disruptions that accompany divorce, death in the family, moving, illness, or even the birth of a new baby may create stress that affects eating. Caregivers need to help children resolve these emotions and find ways to ensure adequate nutrition in the meantime. If children seem seriously affected, caregivers need to communicate this to parents so they can obtain assistance from counselors or psychologists.

The Media

The media, especially television, affect children's eating behavior and attitudes toward food. Television advertisements and programming influence young children even before they have developed their verbal skills. Eventually, children ask for foods they see advertised; as a result, both family food purchases and snacking patterns are influenced. The way people on television relate to food also makes an impression. Attitudes toward obese people, thinness, and the use of food as an emotional tool may come, in part, from role models children see on television shows.

Studies suggest that children from preschool through junior high school watch about 26 hours of television a week, including 3 hours of advertising (Deitz & Gortmaker, 1985). By the time children graduate from high school, they have, on average, spent more hours in front of the television than they have spent in school. Of the 350,000 advertisements children see, about 55 percent promote foods, with the majority being highly sugared foods (Rothenberg, 1983).

Too much television viewing, in itself, may contribute to childhood obesity. Children may not get enough exercise if they spend many hours in front of the television. And advertising cues may encourage nibbling (Deitz & Gortmaker, 1985).

Diversity, Food, and the Child Care Setting

A food environment that builds healthful food patterns considers the full ethnic—religious, racial, and cultural—diversity of the children. Finding their food culture within the center's food experiences helps children develop a strong self-concept and self-esteem. The child care center can encourage this by integrating diverse food patterns into its everyday menus and learning experiences with the children.

The Multicultural Food Experience

A positive learning environment is naturally respectful and thoughtful of multicultural values; it takes each child's culture into account from the beginning (York, 1991). The same is true for multicultural food experiences.

Food experiences that support multicultural education—and at the same time, reinforce healthful eating—should focus on concepts that young children can understand. These include:

- Respect for everyone's food culture
- Similarities and differences in food and the way people eat
- Importance of trying new foods
- Learning about food from our families
- Learning about food from our friends

A center's multicultural food experiences should mainly reflect foods and food patterns of the people in the community today. Activities focusing on foreign foods or holiday food celebrations should be limited; they tend to stereotype and take away the everyday reality of culturally based foods.

Children eat and enjoy familiar foods. A center's breakfast, lunch, and/or snack menus should include foods that children eat at home. For many Asian children, rice helps define a meal. For a Mexican American child, tortillas may be the bread they are accustomed to. Involve both parents and food service staff in planning menus and snacks that represent the children's cultural food preferences.

Through food preparation and tastings, children can share their own foods while they learn about ethnic foods of their peers. Bread tastings, for example, may give them a chance to try tortillas, matzo, pita bread, corn bread, chapati, Mexican sweet bread, black bread, or fried bread. A fruit tasting might introduce mango, papaya, starfruit, guava, mandarin orange, litchi, pomelo, or avocado.

Children usually enjoy exploring food experiences and learning about themselves and one another through dramatic play. Include objects that relate culture to food as an everyday part of the classroom. Include utensils, such as a tortilla press, wok, steamer, rolling pin, mortar and pestle, chopsticks, teapot, rice bowl, whisk, baskets, gourds, and fabrics with ethnic designs (batik, madras).

Children's literature can teach a great deal about food—its variety, where it comes from, and how to eat in a healthful, appropriate way. Books that present the everyday diversity and ethnicity of food also enhance the learning environment.

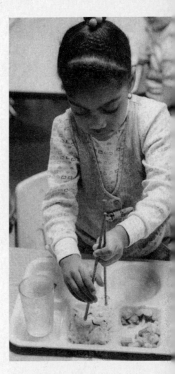

Multicultural food experiences, such as using chopsticks to eat a meal, are fun and can help a child learn about different cultural traditions.

Parent Involvement

Parent involvement is essential if a center's multicultural food experience is to be authentic and relevant. Family contact helps child care professionals learn about the family's culture and its influence on the child's food patterns. It also provides an opportunity for nutrition education.

Through enrollment meetings and home visits, caregivers can gather important information about a child's food sensitivities, the basic staples the family uses, and any religious or health restrictions regarding food. By involving parents from the start, the center can thoughtfully and efficiently handle many food considerations.

During any parent contact, be aware of other concerns—such as money problems, homelessness, neglect—that may affect the development, health, and food behavior of children. Identify social services in the community that address these problems, and refer parents to the appropriate agencies for assistance. For example, food assistance that helps many low-income families comes from the U. S. Department of Agriculture Food Stamp Program; the Special Supplemental Food Program for Women, Infants and Children; and the Child Nutrition Program, which offers free and reduced-priced meals.

Make time to talk regularly with parents about their child's nutrition and eating skills. The child care professional may be the main source of nutrition education to the family. Through parent newsletters, parent programs, and personal contacts, provide nutrition information, including guidelines for healthful meals and snacks.

Encourage parents to add to the food and multicultural experience of the center, too, by sharing typical family recipes. These recipes may be prepared as a learning activity. Or the center's food service staff may adapt them for the children's daily menus. Compiling the recipes into a center cookbook to share with other parents also reinforces multicultural understanding and broadens the families' exposure to foods.

Some states prohibit serving food from home to the class for sanitary or health reasons. However, parent volunteers may prepare foods that represent their family background at the center, perhaps as a food activity. Often raw ingredients—some that may only be available in ethnic markets—can be sent from home if they are properly handled at the center.

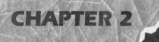

CHAPTER 2 / REVIEW

SUMMARY

- Healthful food patterns, formed during the early years of life, help ensure that children are adequately nourished.
- A positive food environment, which is safe, clean, pleasant, and physically comfortable, promotes a child's enjoyment of food and the development of good eating habits.
- Most young children need regular meal and snack schedules to satisfy their hunger and to provide the nutrients and energy their bodies need.
- Meal and snack planning for young children should take into consideration the children's nutritional needs as well as their food preferences and developmental needs.
- Mealtimes and snack times for young children should be managed to create an atmosphere conducive to positive eating behavior.
- Children learn to enjoy new foods through sensory experiences, careful timing, and positive reinforcement.

- Caregivers—including parents and child care providers—are role models who influence children's food behavior.
- The family is the main influence on a child's early food behavior.
- Ethnicity, or belonging to a group of people with common cultural characteristics, defines many food patterns.
- Food is central to many religious beliefs, and a family's religious practices may influence a child's daily food choices and eating patterns.
- Regional differences in diet and cuisine, caused by the effect of climate and geography on the agriculture and foods of a region, also influence children's food preferences.
- Parents' and caregivers' understanding of food and nutrition can help a child develop healthful food patterns.
- Emotions influence what, when, and how people of all ages eat.
- The media, especially television, affect children's eating behavior and attitudes toward food.
- Food experiences that develop healthful food patterns and self-esteem consider the ethnic diversity of the children.
- Parent involvement is essential to a child care center's multicultural food experiences.

ACQUIRING KNOWLEDGE

1. What is a food pattern? When are food patterns formed?
2. What role does a caregiver play in establishing a child's eating patterns?
3. Describe two characteristics of a positive food environment.
4. What criteria should be used in choosing furniture and eating utensils that are suited to children of a certain age group?
5. How do eating utensils designed for young children differ from adult utensils?
6. Why is cleanliness a priority in the child care setting? How could you help ensure that cleanliness remains a priority?
7. With regard to food preparation and eating, when should hands be washed?
8. What is one way that handwashing supplies and facilities can be made accessible for children?
9. How does appetite differ from hunger?
10. Define *satiety*.
11. How is food intake regulated in most children?
12. What role does timing play when meals and snacks are planned and served to young children?
13. What is the minimum length of time before a meal that a snack should be served?
14. Why is variety important in a child's diet?
15. Name two types of food that most children prefer.
16. Why should cooked foods be served to children warm rather than hot?

17. What is one advantage of serving finger foods to a child?
18. Identify and describe foods that should be avoided for young children because they may cause choking.
19. Why should stories, toys, and television be avoided during children's mealtimes?
20. What should caregivers do when a child repeatedly refuses a food?
21. How do children show independence through food behavior?
22. When is the best time for children to taste and learn about new foods?
23. Describe three major influences on a child's food patterns.
24. How can a child care center encourage the children to learn about the diverse variety of foods eaten by their peers?
25. How can parent involvement make a center's multicultural food experience authentic and relevant?

THINKING CRITICALLY

1. Suppose you work in a child care center where children can serve themselves various ready-to-eat cereals at any time of the day. In your opinion, what effects would this practice have on the children's appetites and food habits?
2. Do you think that positive reinforcement is the best way to teach good food habits? Why or why not? Explain.
3. Children need to try new foods and learn to choose from a variety to develop a balanced, nutritious eating pattern. What are the advantages of a caregiver providing a "guided" choice of foods? Are there any disadvantages to this approach?
4. Television advertisements for low-nutrient, high-calorie foods often lead children to ask for these foods. How might you, as a caregiver, counteract the influence of television commercials on children's eating preferences? How might a caregiver reinforce positive messages about food shown on television?
5. The caregiver often serves as a strong role model to children in the child care setting. With so many food cultures and ethnic backgrounds represented among the children of a class, how might a caregiver's value system and food "etiquette" be at odds with the children's own traditional and individual etiquettes?

OBSERVATIONS AND APPLICATIONS

1. Observe snack time at a child care center. What snacks are served? Are the snacks nutritious? What beverage is served: fruit juice, milk, or sweetened drinks? What is the policy concerning snacks at the center? Are parents responsible for providing snacks on a rotating basis for the whole class, does the center provide the snacks, or do children bring their own? Are there nutritional guidelines for snacks? How are snacks served? Do the children sit and eat the snack at tables? Are they served on plates? Do

caregivers and children wash their hands before handling food? What are the setup and cleanup routines? How many times are snacks served each day? When?

2. Watch an hour of children's programming on commercial television. Count the commercials shown during the hour. How many commercials are for food? How many food commercials are for snack food? How many products advertised are high in sugar or fat? How many commercials are for fruits or vegetables? What kinds of nutritional claims do the advertisements make?

3. Suppose you work with three- and four-year-olds in a child care center. While doing a unit on food, you ask the children to tell you what they ate for breakfast that morning. A surprising number say they did not eat breakfast. Many children say they do not regularly eat breakfast. How might you encourage children to eat breakfast?

4. Suppose you work in a child care center. The mother of one child in your class tells you that her child is used to having rice at every meal. How might you accommodate the child?

FOR FURTHER INFORMATION

Barer-Stein, T. (1991). *You eat what you are: A study of ethnic food traditions*. Toronto: Culture Concepts.

Berman, C., & Fromer, J. (1991). *Teaching children about food*. Menlo Park, CA: Bull Publishing.

Derman-Sparks, L., & the A. B. C. Task Force. (1989). *Anti-bias curriculum: Tools for empowering young children*. Washington, DC: National Association for the Education of Young Children.

Easy menu ethnic cookbooks. (1982). Minneapolis: Lerner Publications. (Cookbooks for these cuisines: African, Caribbean, Chinese, English, French, German, Greek, Hungarian, Indian, Israeli, Italian, Japanese, Korean, Lebanese, Mexican, Norwegian, Polish, Russian, Thai, Vietnamese.)

Kittler, P. G., & Sucher, K. (1989). *Food and culture in America*. New York: Van Nostrand Reinhold.

Lifshitz, F., & Satter, E. (1992, July/August). Nutrition and young children: Issues and challenges. *Dairy Council Digest*, 63 (4).

Lowenberg, M., Todhunter, E. N., Wilson, E. D., Savage, J. R., & Lubawski, J. L. (1979). *Food and people*. New York: Macmillan.

Sanjur, D. (1982). *Social and cultural perspectives in nutrition*. Englewood Cliffs, NJ: Prentice-Hall.

Satter, E. (1986). *Child of mine*. Menlo Park, CA: Bull Publishing.

Satter, E. (1987). *How to get your child to eat . . . but not too much*. Menlo Park, CA: Bull Publishing.

York, S. (1991). *Roots & wings: Affirming culture in early childhood programs*. St. Paul, MN: Toys 'n Things Press.

3 Nutrition Basics

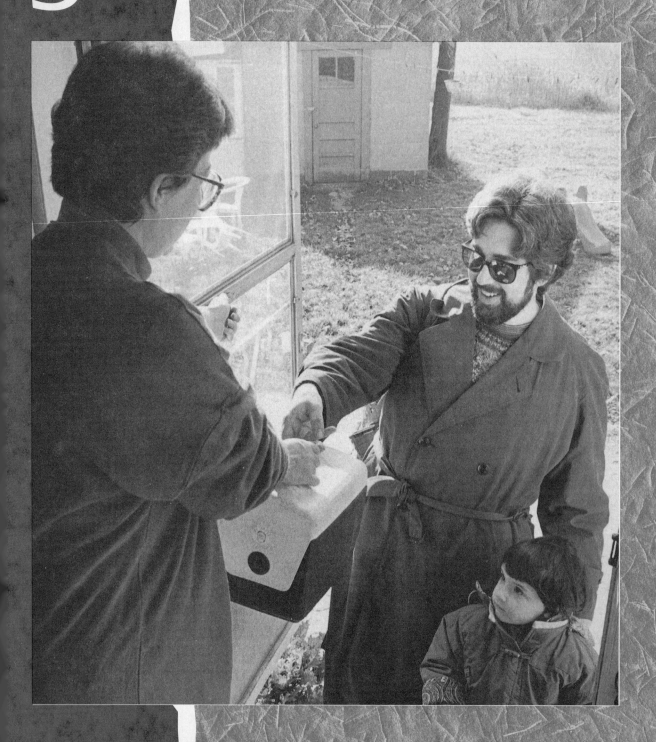

OBJECTIVES

Studying this chapter
will enable you to

- Explain the role of carbohydrates, fats, and proteins in health and list main sources of each nutrient group
- List key vitamins and their main sources, and discuss the role each vitamin plays in health
- List key minerals and their main sources, and discuss the role each mineral plays in health
- Discuss the need for water and its major functions in the body

CHAPTER TERMS

amino acids
antioxidant
calories
cholesterol
complete proteins
complex carbohydrates
dietary fiber
electrolytes
fatty acids
glycogen
HDL cholesterol
LDL cholesterol
legumes
metabolism
minerals
saturated fats
vitamins

IT was 7:30 A.M. Mark walked his four-year-old daughter, Jana, into the ABC Child Care Center. Jana handed her lunch bag to her teacher, Nancy.

Nancy smiled and thanked Jana, then caught Mark's eye. "Is it peanut butter or bologna today?" she asked.

"Today is a peanut butter day," replied Mark.

"If there are any fruits or veggies in here, I'll be glad to put Jana's lunch in the 'fridge," Nancy said in an inquiring tone.

Mark hesitated. "No such luck," he said, "I can never decide what or how much to pack, so it's just the sandwich and some cookies. I figure, with the milk she gets here, it's a pretty good lunch."

"Well," Nancy said, "We've just put together some tips on adding variety and interest to the children's lunches. They include suggestions for colorful, tasty fruits and vegetables and how much to pack. Most of the preparation can be done the night before. Would you like a copy?"

"Sure," Mark replied. He appreciated the thought and knew that it would be a good idea to include fruits and vegetables in Jana's lunch. He glanced down the list of tips. Several looked easy enough. Jana liked carrot sticks, tangerines, and apples. Who would have thought of sprinkling lemon juice on pieces of apple so they would not turn brown?

"Thanks, Nancy," said Mark, heading for the door. "I'll give some of these a try."

The nutrients in fruits and vegetables as well as in milk products, breads and cereals, and meat, poultry, and fish are important for Jana's growth, energy, and overall good health. Because different foods supply different nutrients and each nutrient does different jobs in the body, Jana needs a varied diet with foods from all the groups, including fruits and vegetables. Caregivers and teachers who find ways to help children eat a variety of food can make all the difference.

Nutrients in Food

Metabolism, the whole range of physical and chemical processes that sustain life, requires energy and materials that are supplied by the nutrients in food. Food is composed of more than 40 nutrients, each having specific roles in human health. Because each nutrient has a unique set of functions, no single nutrient can replace another.

Food, rather than dietary supplements, is the body's best source of the various nutrients. Some foods are better sources of specific nutrients than others. During digestion, food breaks down into nutrients, which are absorbed into the bloodstream. The body then transforms these nutrients into thousands of different body chemicals that promote growth and development, provide energy, maintain health, resist infection, and perform the daily functions of life.

Regardless of age, sex, and activity level, everyone needs the same nutrients. However, the amounts of particular nutrients people need change as they grow older and when there are changes in their activity level and lifestyle. Infants and children need an adequate and varied supply of nutrients to grow and develop properly. Adults need these same nutrients, but in different amounts, to keep their bodies in good health over their lifetime.

Nutrients belong in six groups: carbohydrates, fats, proteins, vitamins, minerals, and water. The first three—carbohydrates, proteins, and fats—are often called macronutrients because the body uses them in large amounts. Vitamins and minerals are micronutrients, which we need in much smaller amounts. Water is the most essential nutrient to life; we need this in the greatest amount. By the definition just given, therefore, water is a macronutrient.

Calories are often confused with nutrients, but they are not the same. *Calories* (more accurately called kilocalories) are a measure of energy. They measure both the amount of energy in food and the amount of energy the body uses for its physiological processes, such as the pumping of the heart and breathing, and for physical activity. When caloric intake equals caloric use, body weight remains the same unless the body is in a growth stage. When caloric intake is higher, body fat increases and people gain weight;

TABLE 3.1
Recommended Caloric Intake

Category	Age (years) or Condition	Weight (lb)	Weight (kg)	Average Energy Allowance (kcal)[a] Per lb	Average Energy Allowance (kcal)[a] Per day[b]
Infants	0.0–0.5	13	6	49	650
	0.5–1.0	20	9	44	850
Children	1–3	29	13	46	1,300
	4–6	44	20	41	1,800
	7–10	62	28	32	2,000
Men	11–14	99	45	25	2,500
	15–18	145	66	20	3,000
	19–24	160	72	18	2,900
	25–50	174	79	17	2,900
	51+	170	77	14	2,300
Women	11–14	101	46	21	2,200
	15–18	120	55	18	2,200
	19–24	128	58	17	2,200
	25–50	138	63	16	2,200
	51+	143	65	14	1,900
Pregnant	1st trimester				+0
	2nd trimester				+300
	3rd trimester				+300
Lactating	1st 6 months				+500
	2nd 6 months				+500

[a] A normal variation of +/−20 percent is accepted for younger adults.
[b] Figure is rounded.

Adapted from National Research Council. (1989). *Recommended dietary allowances*. Washington, DC: National Academy Press, p. 33, using weight as basis.

when caloric intake is lower, people lose weight. The number of calories a person needs varies with age, sex, and weight (see Table 3.1) as well as with activity level. Three types of nutrients supply calories: carbohydrates, fats, and proteins.

Carbohydrates: The Body's Main Energy Source

Carbohydrates are the body's main source of fuel. Sugars, starches, and fiber are all forms of carbohydrates. Each has different nutritional benefits.

Sugars are the simplest, smallest form of carbohydrates. They consist of either one or two sugar units. Glucose, fructose, and galactose are one-unit sugars. Sucrose, maltose, and lactose are two-unit sugars. In sucrose, commonly known as table sugar, the two units are glucose and fructose, which are chemically joined to each other.

Complex carbohydrates, such as starches, are made by chemically linking many glucose units together. During digestion, most complex carbohydrates and two-unit sugars break down into one-unit sugars, which are absorbed into the bloodstream. Complex carbohydrates break down more slowly than two-unit sugars, providing a steady supply of glucose. Inside the body, any fructose or galactose from the breakdown of two-unit sugars is changed to glucose before being used.

Fiber, a type of complex carbohydrate, does not break down in the body. During digestion, it is not converted to one-unit sugars. For this reason, fiber is not absorbed and cannot supply energy. Instead, it plays other roles in health, including aiding digestion.

The Role of Carbohydrates in Health

Carbohydrates supply energy for every body function: metabolic processes such as making body proteins, physical activity such as running or jumping, and even breathing. Most of the calories children need to grow, learn, and play should come from carbohydrates. Every gram of carbohydrate in the diet supplies 4 calories. In a healthful diet, 55 to 60 percent of total calories should come from carbohydrates, primarily complex carbohydrates (National Research Council, 1989). If a child requires 1,800 calories a day, 990 to 1,080 calories should come from carbohydrates. At 4 calories per gram, this means that 275 to 300 grams of carbohydrates should be consumed daily.

The sugar glucose, which is the main carbohydrate in the bloodstream, is often called blood sugar. Blood sugar may be transported to cells to be used for energy or changed to either glycogen or body fat. *Glycogen* is a form of carbohydrate that is stored in the muscles, liver, and other body cells. Body fat is stored in the liver and in fat cells. Most excess glucose gets stored as body fat. Glycogen, and then body fat, are changed back to glucose when the blood sugar level gets too low. In that way, the body has energy reserves when the glucose supply from the diet gets low.

Dietary fiber refers to the parts of plants that cannot be fully broken down in the human digestive tract. It plays a special role in health. Although fiber cannot be digested, absorbed, or used for energy, different forms of fiber do perform special functions in the digestive tract. And some fibers offer protection from chronic, or long-term, diseases.

Some fibers, for example, form gels that hold water and make stools softer and bulkier. Other fibers aid the digestive action of bacteria in the colon and help move wastes through the intestinal tract. This latter effect

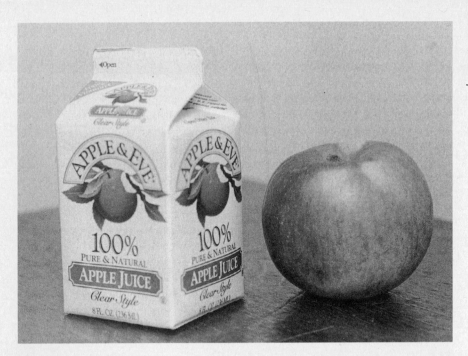

Food processing tends to reduce the fiber content of foods. This apple contains more fiber than the apple juice.

shortens the time that cancer-causing components of food waste come in contact with the intestinal lining. All of these fibers are natural laxatives.

A type of fiber found in foods such as oat bran, beans, and apples may help reduce blood cholesterol because it binds with fatty substances and carries them away as waste. This may help lower the risk of cardiovascular diseases (Wotecki & Thomas, 1992). Fiber also helps stimulate muscle tone in the intestine, offering protection from diverticular disease, in which weakened areas of the intestinal wall balloon out.

While a low-fiber diet is associated with chronic constipation, hemorrhoids, diverticular disease, and even cancer, too much fiber can also interfere with health. Excess fiber may cause diarrhea and hinder nutrient absorption.

Key Sources of Carbohydrates

Carbohydrates come from a wide variety of foods. Grain products, vegetables, fruits, and dry beans are the best sources. These foods, which are naturally rich in carbohydrates, are also good sources of other essential nutrients. In a healthful diet, most carbohydrates are in the form of naturally occurring sugars and complex carbohydrates.

Sugars are a natural component of many foods. For example, fruits and honey are rich in fructose. Milk contains lactose. Sucrose is found in some fruits and vegetables. Sucrose is also processed from sugarcane and sugar beets into table sugar. (Syrup and molasses are two other refined, or processed, sugars.) Foods with processed sugars often have fewer nutrients than foods with naturally occurring sugars.

Enjoying a Varied Diet

Clarisse felt someone tugging on her skirt and looked around to see Michael, a redheaded four-year-old.

"Are we having peanut butter for lunch today?" he asked hopefully.

Clarisse reminded Michael that peanut butter was what they had had yesterday. "We're having tuna salad today, Michael, and it's almost time for lunch. Why don't we wash up so we can sit down together?"

The child care center where Clarisse worked made careful meal plans so that different lunches were served every day of the week. Each day, the children drank a different kind of juice and had a different food for snack too. Most children came to enjoy the variety, even though they didn't like every food that was served. Clarisse encouraged the children by eating with them and letting them see how much she enjoyed the different foods. She always was the first to try a new food, and she had gotten the children to try and appreciate apricots and pears for afternoon snack. Some,

including Michael, had even decided that "cauliflower is pretty good."

Clarisse had been so successful that some parents had commented. She shared her secrets with them. Don't force a food; just show lots of enthusiasm and appreciation for new tastes. Make sure you eat a variety of foods yourself. Clarisse also told parents what she did when a child refused to accept a new food. First, she experimented with preparing it in different ways. Sometimes she allowed children to help her cook the food the next time. Parents thanked her when they, too, were successful in varying the diets of their children.

Clarisse enjoyed seeing the children eat and enjoy new foods. It was rewarding to know that they were building the foundation of a nutritious, balanced diet.

Are there other good ways you can think of to encourage children to enjoy a varied diet? How would you deal with a child who refused to eat more than one or two types of food?

Complex carbohydrates come from several types of foods. Breads, rice, grits, pasta, cereals, and other grains such as oats, barley, buckwheat, rye, triticale, and millet are good sources of complex carbohydrates. Other good sources include starchy vegetables, especially potatoes, corn, beans, peas, yams, and cassava.

Fiber is found in virtually all plant sources of food: grains, nuts, seeds, peas, beans, vegetables, and fruits. Whole grains, especially the bran layer, provide more fiber than refined versions. Food preparation and processing tends to reduce fiber content. An apple, for example, has more fiber than apple juice. Because different foods have different forms of fiber, eating a wide variety of fiber-rich foods is important.

Fats: Enough, But Not Too Much

Nutritionists caution the public that too much dietary fat can compromise good health. Yet fats are nutrients, essential for health. The concern is the amount; many Americans consume more fats than they need.

Fatty acids are the building blocks of fats. Fats contain a mixture of fatty acids: some of these are saturated and some are unsaturated. Those with mostly unsaturated fatty acids tend to be liquid at room temperature, for example, vegetable oil. Fats that are solid at room temperature, such as butter, are considered *saturated fats*—fats that contain mostly saturated fatty acids. Generally speaking, harder fats are more highly saturated.

Cholesterol is a fatlike substance found only in animals. Although it is chemically related to fats, it contains no fatty acids.

The Role of Fats and Cholesterol in Health

Fats have several important functions in human health. They carry fat-soluble vitamins, provide essential fatty acids, and improve the appeal of many foods. Dietary fats yield 9 calories per gram—more than twice the amount of energy provided by a gram of carbohydrate or protein. Excess fat in the diet is stored as body fat.

Body fat is a concentrated source of energy reserves. It is the second energy reserve to be used (glycogen is the first) when blood sugar levels fall because food is not supplying enough glucose for the body's needs. Having some body fat is healthy because it cushions and protects vital organs from injury. The fat layer under the skin is also an insulator from heat and cold. Too much body fat, however, puts an individual at risk for many other health problems.

Fats serve as a carrier for some nutrients—vitamins A, D, E, and K. Because these vitamins dissolve in fats, not water, they can only be carried into the bloodstream by fats. Fat-soluble vitamins cannot be fully used if the diet is too low in fats.

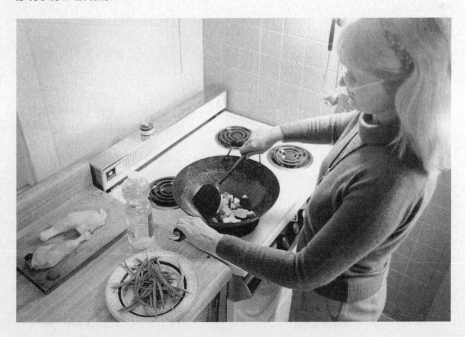

Stir-fry cooking can help keep dietary fats at a healthful, moderate level.

Until they are about two years old, children should receive whole milk, which is high in essential fatty acids. Low-fat dairy foods are preferable for older children and adults.

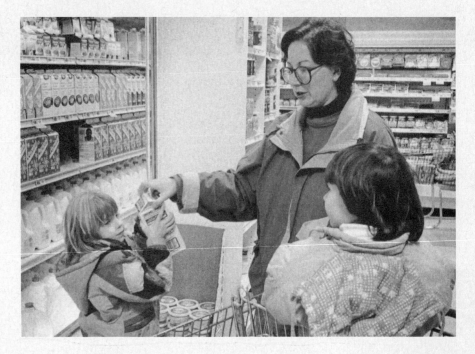

Some fatty acids are essential for health. The body cannot make them; they must come from the diet, mainly from plant and fish oils. Infants and children need the essential fatty acids to grow normally; adults need them to keep skin and other tissues healthy. A diet with moderate amounts of fat provides enough of the essential fatty acids.

Fats in food impart qualities that make eating more pleasurable. When nutritious foods taste good, people are more likely to eat them. Fats add flavor, tenderness, and moisture to food. Fats also help satisfy hunger because they take longer to digest than carbohydrates or proteins do.

While cholesterol is a fatlike substance, its role in health is quite different. Cholesterol is part of the membrane of all body cells and is especially important to the nervous system. Cholesterol is also needed for the production of many hormones, special substances that regulate body processes, and bile, which helps digest fats. And it is used to make a vitamin D precursor that is converted to vitamin D when the skin is exposed to sunlight.

The body makes its own cholesterol, so cholesterol is not an essential nutrient. In fact, too much cholesterol can increase a person's risk of cardiovascular diseases. Dietary cholesterol, or cholesterol obtained from food, is just one factor that affects blood, or serum, cholesterol levels. Other risk factors include smoking, sedentary life-styles, and diets high in fats, especially saturated fats.

Cholesterol and fats are carried through the bloodstream in protein-wrapped packages known as lipoproteins. There are low-density lipoproteins (LDLs) and high-density lipoproteins (HDLs). *LDL cholesterol* is often called bad cholesterol; at high levels, it tends to deposit cholesterol on artery

FOCUS ON ◢ **Cultural Diversity**

Complete Proteins Around the World

Long before scientists had identified the nine essential amino acids, people around the world had figured out many different ways of combining plant foods to obtain these nutrients. One way is to combine a legume (such as peas or beans) with either a grain (such as corn, rice, or wheat) or a seed or nut. Here in the United States, we do this when we make a peanut butter sandwich. Peanut butter is made from the peanut, a legume. When spread on bread made from wheat flour, the result is a complete protein containing all nine essential amino acids.

Legumes, seeds, nuts, or grains can also be combined with eggs or dairy foods to provide complete proteins. Macaroni and cheese and oatmeal with milk are familiar combinations in the United States.

Other cultures have found different ways of combining protein sources. The Mexicans, for example, have a variety of dishes that combine wheat or corn tortillas with cooked beans and other ingredients. Examples include enchiladas and tacos.

In parts of Africa and the Caribbean, cooks often prepare dishes that combine various kinds of peas or beans with rice. Hoppin john, with a base of black-eyed peas and rice, is one such dish that has an African origin.

Hummus, a paste made from chick peas and ground sesame seeds, has long been a favorite in the Middle East. Also popular in that area is falafel, made from chick peas and served with pita bread made from wheat flour. Both dishes contain all the essential amino acids.

Many cultures also use plant proteins to supplement small amounts of animal protein. Rice pudding, a combination of milk and rice that is popular in Western Europe, is an example. Asians stir-fry small amounts of meat, fish, or tofu with vegetables and serve the mixture with rice. And all over the world chicken soup with rice, noodles, or matzo balls is a much-loved way of nourishing the body by combining animal and vegetable proteins.

walls. *HDL cholesterol* is sometimes referred to as good cholesterol since it is associated with a lower risk of cholesterol deposits in the arteries. Raising blood levels of HDLs and lowering LDLs may help lower the risk of cardiovascular diseases.

Too much dietary fat is linked to several health problems, including obesity, cardiovascular diseases, and some cancers. Diets high in saturated fats, as well as cholesterol, are linked to heart disease. For this reason, recommendations have been set for moderating the amount of fat and cholesterol in the diets of healthy people age two and older.

The amount of fat each person needs daily depends on each individual's caloric needs. Health experts advise 30 percent or less of a person's total calories per day should come from fats (National Research Council, 1989). If a person needs 2,000 calories a day, this means that fats should supply no more than 600 calories. Since 1 gram of fat supplies 9 calories, the upper limit on fat would be about 67 grams by this guidance. Less than 10 percent of total calories (in this example, 200 calories) should come from saturated fats. That would mean no more than about 22 grams of saturated fat per day—the amount in about 1½ cups of rich ice cream, which is 16 percent fat (see Appendix B). The guideline for cholesterol is 300 milligrams or less per day for everyone (National Research Council, 1989). This upper limit does not depend on caloric needs.

Key Sources of Fats

Fats come from many types of food. Some have much more fat than others, however. Margarine, butter, lard, shortening, and oil are obvious sources of fat. Foods such as meats, poultry, fish, milk, nuts, seeds, cheese, and chocolate also contain fat. Fruits and vegetables (except avocado and coconut) tend to be low in fat, unless they are fried or served with a cream sauce, salad dressing, mayonnaise, or butter. Grain products may be low in fat, but added ingredients or food preparation can increase their fat and caloric content. Doughnuts, croissants, biscuits, and many muffins and quick breads, for example, are usually high in fat. Rich desserts, such as cakes and pastries, as well as snack chips and cookies tend to be high in fat too.

Different foods have different types of fats. Most vegetable fats, including olive, canola, corn, cottonseed, and soybean oils, have a greater proportion of unsaturated fatty acids. Exceptions are palm, palm kernel, and coconut oils, also called tropical oils, which are high in saturated fatty acids. Animal fats, such as butterfat and beef fat, tend to be high in saturated fatty acids. But seafood is a good source of unsaturated fatty acids.

Cholesterol is found only in animal sources of food, such as meat, poultry, fish, eggs, and dairy foods. Foods with the highest amounts of cholesterol include egg yolks and organ meats. For this reason, most people are advised to eat no more than three to four eggs a week.

Appendix B shows the breakdown of fats, as well as various other nutrients, for specific foods. A comparison of fats in similar foods, for example rich ice cream and ice milk, can provide useful information for people who are concerned about their fat intake.

Proteins: Part of Every Body Cell

The word *protein* means "of prime importance." In fact, protein is part of every body cell, making it essential for life. *Amino acids* are the building blocks of proteins.

Proteins are made of long chains of amino acids. There are 22 common amino acids that combine in different ways to form proteins. There are many thousands of different proteins in the body.

The proteins in food are different from the proteins in the body, but they contain many of the same amino acids. During digestion and absorption, proteins break down into individual amino acids, which are then carried through the bloodstream to body cells. Within the cells, they may be broken down further, then formed into new amino acids. Body cells make new proteins by rearranging amino acids into very precise sequences.

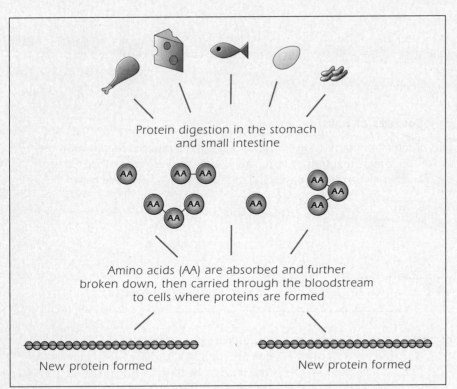

Protein digestion in the stomach and small intestine

Amino acids (AA) are absorbed and further broken down, then carried through the bloodstream to cells where proteins are formed

New protein formed   New protein formed

FIGURE 3.1   Amino Acids: The Building Blocks of Proteins. Digestion breaks proteins down into single amino acids and chains of two or three amino acids. When they are absorbed, the short chains break down, and single amino acids are carried to body cells through the bloodstream. Proteins are made in the cells by linking amino acids in long chains in precise sequences.

The body cannot make nine amino acids. These essential amino acids must be supplied by the diet. If even one of the nine essential amino acids is missing or limited, the body cannot grow or function normally. Dietary proteins that contain all nine essential amino acids are called *complete proteins*. Incomplete proteins lack one or more of the essential amino acids.

The Role of Proteins in Health

Proteins function in three key ways in human health. Their main role is to build and repair body tissue. Proteins also regulate many body processes. Finally, like carbohydrates and fats, proteins are energy nutrients.

Proteins are found throughout the body. Everything external (eyes, hair, nails, skin) and everything internal (muscle, bones, blood, vital organs) contain proteins. Body cells are even held together by the fibrous protein collagen. As body cells wear out, they must be replaced. And new cells are formed as infants and children grow.

The work of making new proteins takes place within each body cell. The code for making each protein is in the genetic material found in the cell. Proteins are synthesized as one amino acid is joined to the next, according to the code (see Figure 3.1).

Proteins help regulate many life processes. Some proteins speed up chemical reactions in the body and stimulate particular tissues and organs to

Peanut butter is a good source of high-quality plant protein.

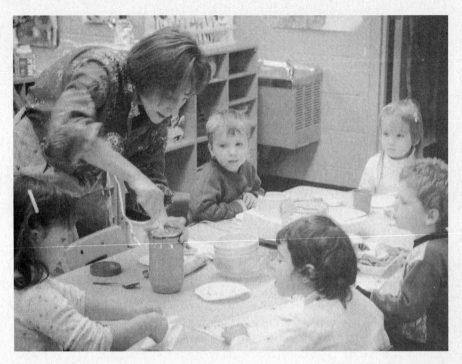

function. Other proteins regulate fluid in body cells, transport minerals across cell membranes, and help maintain a proper chemical balance in the body's systems.

Proteins can also supply energy—4 calories per gram—if the diet has an insufficient amount of carbohydrates and fats for the body's energy needs. When that happens, the unused parts of the protein are disposed of in the urine. When proteins become the main source of energy, for example in a high-protein, low-fat diet, the kidneys must work harder to get rid of these wastes through urine.

There is no specific recommendation for what percent of calories should come from protein. The amount of protein a person needs depends on that person's body size and how fast the person is growing. Infants and children need more protein per pound of body weight than do adults (see chapters 6, 7, and 8). Proteins must be a regular part of the diet because the body does not store excess proteins as reserve amino acids. Instead, extra amino acids are broken down and stored as body fat. Eating too much protein can be as fattening as eating too much fat or carbohydrate.

Key Sources of Proteins

Proteins come from many different foods. Foods from animal sources—meat, poultry, fish, eggs, and most dairy foods—have, from a nutritional standpoint, the highest quality proteins. That is why most meals are planned around these protein-rich foods. Because they have all nine essential amino acids, animal proteins are complete proteins.

Some plant proteins are high quality too. These include proteins in legumes, nuts, and seeds. *Legumes* are seeds found in the pods of certain plants and used for food; beans, peas, lentils, peanuts, and soybeans are all legumes. Yet, plant proteins don't have all of the essential amino acids. For this reason, they need to be combined with other plant or animal proteins. Amino acids in one food can complement those in another; together they may supply complete proteins.

Foods can be combined in these ways to provide a meal with complete proteins:

- Legumes + grains (example: beans and rice)
- Legumes + seeds or nuts (example: mixed peanuts and nuts)
- Legumes, seeds, nuts, or grains + eggs or dairy foods (example: macaroni and cheese)

Vitamins: Vital to Life

Vitamins are substances that help regulate body processes. There are two categories of vitamins: water-soluble and fat-soluble. The terms refer to the way in which they are dissolved in food and transported within the body. Water-soluble vitamins (B vitamins and vitamin C) move through the body dissolved in water; fat-soluble vitamins (vitamins A, D, E, and K) are carried by fat.

Vitamins are needed in very small amounts. A varied diet generally supplies all the vitamins a person needs. However, vitamin-rich foods need to be carefully prepared. Excessive cooking, especially at high temperatures, can destroy many vitamins.

Three vitamins—C, E, and beta carotene (a form of vitamin A)—also work as antioxidants. An *antioxidant* is a substance that removes certain by-products of metabolism. These by-products, known as free radicals, can damage cells and their genetic material, increasing the risk for some chronic diseases. Antioxidants may offer protection against some chronic diseases, including some cancers, heart disease, and cataracts.

Water-Soluble Vitamins

The B vitamins and vitamin C are water-soluble. Water-soluble vitamins can be lost from food if the food is cooked for too long in too much liquid. There is generally little risk of toxicity with water-soluble vitamins because they are not stored in the body. They are carried in the bloodstream and excess amounts are excreted with the urine. For this reason, deficiencies can develop quickly if the diet does not regularly supply the necessary amounts of these vitamins.

B Complex Vitamins.   The B vitamins are not one nutrient, but a group of eight nutrients with specific, interrelated roles in human health. Most B vitamins help the body produce energy within the cells. The amount of B vitamins needed relates to the amount of energy the body uses. B vitamins are also important in the manufacture of some materials, the multiplication of cells, and the function of nerves.

Thiamin (vitamin B_1) helps the body produce energy from carbohydrates. It is found in meat, eggs, beans, whole grains, and enriched breads and cereals.

Riboflavin (vitamin B_2) helps the body produce energy from carbohydrates and helps regulate many other body processes. It is found mainly in liver, milk, and dark-green leafy vegetables; whole grains and enriched breads and cereals are other good sources.

Niacin helps produce energy from fats, proteins, and carbohydrates and helps the body manufacture fatty acids. Niacin is found in grain products, nuts, beans, meat, poultry, and fish.

Folic acid, also known as folacin, helps the body make the genetic material in the cells and helps produce amino acids. Some forms of anemia are related to a low intake of folic acid. Dark-green leafy vegetables, liver, and fruits are good sources of folic acid.

Cobalamin (vitamin B_{12}) is needed for folic acid activity and to maintain the function of nerves. It is found only in foods of animal origin, such as meat, milk products, and eggs. Children on strict vegetarian diets may not consume enough of this nutrient to grow properly.

The remaining three B vitamins are pyridoxine (vitamin B_6), biotin, and pantothenic acid. They play various roles in breaking down foods for energy and helping to produce other molecules.

Vitamin C.   Vitamin C, also called ascorbic acid, has several roles in the human body. Vitamin C helps form connective tissue and strengthens the walls of blood vessels, protecting them from bruising. Vitamin C aids in the healing of cuts and wounds, helps the body use calcium and iron, and helps in the production of some proteins. The body needs vitamin C to synthesize and maintain collagen, the protein that is part of all connective tissue.

Vitamin C is also an antioxidant. In that role, it may offer protection from high blood pressure, heart disease, cataracts, and cancers of the mouth, throat, pancreas, and stomach.

A relatively small amount of vitamin C each day (the amount provided in a 6-ounce glass of orange juice) is sufficient for the functions it performs. It is sometimes said that large doses of vitamin C will prevent or cure the common cold; however, there is no scientific evidence to confirm this.

Many fruits and vegetables are rich in vitamin C. The best sources are citrus fruits: lemons, limes, oranges, grapefruits, and tangerines. Other good fruit sources of vitamin C include strawberries, papaya, pineapple, and cantaloupe. Tomatoes, broccoli, green pepper, cabbage, turnips, and collard greens are among the many vegetables that are good vitamin C sources. People who make a habit of consuming citrus fruit or juice for breakfast get plenty of vitamin C in their diets.

Fat-Soluble Vitamins

Vitamins A, D, E, and K are fat-soluble. Fat-soluble vitamins must be carried into and through the body by fat. Therefore, it is important that the diet include a moderate amount of fat.

In the United States, severe deficiencies of fat-soluble vitamins are not common. Because these vitamins are stored in body fat, consuming too much of them, perhaps from a large dose of a vitamin supplement, could be toxic, however.

Vitamin A and Beta Carotene.   Vitamin A is found in two forms in food. One form, retinol, is found primarily in liver and fish liver oils. The

---

FOCUS ON **Communicating with Children**

Importance of Drinking Water

Donna and Ricky put the finishing touches on the parking garage they had been working on for half an hour in the block area. Donna parked two cars, and Ricky parked the truck he had brought from home. They ran over to Margie, the teacher of the four-year-old group at the Red Bank Learning Center.

DONNA: Can we have some juice?

MARGIE: You know what? We used up all the juice at snack time. How about some nice cold water?

RICKY: Yuck, I don't want water.

MARGIE: Hey, you two. Remember what happened to our geranium plant when we forgot to water it?

DONNA: Yeah, it got all like this. (She made herself limp like a rag doll.)

MARGIE: And it dried up, right? The flowers started turning brown. You know, people need a whole lot of water, too, just like the geranium. In fact, people need water every day. Do you know how water helps you inside? (She put her hand on her own stomach.)

DONNA: Nope.

MARGIE: You know when you throw a stick in the stream behind the school, the water carries it away? Well, the water inside you carries some of the vitamins from the food you eat all over your body. That helps keep you healthy.

RICKY: Like a little river inside you?

MARGIE: Yes. But just by playing and running, you use up a lot of water every day. That's why you have to drink so much water—to put back the water you use up.

RICKY: Hey, I know! Just like a gas station. Fill 'er up! (He tipped his head back, opened his mouth wide, and pointed inside.)

MARGIE: Okay, sir! Let's go to the 'fridge. (She poured two glasses of water from a pitcher and handed them to Donna and Ricky.) I'll take a glass too.

What other messages about water are important for young children to know? How else might Margie have explained what water does for the body?

Playing outdoors can help children produce vitamin D, which is synthesized by the body in the presence of sunlight. Vitamin D is involved in many body processes, including forming healthy bones and teeth.

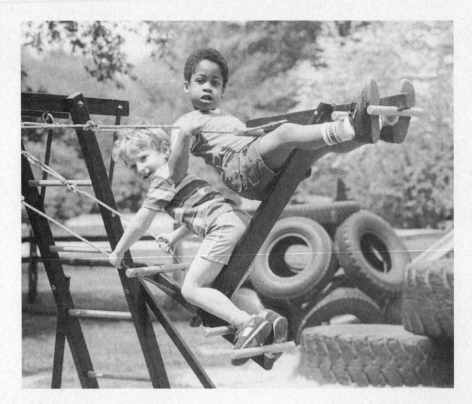

other, more familiar, form is beta carotene, present in foods such as carrots and sweet potatoes. Unlike retinol, beta carotene must be converted to vitamin A in the body.

Vitamin A serves several purposes as a regulator in human health. It helps maintain normal vision at low light levels. Night blindness, which is the inability of the eye to adjust well to darkness, can be caused by a deficiency of vitamin A.

Vitamin A helps maintain healthy skin and mucous membranes. Mucous membranes line the mouth, nose, throat, and digestive tract. When these membranes are moist and healthy, they help protect the respiratory and digestive systems from infection. Vitamin A also helps white blood cells fight infection, and it is necessary for normal growth and the development of bones and teeth. Beta carotene is an antioxidant, and it may help protect against some forms of cancer and heart disease.

Vitamin A is stored mostly in the liver. Small amounts in storage are useful, allowing a constant supply of vitamin A when the dietary contribution is low. While toxic levels of beta carotene have not been identified, large doses of retinol can be toxic and may cause headaches, nausea, dry and itchy skin, and pain in the bones and joints. In extreme cases, toxic levels of vitamin A can retard growth and cause birth defects.

Vitamin A comes from both animal and plant sources of food. Liver and fish liver oils are especially rich sources of vitamin A. Eggs, butter, vitamin

A-fortified milk, and meats supply some vitamin A too. Dark-green leafy vegetables and deep yellow or orange fruits and vegetables are good sources of beta carotene. These include broccoli, spinach, turnip greens, squash, carrots, sweet potato, apricots, and papaya.

Vitamin D.   Vitamin D is often referred to as the sunshine vitamin because the body synthesizes vitamin D when skin is exposed to sunlight. When the body doesn't have enough contact with ultraviolet light from the sun, vitamin D must be obtained from food. People who stay indoors too much or who live in locations with very short winter days may not get enough exposure to sunlight to supply their vitamin D needs.

Vitamin D is stored primarily in the liver. It works in partnership with calcium and phosphorus in many body processes: to form and maintain bones during growth and throughout life; to build strong, healthy teeth; and to help muscles contract and relax.

Varying amounts of vitamin D are found in liver, eggs, and some fish, but it is not as common as other nutrients in food. For this reason, milk (which contains both calcium and phosphorus) is fortified with vitamin D. Drinking milk daily helps children get the vitamin D they need to grow. Breakfast cereals may also be fortified with vitamin D.

Vitamin E.   Vitamin E works mainly as an antioxidant in the body and in food. It keeps oxygen from destroying fatty acids. This may not sound very important. However, by preventing oxidation of fatty acids, vitamin E helps keep all the membranes in every cell of the body intact. Vitamin E also protects the other fat-soluble vitamins from oxidation and may help lower the risk of fatty deposits that can clog arteries. Vitamin E is stored wherever there are fats in the body. Vegetable oils, nuts, seeds, wheat germ, and dark-green leafy vegetables are all good sources of vitamin E.

Vitamin K.   Vitamin K is necessary for making certain proteins, including six that are essential to blood clotting. It is synthesized by bacteria normally present in the intestinal tract. The body doesn't need much vitamin K from food unless an intestinal infection or antibiotic treatment temporarily destroys the helpful bacteria. Vitamin K is stored in the liver. The best food source of vitamin K is dark-green leafy vegetables. It is also found in cereals, dairy foods, meat, eggs, and fruits.

Vitamin Supplements

Since vitamins are so vital to health, aren't vitamin supplements a good idea? With the exception of certain health conditions, such as pregnancy, food is the best source of nutrients, including vitamins. That's because food has the 40 or more nutrients that the body needs for health; nutrient supplements do not. Nutrients that occur naturally in food are often better absorbed than nutrients in supplements. A balanced and varied diet can supply all the nutrients needed for growth, energy, and health (Institute of

Medicine, 1991). Unless vitamins are prescribed by a physician because particular foods are not included in the diet or certain health conditions are present, there is no reason to spend money on vitamin pills.

Minerals: To Regulate Body Processes

Minerals are substances that help regulate body processes. Unlike many vitamins, minerals are not destroyed by heat.

Minerals make up 3 to 4 percent of the body's total weight, contributing to skeletal and dental structures, blood, muscle, and other body tissues. Minerals also help regulate a wide variety of metabolic processes, including maintaining the chemical balance of body fluids.

Compared with carbohydrates, fats, and proteins, we need relatively small amounts of minerals. However, the body does need some minerals in significantly larger amounts than others. These major minerals include calcium, phosphorus, magnesium, sodium, chloride, and potassium. Trace minerals are needed in smaller amounts. Most people know about the trace mineral iron. Other trace minerals include chromium, copper, fluoride, iodine, manganese, molybdenum, selenium, and zinc. The importance of a mineral to the health of the body is not always reflected by the amount of that mineral the body needs.

Calcium and Phosphorus

The body contains more calcium than any other mineral. The amount of phosphorus in the body runs a close second to calcium. Calcium and phosphorus work together to help build and maintain bones and teeth. About 99 percent of the calcium in the body is found in bones and teeth. For phosphorus, this figure is about 85 percent.

Even after people stop growing, calcium and phosphorus are important. Like every other body tissue, bone tissue requires constant maintenance. Calcium and phosphorus are needed to maintain bones and teeth. If the diet is deficient in these two minerals for long enough, bones and teeth lose density and strength as calcium and phosphorus are removed from them and used for other functions in the body. Ultimately, this may lead to a condition known as osteoporosis, or brittle bone disease.

Calcium is important to muscle contraction, including the action of the heart muscle. It also helps transmit nerve impulses, thereby sending messages throughout the body. Blood clotting requires the presence of calcium as well. New research also suggests that calcium has a role in protecting against colon cancer and cardiovascular disease (McBean, 1993).

Phosphorus is essential for growth and maintenance of every tissue in the body. Every cell contains genetic material and phosphorus is a key element in the structure of the genetic materials DNA and RNA. Phosphorus plays a central role in the body's energy production in the body cells. Phosphorus is needed to form phospholipids, substances that allow fats to move through the blood and across cell membranes.

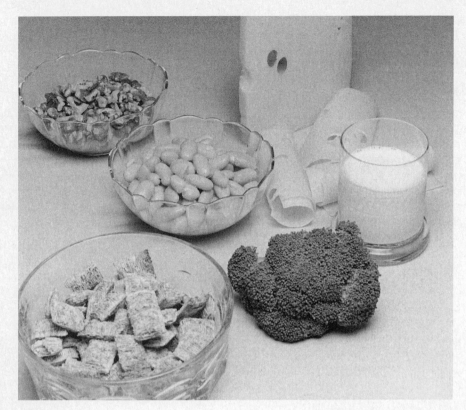

Calcium and phosphorus help the body build and maintain bones and teeth. The foods shown here are good sources of these minerals.

Daily foods such as milk, cheese, and yogurt are some of the best sources of calcium. Fish with edible bones (such as sardines), broccoli, spinach, and other dark-green leafy vegetables supply calcium too, but in much smaller amounts. Phosphorus comes from milk, legumes, meat, fish, cereals, nuts, and the phosphates in soft drinks.

Magnesium

As with calcium and phosphorus, much of the body's magnesium is found in bones. Most of the remainder is found in blood and softer tissues. Magnesium is essential to proper muscle and nerve function and is involved in bone formation. Magnesium also helps the body produce energy and plays a critical part in all of the body's synthetic processes such as making new protein. The best sources of magnesium are grain products, seeds, nuts, green vegetables, and legumes.

Sodium, Chloride, and Potassium

Three minerals—sodium, chloride, and potassium—work together as electrolytes. *Electrolytes* maintain the proper water balance within the body, regulating fluids that move into and out of every cell. Electrolytes are needed to send nerve impulses throughout the body and to maintain the body's fluid balance.

All three minerals are widely available in food. Common table salt is sodium joined to chloride. Sodium is also present in many processed foods, monosodium glutamate (MSG), and soy sauce. Chloride is typically found with sodium in processed foods. And potassium is found in fish, meat, citrus fruit, bananas, mushrooms, legumes, yogurt, and potatoes.

The kidneys help regulate electrolyte levels by excreting the excess through urine. The body also loses these minerals in sweat. A normal diet provides enough to replace them, so electrolyte supplements or drinks aren't generally necessary for healthy people, even those who work out strenuously. Severe diarrhea, however, can produce an electrolyte imbalance that may necessitate electrolyte replacement, particularly in infants.

Iron

Iron helps the body get the energy it requires. Iron doesn't supply calories, but it does join with protein to make hemoglobin. Hemoglobin carries oxygen to the cells for the production of energy.

Iron is found in many different foods. Except for liver and other organ meats, no one food has a large amount of iron. But meats, egg yolks, legumes, dark-green leafy vegetables, and whole grain and enriched breads and cereals are good sources. For some people, iron supplements are also recommended.

Other Minerals

Most people are familiar with calcium and phosphorus, even magnesium. Sodium, chloride, potassium, and iron are also known to most consumers. Some less familiar minerals that are equally important for health are listed and described below.

- **Chromium**. Chromium works with insulin to aid the metabolism of carbohydrates and regulate blood sugar levels. Sources of chromium include organ meats, whole grains, nuts, and brewer's yeast.
- **Copper**. Tiny amounts of copper help in energy production. Copper also helps the body use iron to form hemoglobin. Meat, liver, seafood, nuts, seeds, and whole grains supply copper.
- **Fluoride**. As a nutrient in food, fluoride hardens and strengthens both tooth enamel and bones. Fluoridated toothpaste provides topical, or surface, protection to teeth. Dietary sources of fluoride include some natural water, fluoridated drinking water, and tea.
- **Iodine**. Iodine is part of the structure of regulatory substances made by the thyroid gland. These thyroid substances control functions ranging from body temperature to growth and reproduction. Good sources include saltwater fish and iodized salt. Because iodine is added to salt, deficiencies are uncommon in the United States.

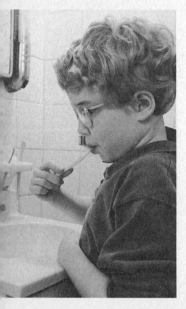

The fluoride found in toothpaste, drinking water, and some foods is good for teeth and bones. Too much of it, however, can discolor a child's teeth.

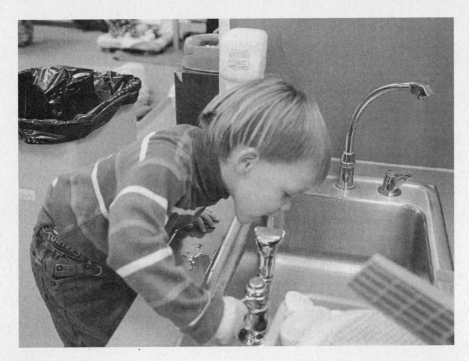

Water plays an essential role in many of the body's functions, including metabolism, nutrient transport, and temperature regulation. Children should have access to good drinking water at all times.

- **Manganese**. Manganese is needed for the activity of a variety of proteins involved in regulating important body processes. It is widely available in food, especially whole grains, cereal products, fruits, and vegetables.
- **Molybdenum**. The presence of molybdenum allows certain proteins to function properly in the body. Milk, beans, and grain products are generally good sources.
- **Selenium**. Besides other, less understood functions, selenium is part of a regulatory protein that acts as an antioxidant; however, excessive amounts can be toxic. Seafood, kidney, liver, and other meats are good sources of selenium. Grains also provide selenium in the diet.
- **Zinc**. Essential for growth, zinc promotes cell reproduction and tissue growth and repair. Zinc also helps the body use carbohydrates, fats, and proteins. A zinc deficiency during pregnancy can cause birth defects, and during childhood it can cause retarded growth. Too little zinc also can change the way food tastes to a person and affect the immune system. Zinc comes from a wide variety of foods, including meat, seafood, milk, legumes, poultry, eggs, and whole grains.

Water: The Forgotten Nutrient

Every nutrient has a number of essential roles to play in maintaining the health of the body. However, water is uniquely important since more than half of the body (about three-quarters for an infant) is water. Found both inside and outside of body cells, water is a key factor in the body's chemistry.

Metabolism takes place in a watery medium; it could not proceed without water. Yet many of us forget that water is a nutrient.

Many body functions depend on water. As part of blood, water helps carry nutrients to the cells where they are used, and it takes away the by-products of metabolism, eliminating them through the urine. Fluids also help control the internal thermostat by cooling the body through perspiration.

To maintain the proper fluid balance in the body, adults are advised to consume about 8 cups of fluids each day. That amount replaces fluids lost daily through urine, feces, respiration, and sweat. When sweating heavily, a person needs more water to maintain the body's water balance. Serious water loss can cause death more quickly than any other nutrient deficiency.

Fluid replacement can come from many sources besides water itself, including milk, juice, and other beverages. Even solid foods contain water, although some foods have more water than others. Lettuce, for example, is about 95 percent water. Meat and grains have much less. Regardless of the source, water in the diet helps to maintain good health.

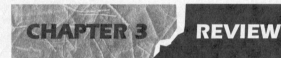

CHAPTER 3 / REVIEW

SUMMARY

- Food is the body's best source of nutrients. Different foods supply different nutrients.
- All people need the same nutrients, but particular nutrients are needed in different amounts at different ages.
- Carbohydrates, fats, and proteins supply energy, or calories, to the body.
- Carbohydrates include starches and sugars that are the body's main energy sources. Fiber is a type of carbohydrate that cannot be digested.
- Most calories in the total diet should come from carbohydrates, mostly complex carbohydrates or starches.
- Dietary fiber promotes digestion by increasing bulk and reducing transit time of wastes in the intestine, softening stools, and aiding bacterial action in the colon.
- Carbohydrates are found mainly in foods from plant sources. Many dairy foods also have carbohydrates.
- Fats are an essential nutrient containing saturated and unsaturated fatty acids. While fat is an energy nutrient, it has several other functions in human health.
- Fats carry the fat-soluble vitamins through the body and provide essential fatty acids. Fats add flavor, tenderness, and moisture to food. Because fats take longer to digest, they make foods more satisfying.

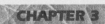
- Cholesterol forms part of the structure of cell membranes, many hormones, and the fat-digesting substance known as bile. The body makes all the cholesterol it needs.

- Too much fat in the diet is linked to several health problems. On average, 30 percent or less of total calories should come from fats.

- Many foods contain fats, including dairy products, oils, nuts, seeds, meats, poultry, fish, and baked goods.

- Proteins build and repair body tissue. Proteins are made of many different combinations of amino acids. Nine amino acids are essential in the diet because the body cannot make them.

- Proteins from animal sources such as meats, eggs, and dairy products are complete proteins. Incomplete proteins are found in plant foods such as legumes, grains, nuts, and seeds. These can be combined to form complete proteins.

- Vitamins are either water-soluble (B vitamins and C) or fat-soluble (A, D, E, and K). Vitamins are regulators of body processes; each has unique functions.

- Food sources of fat-soluble vitamins vary. Liver, fish liver oils, eggs, butter, and some fruits and vegetables provide vitamin A. Vitamin D is added to milk and some breakfast cereals. Vitamin E is found in oils, nuts, seeds, and whole grains. Some vegetables, cereals, dairy foods, meat, egg yolks, and fruits are among the food sources of vitamin K.

- Major minerals are needed in relatively large amounts for vital functions in the body. Trace minerals are required in quite small amounts but also have very important roles in health.

- Among the major minerals, calcium and phosphorus are required in the formation of bones and teeth. Magnesium is essential to proper muscle and nerve function and is involved in bone formation. Sodium, potassium, and chloride act as electrolytes. Iron, a trace mineral, is essential to the formation of hemoglobin.

- Water, which makes up more than half of the human body, is a nutrient too. The adult body should have at least 8 cups of fluids daily to replace losses and to avoid dehydration.

ACQUIRING KNOWLEDGE

1. Define *metabolism*.
2. List the six groups of nutrients.
3. What do calories measure?
4. What is the role of carbohydrates in the body?
5. Explain the role of dietary fiber in the body.
6. What are the best food sources of carbohydrates?
7. What role do fats and cholesterol play in health?
8. According to health experts, what percentage of a person's daily calorie consumption should be made up of fats? What health conditions are linked with high levels of dietary fat?

9. Name three food sources of fats.
10. What are amino acids and how are they supplied to the body?
11. What is the role of proteins in good health?
12. Describe the difference between animal and plant proteins and tell how plant foods can be combined to produce complete proteins.
13. What are vitamins and what are the two categories of vitamins?
14. Which three vitamins are antioxidants and how do antioxidants work?
15. List the B vitamins and explain their major role in human health.
16. List two fruit and two vegetable sources of vitamin C and summarize the role of vitamin C in human health.
17. List two ways vitamin A aids human health and name five food sources of this vitamin.
18. What is the function of vitamin D in the body?
19. What are minerals and how do they differ from vitamins?
20. Which of the minerals are needed by the body in the largest amounts?
21. How do calcium and phosphorous work together in the body? Name two food sources for each mineral.
22. What are electrolytes and how do they help the body?
23. What foods are good sources of iron?
24. List three trace minerals, other than iron, that are needed by the body.
25. How does water help the body remain healthy?

THINKING CRITICALLY

1. Suppose a three-year-old child has a favorite meal consisting of a cheese sandwich on whole wheat bread, a sliced tomato, and a glass of orange juice. For a month, she eats her favorite meal three times a day with no other foods in her diet. Will she take in a sufficient variety of nutrients over the course of the month? Why or why not?
2. Nutritionists recommend that 55 to 60 percent of a person's caloric intake should come from carbohydrates and that most of these should be complex carbohydrates. Why do they recommend more complex carbohydrates than sugars? What particular health benefits does fiber provide?
3. Compare the nutritional value of eating a fresh orange, a glass of bottled orange juice, or a vitamin C supplement tablet. What are the differences?
4. Many commercial snack foods contain considerable amounts of fat. Medical professionals advise against eating too much fat because it increases the risk of various health problems, including cardiovascular disease. What nutrients do you think should be emphasized in snack foods for children in place of fat? Why?
5. Processed foods tend to have less fiber than fresh foods. Suggest ways to add fiber to a diet containing large amounts of processed foods.

OBSERVATIONS AND APPLICATIONS

1. Observe customers ordering food at a fast-food restaurant. Write down the selections made by five customers. Note which foods are fried, which

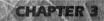

are broiled, and which are served uncooked. What sauces and dressings are added or come with the order? What sources of carbohydrates are selected? Proteins? Fats? Other nutrients?

2. Write down five of your favorite foods. What nutrients do your favorite foods provide? Write down three liquids you like to drink. Identify the nutrients supplied by these drinks. Do your favorite foods and beverages offer a wide variety of nutrients?

3. Fiber is an important part of a healthful diet. Products that contain bran are good sources of fiber. Bran occurs naturally in some foods and is available in many forms in commercially manufactured foods. Go to a grocery store. Find ten products that contain bran in the product name (Oat Bran Bagels, for example). List the names of the products.

4. A friend tells you he is on a new diet. To lose weight, he is cutting out most carbohydrates, particularly starches, until he loses 15 pounds. Do you think this is a good way to lose weight? Why or why not?

FOR FURTHER INFORMATION

Deutsch, R. M., & Morrill, J. S. (1993). *Realities of nutrition*. Menlo Park, CA: Bull Publishing.

Hamilton, E. M. N., Whitney, E. N., & Sizer, F. S. (1988). *Nutrition: Concepts and controversies*. St. Paul, MN: West Publishing.

Pipes, P. L., & Trahms, C. M. (1993). *Nutrition in infancy and childhood*. St. Louis: C. V. Mosby.

Wotecki, C. E., & Thomas, P. R. (1992). *Eat for life*. Washington, DC: National Academy Press.

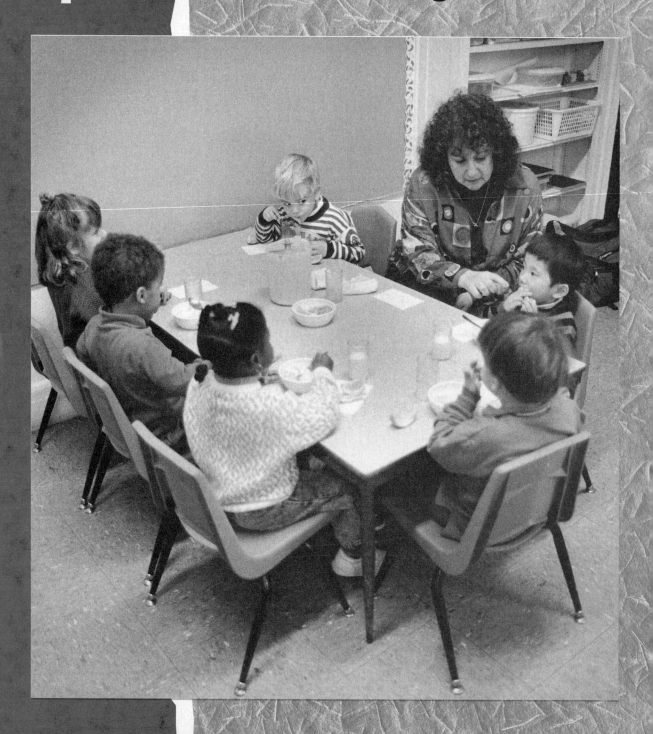

OBJECTIVES

Studying this chapter
will enable you to

- Explain how the Recommended Dietary Allowance and various dietary guidelines can help caregivers plan for healthful eating
- Use the Food Guide Pyramid to plan a varied, nutritionally balanced, and moderate diet for children
- Describe specific methods for planning healthful meals and snacks in a child care setting
- Describe how food labels can help caregivers choose foods wisely
- Explain how to select and prepare foods for children in ways that retain nutrients; moderate fat and cholesterol; control salt, sodium, and sugar; and help increase their consumption of fruits, vegetables, and grains
- Discuss methods for safe food handling in the child care setting

CHAPTER TERMS

cross-contamination
dental caries
enriched
food-borne illness
Food Guide Pyramid
hypertension
nutrient density
Percent Daily Value
Recommended Dietary Allowances
vegetarian

"MISS Delgado, are we going to have 'psketti' for lunch today?" asked Drew as he finished his breakfast of orange juice, cereal, and milk.

Maria Delgado smiled at Drew's pronunciation of his favorite food—spaghetti. Drew was one of Caldwell Head Start's early arrivals. His mother dropped him off at 7:30 each morning, and every morning he had breakfast at the center. Drew's mother knew he got fussy when he had to eat quickly, and he just wasn't ready to eat before they left the house. So eating at the center was the perfect solution.

"Drew, it's fun to cook for someone who enjoys his food as much as you do. Let's see what we planned for lunch today. Yes, we are having spaghetti and meatballs with spinach, a banana, and milk. How did you know that?"

"Remember? You wrote it on a paper. And you gave it to Mommy. She told me. She always tells me!" Drew said proudly.

Maria was pleased that Drew's mother reviewed and reinforced the menus she sent home each week. Drew's mother also planned family menus to add variety and balance to what he ate at the center.

Drew ate a number of meals and snacks at Caldwell. At midmorning, all the children would enjoy a snack of applesauce and milk. After lunch was nap time and, after that, he and the other children ate a midafternoon snack. Today they would help make cheese sandwiches for the snack. Maria knew that the children needed small, frequent meals and snacks spaced throughout the day.

As part of the government-sponsored Head Start program, Maria and the other staff members were very careful to provide meals and snacks that matched the pattern set by the government. That way, the children would be more likely to get the nutrients and calories they needed to grow, have energy, and stay healthy.

Guidelines for Good Nutrition

Early childhood professionals like Maria Delgado play an important role in promoting good health. Today's definition of good health involves more than not being sick. It means overall fitness, or an optimum physical, mental, and psychological condition. Health promotion, along with disease prevention, is the strategy for health care, and health promotion includes nutrition education. By planning nutritious meals and snacks and guiding children toward healthful food choices, caregivers can make a lasting difference in the lives of children and families.

There are a number of guidelines and tools to help early childhood professionals plan meals and snacks that promote health. Many are available from government sources. Among these planning aids are the Recommended Dietary Allowances, dietary guidelines, and the Food Guide Pyramid.

Recommended Dietary Allowances

What does Drew need to eat daily to maintain his rate of growth, energy level, and overall health? How much do you need? The *Recommended Dietary Allowances* (RDAs), established by the Food and Nutrition Board of the National Research Council (National Academy of Sciences), offer advice for diet planning. They suggest how much of many key nutrients an average healthy person needs each day for optimum health. The RDAs also provide calorie recommendations based on normal growth needs and moderate activity levels. The RDAs, updated every five to ten years, reflect the most current nutrition research.

Everyone needs the same nutrients, but in different amounts. Because nutrient needs change throughout life, the RDAs are age and gender specific. Infants and young children, for example, gradually need more nutrients as their bodies grow and develop. Specific guidelines are provided, therefore, for newborns; older infants; and children ages one to three years and four to six years. Appendix A shows these RDAs.

By consuming a diet that meets the RDAs, most healthy children can obtain the nutrients they need for their growth and their health. The RDAs

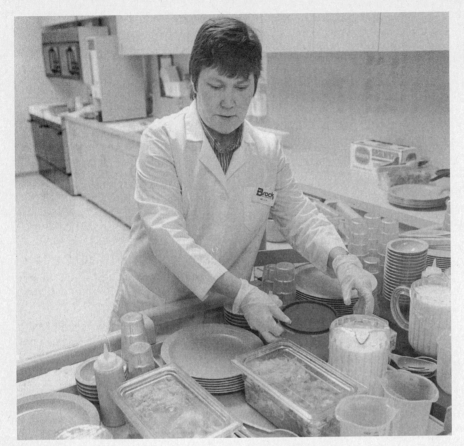

Providing children with a variety of foods helps ensure that they receive all the necessary nutrients.

allow for a safety margin for those who need a little more on an everyday basis and for times of stress or illness when additional nutrients are required (National Research Council, 1989). RDAs are useful for planning daily menus at home and in child care and school settings.

Dietary Guidelines

Dietary guidelines have been established by the U. S. Department of Agriculture as well as by health agencies and organizations such as the American Heart Association and the American Cancer Society. These guidelines offer nutritional advice for consumers and health professionals.

For example, the dietary guidelines established by the U. S. Department of Agriculture make the following recommendations for people age two and over: eat a variety of foods; maintain healthy weight; choose a diet low in fat, saturated fat, and cholesterol; choose a diet with plenty of vegetables, fruits, and grain products; use sugars only in moderation; use salt and sodium only in moderation; if you drink alcoholic beverages, do so in moderation (children and teens are advised to avoid alcohol) (U. S. Department of Agriculture and U. S. Department of Health and Human Services, 1990).

Although the guidelines from different organizations differ in details, they reflect a consensus among nutrition experts in many areas. The consensus covers the following principles.

Variety.   A varied diet is important since no one food can supply all the nutrients that children need. The exception is young infants, who can get enough nutrients and calories from breast milk or iron-fortified formula.

Although any food that provides nutrients and calories can fit in a healthful diet, each type of food contains different nutrients. Many dairy foods, for example, are good sources of calcium, whereas meats are good sources of iron; both supply protein. Even among foods in the same general group, nutrients vary. For example, apricots are high in beta carotene, which turns into vitamin A; oranges are an excellent source of vitamin C.

Variety in the child care setting is crucial. Children tend to have very strong opinions about food, and they may not want to try new foods on their own. When caregivers offer a variety of foods—as Maria Delgado did in the opening story—they introduce new foods to both children and parents, and they increase the chances that children will consume all the nutrients they need to grow and develop properly. Variety promotes healthful eating habits that can be carried out of the classroom and throughout life.

Balance.   Nutrition experts agree on the need for a diet to be balanced as well as varied. A balanced diet includes adequate, but not excessive, amounts of foods from the five major food groups. The food groups are discussed in this chapter. Certain foods should be eaten more frequently than others, forming the basis on which a healthful diet is built.

Many Americans eat unbalanced diets with too much fat and sugar and not enough fruits, vegetables, and grain products. Nutritionists point out that fruits, vegetables, and whole grains provide complex carbohydrates, including fiber, which are needed for good health. These foods also provide plenty of vitamins and minerals. In addition, they are generally low in fat (Institute of Medicine, 1991).

For young children, eating fruits, vegetables, and grain products supplies nutrients and energy needed for growth, development, and physical activity. Eating these foods also establishes a lifetime habit that promotes health.

Moderation.   All the guidelines agree on moderation of caloric intake and of certain dietary components: fats, cholesterol, sugars, and sodium. For infants and children, however, diets that limit fats severely, as well as those that are high in fat, can be harmful to health. For infants and toddlers up to age two, restricting dietary fat is not advised. The body and brain require an adequate supply of calories and essential fatty acids from fat for normal cell growth, development, and multiplication.

A moderate sugar intake poses no health risk to children. In fact, sugars are a source of energy. Many sugary foods, however, such as sweet snacks, desserts, and soft drinks, supply calories with few nutrients or little fiber. Moreover, sugar, especially when consumed frequently, is linked to *dental caries*, or tooth decay. Children who fill up on sugary foods may have no appetite later for more wholesome, nutritious foods. Naturally sweet foods, such as fruit, are good choices for children since they provide essential nutrients as well as an appealing taste.

Sodium has gotten a great deal of attention in the media because of its association with *hypertension*, or high blood pressure. High blood pressure is a risk factor for cardiovascular disease. However, there is no indication that strictly limiting salt and sodium during early childhood prevents high blood pressure later in life. But some people are sodium sensitive—their blood pressure is affected by a diet high in sodium (National Research Council, 1989). Cutting back on sodium helps lower their blood pressure. No one can predict which children will develop sodium sensitivity or who will benefit by reducing sodium intake; moderation, therefore, is a wise choice for

FOCUS ON *Promoting Healthful Habits*

Food Groups Game

For about two weeks, Rose Chen had been planning activities around the food groups with her five-year-old class at the Harborside Preschool. She made snacks from the five food groups—bagels on Monday; carrot sticks on Tuesday; apple slices on Wednesday; tuna fish on Thursday; and strawberry yogurt on Friday. But Rose wanted the children to understand that it is important to eat food from all five groups *every day*. Then she hit on it—a food groups game! On Monday before the children arrived, Rose set up three picnic baskets and made a sign for each: breakfast, lunch, and dinner. She gathered play foods such as fruits, vegetables, cottage cheese, steak, chicken soup, peanut butter, and bread from the dramatic play area. She took empty egg containers, cereal boxes, milk cartons, and some real food—potatoes and plastic bags of rice and beans. Then she made up five boxes of food, one for each food group.

Rose addressed the class, "Remember last week when we talked about eating at least three meals every day? Today we're going to play a game. Each picnic basket is one meal." Rose pointed to the baskets. "Breakfast, lunch,

and dinner. We're going to fill them with all kinds of foods from all five food groups. When we're done, all the foods should be gone. What might we put in the breakfast basket?"

"Bread" "Cereal" "Milk" "Cottage cheese," the children answered.

"Great!" encouraged Rose. "But what about a fruit or vegetable?" she added, pointing to those two boxes.

"I know what I like to have for breakfast," Wan Li said as he grabbed a plastic grapefruit and the potatoes and dropped them in the basket.

"Hmmm. It doesn't look like we got anything from this box," Rose said, pointing to the meat group box. "What food would you eat for breakfast from that box?" Rose asked.

"Peanut butter or chicken soup!" yelled Cara.

"Okay, you can eat any of these foods for breakfast if you'd like to. Now who can find some food for the lunch basket?"

What other questions would help the children to think about combining food from the different groups?

everyone. Moderation of sodium intake may help limit the development of a lifelong preference for salty foods. For infants and children, formula, breast milk, baby food, and, later, table food supply enough sodium. Adding extra salt is unnecessary and inappropriate.

Food Guide Pyramid

The *Food Guide Pyramid*, shown in Figure 4.1, is a practical tool that takes commonly accepted dietary guidelines and translates them into daily food selection advice. Designed for healthy people ages two and above, it offers a general guide for making smart food choices. By selecting foods as the pyramid suggests, people eat a varied and balanced diet with enough nutrients yet not too many calories, added sugars, or fats—especially saturated fat.

The Five Food Groups and Pyramid Tip. In the Food Guide Pyramid, nutrient-rich foods fit into five major food groups. Each group supplies some, but not all, of the nutrients a person needs. For that reason, foods in

FIGURE 4.1 Food Guide Pyramid. The pyramid categorizes foods into five major groups and shows the relative contribution of each group to a balanced diet.

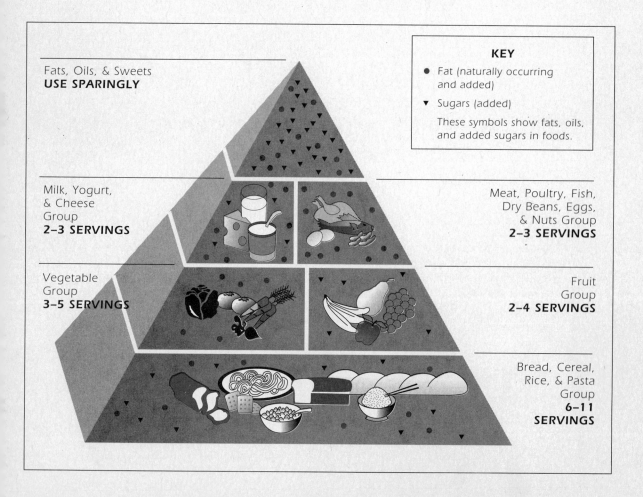

KEY
● Fat (naturally occurring and added)
▼ Sugars (added)
These symbols show fats, oils, and added sugars in foods.

Fats, Oils, & Sweets
USE SPARINGLY

Milk, Yogurt, & Cheese Group
2–3 SERVINGS

Meat, Poultry, Fish, Dry Beans, Eggs, & Nuts Group
2–3 SERVINGS

Vegetable Group
3–5 SERVINGS

Fruit Group
2–4 SERVINGS

Bread, Cereal, Rice, & Pasta Group
6–11 SERVINGS

one food group cannot replace those in another. No one food group is more important than another. All five food groups are needed in the diet to promote good health.

- **The Bread, Cereal, Rice, and Pasta Group.** This group includes foods made from grains: breads, waffles, pancakes, muffins, bagels, noodles, and rice, among others. These foods form the base of the pyramid and the foundation of a healthful diet. Many are good sources of complex carbohydrates, B vitamins, and iron. Because they come from plants, most grain products are naturally low in fat.
- **The Vegetable Group.** This group is naturally low in fat as well, and contains a wide variety of foods including broccoli, carrots, collard greens, potatoes, and squash. Foods in this group are good sources of vitamins A and C, potassium, complex carbohydrates, and iron.
- **The Fruit Group.** This group includes plant foods with many of the same benefits as those in the Vegetable Group. Oranges, cantaloupe, strawberries, apples, bananas, and plums are among the many foods in this group. These foods provide vitamins A and C, potassium, and complex carbohydrates, including fiber.
- **The Milk, Yogurt, and Cheese Group.** This group consists of several dairy products. Although some foods in this group are higher in fat than many fruits, vegetables, and grain products, most milk products are a good source of protein, calcium, and riboflavin.
- **The Meat, Poultry, Fish, Dry Beans, Eggs, and Nuts Group.** Both animal and plant food sources, including beef, pork, poultry, fish, eggs, and legumes fit in this group. These foods supply protein, iron, thiamin, niacin, and zinc. Legumes tend to be lower in fat than the animal food sources in this group.

The pyramid tip—Fats, Oils, and Sweets—includes foods with calories but few nutrients. These foods are not considered a "food group" and should be used sparingly. Salad dressings and oils, cream, butter, margarine, sugars, soft drinks, candies, and many rich desserts belong here. Although fats and added sugars come mainly from the pyramid tip, smaller amounts also come from the five major food groups. Two icons, or symbols, on the pyramid—circles that represent fat and upside-down triangles that represent added sugars—indicate food groups with these substances.

When planning menus for children, it is important to consider the *nutrient density* of different foods. Nutrient-dense foods supply plenty of nutrients for their calories. In contrast, calorie-dense foods supply few nutrients, but plenty of calories. Consider this example. A serving of ready-to-eat cereal and a brownie both have about 110 calories. But the brownie provides only small amounts of four nutrients (protein, thiamin, riboflavin, and iron) for its 110 calories. Cereal provides twice as much protein and significant amounts of thiamin, riboflavin, iron, vitamins A and C, and niacin.

Even within a group, the same food prepared differently—a baked potato and french fries, for example—may differ in nutrient density. French fries have more fat and calories. The meals you plan for children should include mostly nutrient-dense foods.

How Much from Each Food Group?   The Food Guide Pyramid indicates a range of servings for each of the five food groups. Age, gender, body size, and activity level determine how many calories people need and, therefore, how many servings from each food group can supply their nutrient and caloric needs. To consume enough nutrients, most people over the age of two need at least the minimum servings from each food group daily.

No serving amounts are recommended from the pyramid tip. Everyone is urged to eat fats, oils, and sweets sparingly to avoid consuming too much fat and too many calories.

Table 4.1 suggests the number of child-sized servings children might consume daily from each of the food groups in the Food Guide Pyramid. Young children can meet their nutrient and energy needs by consuming the total servings shown on the chart.

Servings: What Size?   Serving sizes differ, depending on both the food group and the specific foods. The amounts shown in Table 4.2 count as a single serving for children. A smaller portion counts for less; a larger portion, for more. Typically, nutrition information is given in terms of adult-sized servings. Children, because of their smaller stomachs, need smaller amounts of food served more frequently in the course of a day. Table 4.2 gives typical serving sizes for toddlers and preschoolers. They are about half the adult serving size in most cases. When a range is given, the smaller amount is for one- to two-year-olds or reflects different recommendations for amounts to be served at meals or snacks.

TABLE 4.1
Servings from Each Food Group

Food Group	Servings for Children Ages One to Two	Servings for Children Ages Three to Five
Bread, Cereal, Rice, and Pasta Group	5	5–6
Vegetable Group	3–4	4–5
Fruit Group	3	3
Milk, Yogurt, and Cheese Group	4–5	4–5
Meat, Poultry, Fish, Dry Beans, Eggs, and Nuts Group	2–3	2–3

Based on meal patterns and suggested menus from the Child Care Food Program.

TABLE 4.2 Serving Sizes for Each Food Group	
Food Group	**Typical Serving Sizes for Children**
Bread, Cereal, Rice, and Pasta Group	½ slice bread ½ muffin or bagel ¼ to ⅓ cup (⅓ to ½ ounce) ready-to-eat cereal ¼ cup cooked cereal, rice, or pasta
Vegetable Group	¼ to ½ cup cooked vegetables ¼ to ½ cup chopped, raw vegetables ¼ to ½ cup vegetable juice
Fruit Group	½ medium apple, banana, orange (½ cup) ¼ to ½ cup cut-up, canned, or cooked fruit ¼ to ½ cup berries ¼ to ½ cup fruit juice
Milk, Yogurt, and Cheese Group	½ to ¾ cup milk ¼ to ½ cup yogurt 1 to 1½ ounces natural cheese 1 ounce processed cheese
Meat, Poultry, Fish, Dry Beans, Eggs, and Nuts Group	½ to 1½ ounces cooked lean meat, poultry, or fish ½ egg ¼ to ⅜ cup cooked dry beans 2 to 3 tablespoons peanut butter

Based on meal patterns and suggested menus from the Child Care Food Program.

Many mixed foods, or combination foods, belong in two or more food groups. Pizza, macaroni and cheese, and chicken and vegetable stir-fry dishes are three examples. You can figure out how many servings they supply by estimating the amount of their total ingredients. Macaroni and cheese made with ¼ cup of cooked pasta and 1 ounce of cheddar cheese has one bread group serving and one milk group serving.

Planning Healthful Meals and Snacks

A healthful diet is varied, balanced, and moderate over time. In other words, what a child eats at one meal or in one day is not as important as what that child eats over the course of several days or a week. Using the recommendations of the Food Guide Pyramid as a planning tool helps ensure a healthful diet for children in your care.

Planning Meals for Child Care Settings

The child care center has a major responsibility for children's nutrition, especially for those infants and children—like Drew in the opening story in this

FOCUS ON   Communicating with Children

The Food Guide Pyramid

Nan wanted to talk about the Food Guide Pyramid with her five-year-olds—Katie, Ahmed, Matt, Adena, and Yung. She had drawn a food pyramid on a large piece of poster board. In each section of the pyramid, she had pasted magazine pictures of appropriate foods. She propped the chart on an easel and invited the children to sit around it. Although she had prepared a zippy introduction, she didn't get to use it. Katie, frowning, spoke up first.

KATIE: What's that?

NAN: That's what I call a food triangle. Some people call it a food pyramid. It is a picture that helps us see what foods we need to help us grow and have energy. What do you notice about the size of the spaces in the triangle?

AHMED: Some of the spaces are bigger than others. The one at the top is really small.

NAN: Very good, Ahmed. The spaces are different sizes for a reason. The size of the space for each kind of food tells you how much of that food you should eat each day. The bigger the space, the more of that food you should eat. The smaller the space, the less you should eat.

ADENA: So you mean we should be eating lots of bread and rice and spaghetti?

NAN: Yes, that's right. But what else is important?

SEVERAL CHILDREN: Apples! Green peppers! Carrots! Oranges!

NAN: Yes. And you can see that milk and cheese and meats are important too. But what kinds of foods should we eat less of?

YUNG: (looking sheepish) Candy and cake and cookies. But I *like* those things!

NAN: I like those things, too, Yung. And we *can* eat them. But we should eat less of them than we eat of the other kinds of food, like fruits and vegetables, bread, milk, and eggs. They can be yummy too. Remember the fruit salad we had for lunch yesterday?

MATT: Yeah! That was good! And I *love* carrot sticks!

NAN: Me too. You know, it's almost snack time and I'm getting hungry. I'm going to put this food triangle up on our bulletin board now. Whenever we eat a meal or a snack, let's see which kinds of foods we're eating. Then we can see whether we're eating enough of the right foods every day.

Did Nan's explanation and poster help the children understand the basic meaning of the Food Guide Pyramid? Is there anything you would have added or done differently?

chapter—who eat one or more meals at the center. One meal and one snack should provide two-thirds of the RDAs of all nutrients for children (American Public Health Association and the American Academy of Pediatrics, 1992). U. S. Department of Agriculture guidelines call for child care centers to serve either one meal, or one meal and one snack, to children who stay at the center for four to six hours.

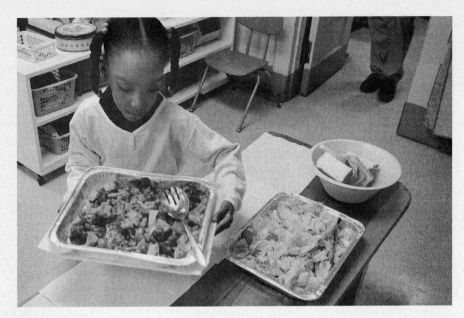

Vegetables and bread are important components of a nutritionally sound meal for young children.

The Child Care Food Program, administered by the U. S. Department of Agriculture, has established a meal pattern for infants in child care settings showing the types and minimum amounts of foods for the first year of life. The pattern, which changes with the child's age at three- or four-month intervals, specifies breakfast, lunch, supper, and snack. This guideline recognizes that babies' feeding schedules must be flexible and that babies should be fed when hungry. The menu pattern from *Feeding Infants: A Guide for Use in the Child Care Food Program* is shown in Chapter 6.

With careful planning, sufficient nutrient and caloric levels can be achieved for young children who eat several meals and snacks at the child care center. The U. S. Department of Agriculture also has published *A Planning Guide for Food Service in Child Care Centers*, which helps child care providers plan nutritionally sound menus for young children, ages 1 through 12. To receive federal subsidies and participate in the Child Care Food Program, these guidelines must be followed. Many privately funded child care programs use the planning guide to ensure that menus are nutritious. These same meal patterns may be adapted for various ethnic food preferences or to introduce a variety of new foods to children.

The meal patterns recommended for toddlers and preschoolers who are in child care centers are shown in chapters 7 and 8, respectively. Sample menus for children in those age groups also appear in those chapters. Foods high in calcium, vitamin A, vitamin C, and iron are recommended daily.

Breakfast. Breakfast has been described as the most important meal of the day. A good breakfast prepares children to learn about and explore their environments (McBean, 1993). While adults may be able to compensate for symptoms brought on by skipping breakfast, children usually cannot. A

FOCUS ON / **Cultural Diversity**

Keeping Kosher

Some Conservative and many Orthodox Jews adhere to a strict kosher diet. *Keeping kosher* does not mean merely eating certain foods and not eating others. It also means that the kitchen and its utensils are arranged and segregated according to the food being prepared and eaten.

The kosher diet prohibits eating of any products coming from the pig: pork, ham, bacon, and foods made from these products. It also prohibits the eating of shellfish. Animals used for meat must be vegetable eaters, have cloven hooves, and chew their cud (cows, for example). They must be ritually slaughtered by a trained kosher butcher or in a kosher slaughterhouse.

People who eat according to kosher rules never mix meat and milk or any dairy products. If both of these types of foods are part of a meal, the dairy products are eaten first and separately. Several minutes later, meat may be eaten. If meat is eaten first, the dairy part of the meal can only be served and eaten several

hours later. If there are children in your care who keep kosher, offer them a glass of juice with their kosher meat sandwiches.

The prohibition about mixing milk and meat applies in the kitchen as well. Strictly kosher households keep two sets of dishes, pots and pans, and utensils. One set is used for cooking meat. The other set is used solely when dairy foods are prepared. The two are never interchanged. If you are caring for Jewish children from kosher homes, you may need to keep two basic sets of strictly separate cooking utensils, one for each type of food.

During the holiday season called Passover, a Jewish child may refuse leavened bread, or bread made with yeast. A Jewish child may bring in his own lunch made with unleavened bread called matzo. If not, have some matzo on hand for the child to eat. Egg matzo is very tasty and low in calories and fat. This might be a good time to introduce other children to this healthful ethnic food.

child's small stomach empties quickly and if she has skimped or missed breakfast, she may have midmorning stomachaches that are really hunger pangs. Other children who haven't eaten a healthful breakfast may be sleepy, irritable, or have a very short attention span.

For young children, a healthful breakfast includes milk; juice, fruit, or a vegetable; and bread or cereal. Occasionally, meat or an egg might be included in the meal.

Snacks. Snacks can be part of a healthful diet for people of all ages. For young children, who have small stomachs and greater caloric needs per pound of body weight than adults, snacks help supply the nutrients and calories they need each day. They may not be able to consume enough nutrients at three meals alone.

In the child care environment, midmorning or midafternoon snacks are an important part of food service. Regular snack times, rather than all-day

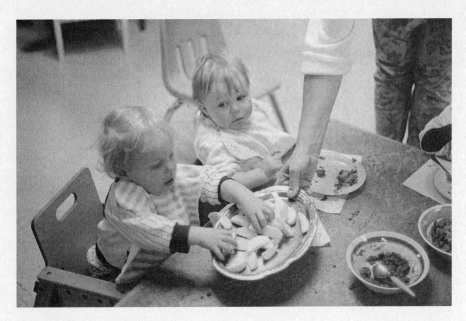

Most toddlers enjoy fresh fruit slices with any meal or snack.

nibbling, help establish good food habits. For toddlers and preschoolers, snacks should be scheduled at least two hours before mealtime so the children have an appetite for lunch or dinner. Caregivers can use snacks to teach about nutrition, explaining which food groups the snacks belong to and how these foods fit into a healthful diet. Snacks also provide an opportunity for children to help with simple food preparation.

For infants, breast milk or formula is the suggested snack through seven months of age. After that, breast milk, formula, or fruit juice and bread or crackers are recommended. The Child Care Food Program guidelines suggest whole milk as a possible snack for infants 8 through 11 months old. It is important, however, to check facility policies and parent instructions on this subject. Many pediatricians suggest withholding cow's milk from infants until they are over one year old because the high protein content of cow's milk makes it difficult for infants to digest. Also, introducing cow's milk too early may trigger an allergic reaction.

Nutritious snacks for preschool and older children often include foods from at least two food groups. Children of this age enjoy snacks such as:

- Cheese on a whole wheat cracker
- Peanut butter on a celery stick
- Cold cereal with fruit and milk
- A tortilla with melted cheese
- Raw broccoli with cottage cheese dip
- Orange slices on a graham cracker
- Apple slices spread with peanut butter
- Unsweetened applesauce blended with plain yogurt
- Frozen bananas coated with yogurt

Some people choose to follow a vegetarian diet for religious reasons. With careful meal planning, such diets can provide all necessary nutrients.

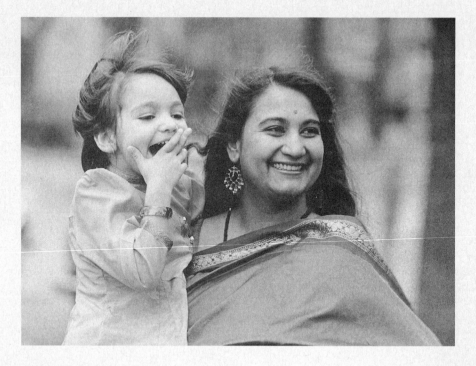

Vegetarian Diets.   For a variety of reasons—religious, ethical, economic, and health-related—some people choose to follow a vegetarian diet. *Vegetarian* refers to a variety of eating styles in which plant sources of food are central. Lacto-vegetarians consume dairy foods as well as plant foods. Lacto-ovo-vegetarians eat dairy foods, eggs, and foods from plant sources. Neither lacto-vegetarians nor lacto-ovo-vegetarians eat any animal flesh. Other vegetarians include fish or poultry (but no red meat) in their diet. Very strict vegetarians, called vegans, eat no animal-derived foods at all. All of their proteins, fats, and carbohydrates come from combinations of foods from plant sources.

With careful planning, vegetarian diets that include some animal products can supply enough complete protein and other essential nutrients to promote growth and overall good health. Vegan diets, however, are not recommended for infants and children because they may not supply enough complete protein for growth (Farley, 1992). Other nutrients, including iron, calcium, and vitamin B_{12}, may be undersupplied as well. If a family does choose to follow a strict vegetarian diet, parents and other caregivers should seek advice from a physician or registered dietician to plan a diet that supports normal growth.

To ensure that vegetarian meals are balanced, include:

- Plenty of iron-rich legumes and fortified grain products to compensate for iron from animal flesh. Meat, poultry, and fish are the best iron sources; iron from meat, poultry, and fish is better absorbed than iron from plant sources.

- Milk, cheese, and yogurt for calcium, protein, and vitamin B_{12}, a vitamin that is vital for growing infants and children. Plant sources cannot supply all the calcium that growing infants and children need for strong, healthy bones and teeth.
- Eggs, which supply iron, protein, and vitamin B_{12}.
- Protein-rich meat substitutes, such as eggs, cheese, legumes, seeds, nuts, poultry, or fish. Consuming enough complete protein can be a challenge for vegetarians who avoid meat, poultry, and fish. Some food combinations supply complementary amino acids that together provide complete protein—for example, milk, cheese, or yogurt plus grains; grains plus legumes; and legumes plus seeds or nuts. Chapter 3 discusses essential amino acids and complete protein.

Fast Foods

Many families make fast foods a regular part of their weekly diet. When children eat out, they are more likely to go to a fast-food establishment than a traditional restaurant. Learning to make smart fast-food choices is part of eating in a healthful way. Caregivers can help with this process.

Typically, fast-food meals are high in fat, calories, and sodium, and they don't include many fruits or vegetables. However, these meals can be nutritious if chosen with variety, moderation, and balance in mind. Caregivers can help parents and children to use fast foods wisely by choosing carefully and by considering fast food meals as part of the day's or week's eating plan. If a fast-food meal is short on vegetables, additional vegetables can be eaten at another meal or on another day.

Encourage children to drink milk or juice with fast-food meals instead of soft drinks. They can cut down on fats by sharing a large order of french fries among the whole family. When ordering pizza, families can include extra vegetable toppings, such as green pepper or broccoli instead of meats high in fat. Salad bars are an excellent way for children to add vegetables and fruits to their meals while enjoying a chance to choose for themselves from a variety of nutritious foods. Teachers can reinforce such healthful food choices through a field trip with children to a fast-food restaurant.

Using Food Labels Wisely

Food labels do not offer nutrition guidelines. However, labels on food packages can help consumers make food decisions that contribute to their good health. Information on food labels can help caregivers compare foods, make informed food choices, and plan nutritious meals and snacks for children in their care.

Nutrition labeling has appeared on food packages since the 1970s. However, the Nutrition Labeling and Education Act, which became law in 1990, mandated changes in the labeling format. The deadline for full implementation of the new regulations was set at May 1994 for processed foods and at July 1994 for processed meat and poultry items.

WHOLESOME SNACKS

Pineapple Freeze

Ingredient:

One 16-ounce can crushed pineapple, packed in own juice

Directions:

1. Place unopened can of pineapple in freezer until hard.

2. Place under hot running water for 30 seconds and remove from can.

3. Place in blender or food processor and blend to slush consistency.

4. Spoon into serving dishes or allow children to serve themselves from a serving bowl.

Yield: 4 servings

Each serving contains:

Calories: 74
Protein: 1 g
Fat: 0.2 g
Carbohydrates: 19 g

Source: DeBakey, M. (1984). *The living heart diet.* COPYRIGHT © 1984 by Raven Press Books, Inc. Reprinted by permission of Simon & Schuster, Inc.

Nutrition Facts.   As a result of the new law, almost all packaged foods have nutrient labeling. Although not required, many fresh fruits, vegetables, meat, poultry, and fish have nutrition labeling too.

"Nutrition Facts" on the label help consumers compare the nutrients and calories in a standard serving. Both the serving size and servings per container are listed. Certain nutrition information is required: calories and calories from fat; amounts of total fat, saturated fat, cholesterol, sodium, total carbohydrate, fiber, sugars, and protein; and amounts of vitamins A and C, calcium, and iron. Other vitamins and minerals may be listed as well.

Information about most nutrients is given as a percent of the Daily Value. The Daily Value is the amount of a nutrient that an average person needs for a 2,000- or 2,500-calorie-a-day diet. The government sets Daily Values on the basis of current nutrition information and advice. Daily Values are used as reference amounts for food labeling. The *Percent Daily Value* helps consumers see how a single serving of the food fits into a 2,000-calorie-a-day diet. (Some labels also list information for a 2,500-calorie diet.) Children's overall nutrient needs are lower because their bodies are smaller, although they need more nutrients per pound of body weight than adults do. While labeling information is not based specially on a child's nutrient needs, it does allow caregivers to compare foods.

Descriptors, Label Terms, and Health Claims.   Many food labels carry nutrient content claims, or descriptors, such as *low sodium*, *fat free*, or *low cholesterol*. In the past, these terms were confusing and often misleading because no standard definitions existed. Now laws strictly define these nutrient content claims, so consumers can better judge the nutritional value of a food by its label.

The descriptor *enriched* for grain products is one that has been regulated for some time. An enriched product must include such vitamins and minerals as niacin, thiamin, riboflavin, and iron to replace what is lost by processing. Under new rules, enriched grain products must also include set amounts of folic acid.

Health claims on some food packages suggest a relationship between the food or its components and a disease or health condition. For example, a food may claim to be high in fiber and claim, on this basis, to prevent heart disease. Such claims are now regulated as well. To make a claim, the food must contain certain nutrient levels. And only certain types of health claims can be made.

Other Information.   An ingredient list on food packages informs consumers of the composition of processed foods, such as canned soups, frozen dinners, canned and frozen vegetables, packaged mixes, combination foods, and condiments. Ingredients must be listed in descending order by weight.

Other information found on food packaging that may be useful includes cooking and heating instructions, freshness dating, recipes, and warnings for people with phenylketonuria who cannot tolerate the amino acid phenylalanine, which is present in most proteins.

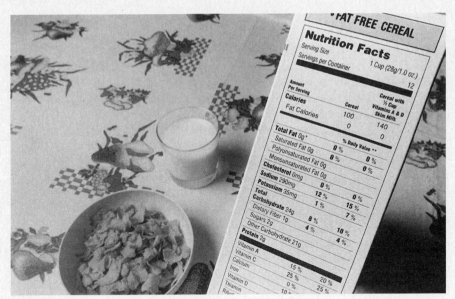

This label meets the regulations established by the Nutrition Labeling and Education Act. Under this law, food labels must now include nutrition facts, such as fat and sodium content, and percentages of recommended Daily Values for important vitamins and minerals.

Preparing Food the Healthful Way

When meals and snacks are prepared in the child care setting, caregivers should use techniques that maximize nutrient content while controlling fat, cholesterol, sugar, and sodium. Refer to Chapter 6 for guidelines on preparing bottles, commercial baby food, and "homemade" baby food for infants.

Retaining Nutrients

Proper food preparation and storage techniques can help preserve important nutrients in the food caregivers serve to children. Fruits and vegetables are especially vulnerable to nutrient loss. Some nutrients dissolve in water and escape with steam. When cooking vegetables, cook them covered, in a small amount of water or steam them. Water-soluble vitamins—the B vitamins and vitamin C—can be destroyed by heat. Avoid overcooking both vegetables and fruits. Instead, cook them only until they are tender, or enjoy them raw. Don't cut vegetables into small pieces before cooking them. The more surfaces that are exposed, the more nutrients may be lost. Cut children's portions into small pieces just before the food is served.

Store foods properly so they stay in their peak condition. Keep perishable foods in the refrigerator or freezer. Avoid storing milk in a clear pitcher; riboflavin is destroyed by light. Store dry foods in a cool, dark place.

Cutting Fat and Cholesterol

Most children get more than enough fat in their diets. Good menu planning and food preparation techniques can reduce excess fat and cholesterol in the food you serve. Serve lean meats and poultry as often as possible. Always trim visible fat, gristle, and skin from meat, poultry, and fish. Be careful to limit processed meats—hog dogs, luncheon meats, and sausages—because they tend to be high in both fat and sodium, or choose those with less fat and sodium. Offer low-fat dairy foods as well: low-fat milk, yogurt, and cottage cheese. Because egg yolks are high in cholesterol, moderate the amount of them to no more than four per week, including those children eat at home. This amount includes egg yolks in baked and prepared foods. Caregivers can use food labels on packaging to compare the fat and cholesterol in various foods.

When food preparation requires fat, use mostly liquid vegetable oils, which have less saturated fat than stick margarine or butter. Use low-fat cooking methods when you can: bake, roast, boil, broil, steam, or stir-fry instead of pan- or deep-frying. Skim off visible fats from soups and gravies. Drain fat after cooking ground meat.

You can control added fats in uncooked foods as well. For example, when making sandwiches, spread only a little mayonnaise, butter, or margarine on the bread.

Controlling Salt and Sodium

The benefits of controlling salt and sodium intake have already been discussed. Caregivers have several options for controlling sodium in food. If there is a saltshaker on the table, remove it. Pasta, rice, cereal, and vegetables can all be prepared without adding salt to the cooking water. Caregivers should encourage children to enjoy the natural flavors of food, particularly by their examples. For infants, foods should always be prepared without added seasoning. For toddlers, preschoolers, and older children, caregivers may use herbs, spices, and lemon juice rather than salt to enhance the flavor of food. Keep in mind, however, that many young children prefer their food unseasoned or very lightly seasoned. Quick cooking of vegetables—stir-frying and steaming—brings out the flavor because foods are not overcooked.

As noted earlier, caregivers should limit the use of processed meats because they are usually high in salt. Try to prepare mostly fresh meat, poultry, and fish. Provide low-sodium or lightly salted pretzels and crackers as snacks. Use the information on food labels to choose processed foods that do not contain large amounts of sodium.

Controlling Added Sugars

Fruits are naturally sweet and offer important nutrients. Use fresh fruit for snacks and desserts. When buying canned fruit, choose fruit packed in natural juices or water rather than syrup. Instead of spreading jams and jellies on toast and sandwiches, offer pureed fruit and applesauce.

Cut back on sugar in food preparation; when appropriate, use spices that offer a perception of sweetness, such as allspice, cinnamon, ginger, and nutmeg. Check food labels for added sugars. Processed foods that are high in added sugars often list these ingredients: sucrose (table sugar), brown sugar, raw sugar, dextrose (glucose), fructose, maltose, lactose, honey, syrup, corn sweetener, high-fructose corn syrup, molasses, or fruit juice concentrate. Restrict the use of heavily sugared foods. Offer only 100 percent juice or 100 percent juice blends. Drinks with added sugar are not acceptable in a child care setting.

Offering Fruits, Vegetables, and Grains

Caregivers can add nutrient-dense fruits, vegetables, and grains to children's diets in many enjoyable ways. Fresh fruits, raw vegetables, crackers, bagels, and whole grain or enriched breads make delicious snacks. A variety of grain products can include breads that may be new to children, such as corn bread, enriched pita bread, and tortillas. Serving a variety of fruits and vegetables with meals helps children learn to try and enjoy new foods. Caregivers also can add extra vegetables to soups and pizza and serve fresh fruit on breakfast cereal, pancakes, waffles, and on ice cream and frozen yogurt.

When serving fruits and vegetables to young children for the first time, however, remember to serve them simply. It is often helpful to separate foods from each other, since many children object to having one food touch another.

Safe Food Handling

Proper food handling is important because food offers the perfect medium for spreading certain diseases. Some illness is spread when disease-causing

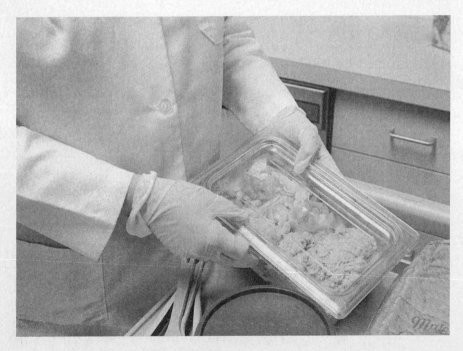

Food preparers in child care facilities should avoid touching foods with their hands. Tongs, serving spoons, or disposable gloves should be used instead.

microorganisms from caregivers or children are transferred to food and then ingested by other children or adults. Streptococcus (strep) and staphylococcus (staph) are two common bacteria that can be passed in this way.

Food-borne illness, or food poisoning, is the result of eating food that has been contaminated by bacteria or the poisons they produce. Harmful bacteria usually cannot be seen, smelled, or tasted. Flulike symptoms—nausea, vomiting, diarrhea, fever, and body aches—result from bacteria that have multiplied in food.

Food poisoning is not the only food preparation hazard to be avoided in the child care setting, however. Kitchen areas present many safety hazards, too, especially for young children. The dangers of slips, burns, and cuts and the safety rules to help prevent these injuries are discussed in chapters 12 and 13.

Food Sanitation

Cross-contamination occurs when bacteria present in one food spread to another food, for example, when drippings from meat are left on a cutting board used for preparing vegetables. Bacteria can spread to food if people handle it directly or sneeze or cough nearby. Colds, flus, and other contagious diseases can be passed from one person to another in this way. Food sanitation and safety must be a high priority in child care settings, especially since young children have not built up immunities to many infections.

Children, staff, and volunteers should always wash their hands with soap and water before and after meals, snacks, and learning activities that involve food. Caregivers should wear clean clothes and aprons when handling food; their hair should be clean and tied back. Food preparers should avoid touching foods with their hands; tongs, disposable gloves, scoops, or serving spoons should be used instead. A staff member who is ill or has an open sore or cut must not handle food.

A spoon that is used for tasting should never be used to stir food during cooking or to serve food. When children help with food preparation, watch out for finger-licking, a practice nearly irresistible to young children. When it happens, see that children wash their hands before they handle food, dishes, or utensils again. Once the food is served, make sure that children do not share utensils or food.

Cutting boards, slicers, knives, and other utensils must be thoroughly cleaned between each use and at the end of the day to avoid cross-contamination. For example, after you slice raw chicken or chop a green pepper, wash the knife, the cutting board, and your hands with hot water and soap or detergent. All food preparation surfaces, work areas, and eating areas must be kept clean.

Dishes, utensils, and food preparation equipment must be washed and sanitized with soap and water hot enough to kill bacteria. Freshly laundered towels and dishcloths and clean sponges may be used for these tasks if an automatic dishwasher is not available. Clean dishes should be handled by the rims; flatware or chopsticks by the handles; and glasses by the outside.

Food Storage

Many foods contain some bacteria, but at levels that are not dangerous. Bacteria need nutrients, warmth, and moisture, along with sufficient time, to grow to dangerous levels. Temperatures between 40° and 140° F (4.4° and 60° C) are ideal for bacterial growth. The moisture and nutrients that bacteria need for growth may be present in food. If these three factors—warmth, moisture, and the nutrients from food—are present for long enough, bacteria will multiply to dangerous levels. Proper food storage slows the process of bacterial growth by keeping food cool and dry and limiting storage time. Proper storage also protects food from chemical contamination, insects, and rodents.

Foods should be stored as soon as they are received. Proper storage involves dating, labeling, and storage off the floor. Perishable foods must be refrigerated between 32° and 40° F (0° and 4.4° C), or frozen at 0° F (-17.8° C) or less. Dry foods should be stored in a cool, dark area, such as a storeroom, pantry, or cabinet, preferably below 65° F (18.4° C). All foods need to be well covered or sealed in airtight containers.

Food preparation should start with good quality food—fresh whenever possible. Any spoiled food must be immediately discarded or rejected at the time of delivery.

Hot foods should be kept at 140° F (60° C) or above until serving time (Edelstein, 1992). Meat, poultry, fish, and eggs should be cooked through—for meat, to an internal temperature of 160° F (71.4° C), and for poultry, to 180° F (82.2° C) (USDA, 1990).

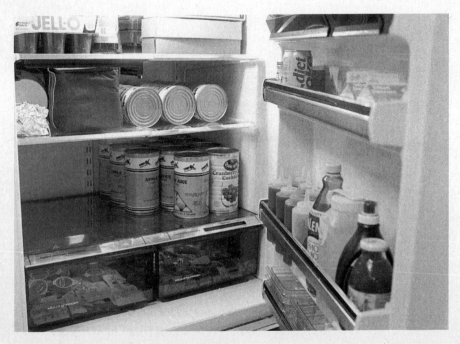

Proper food storage slows bacterial growth. All foods need to be well covered or sealed in airtight containers.

Leftovers need to be covered and refrigerated immediately, then used within 72 hours. Discard uneaten food on children's plates. Food should be thawed in the refrigerator or microwave oven, not on the counter.

A child care facility should provide adequate refrigerator space for perishable foods, such as sandwiches or bottles with formula, that children bring from home. Bottles and containers must be labeled with children's names. Refrigerate food as soon as the child arrives.

"Use by" and "sell by" dates indicate the freshness of packaged foods. Food packages with cracks, leaks, bulging lids, or popped-up safety buttons must be discarded. When in doubt, throw it out; do not taste first.

To avoid chemical contamination, food and cooking equipment should be stored away from chemicals and cleaning supplies. Refuse, diapering, and toilet areas as well as pets need to be located well away from places where food is stored, prepared, and eaten.

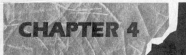

CHAPTER 4 REVIEW

SUMMARY

- The Recommended Dietary Allowances, categorized by age and gender, indicate how many calories and how much of many key nutrients an average healthy person needs daily.

- Dietary guidelines have been established by the government and other sources. They reflect an emphasis on variety, balance, and moderation.

- The Food Guide Pyramid translates commonly accepted dietary guidelines into daily food selection recommendations.

- The five major food groups are the: 1) Bread, Cereal, Rice, and Pasta Group, 2) Vegetable Group, 3) Fruit Group, 4) Milk, Yogurt, and Cheese Group, 5) Meat, Poultry, Fish, Dry Beans, Eggs, and Nuts Group. All of the food groups are important for health and growth.

- The pyramid tip includes foods with calories but few nutrients. These foods should be eaten sparingly.

- When planning meals for children, caregivers should choose foods with high nutrient density, that is, foods with a high percentage of nutrients for their calories.

- The child care center has a major responsibility for children's nutrition. Government publications can help child care providers plan nutritionally sound menus for young children.

- A good breakfast prepares children to learn and explore their environments.

- Snacks are important for children because they need smaller, more frequent meals. Nutritious snacks come from the five major food groups.

- Vegetarian diets must be carefully planned to provide essential nutrients for good health.
- Fast foods can be selected to minimize fat and calories while providing nutrients for a healthful diet.
- Food labels provide information that helps caregivers make food comparisons and informed food choices.
- Food preparation techniques can minimize nutrient loss.
- Food selection can moderate the amount of fat, cholesterol, salt, sodium, and sugar in the diet.
- Caregivers should offer children plenty of fruits, vegetables, and grain products.
- Proper food handling is critical to the prevention of food-borne illness.

ACQUIRING KNOWLEDGE

1. What information is given in the Recommended Dietary Allowances (RDAs)?
2. Why do RDAs differ depending on age?
3. Nutritional guidelines established by various health agencies and organizations agree that diet choices should be based on three principles. What are they?
4. The chapter states that many Americans eat unbalanced diets. Explain this statement.
5. Why should the fat intake of infants and children up to the age of two *not* be restricted?
6. Why should children's sugar intake be moderated and why are some sources of sugar preferable to others?
7. What is a wise policy regarding the intake of sodium in the diet of children?
8. Name the five food groups in the Food Guide Pyramid.
9. What does nutrient density refer to?
10. What factors determine how many servings a person should have from each food group?
11. What are the components of a healthful breakfast for young children?
12. Distinguish between the types of vegetarian diets explained in the text.
13. Why is a strict vegan diet *not* recommended for young children?
14. Why is it difficult to make wise food choices when eating at a typical fast-food restaurant? Without eliminating fast foods completely, how can parents use fast foods wisely as part of a child's overall diet?
15. What information is contained on a nutrition label?
16. In what order are ingredients listed on food packages?
17. How should vegetables be cooked so that they retain as much of their nutrient value as possible?
18. List three ways to reduce excess fat and cholesterol in the diet.
19. List three ways to reduce salt and sodium in the diet.
20. List three ways to reduce your intake of sugar.

21. Why is it important to follow proper precautions when handling food?
22. What are three ways to limit cross-contamination when preparing and serving food?
23. What are the ideal conditions for growth of bacteria in food?
24. How should food be stored so that bacteria will not grow in it and it will be protected from chemical contamination, insects, and rodents?
25. How quickly should leftovers be eaten?

THINKING CRITICALLY

1. Your friend Alice tells you she is trying to lose weight by watching the number of calories in the food she eats. She limits herself to 1,200 calories a day. Today she had a doughnut and cup of coffee for breakfast. This adds up to a breakfast of 400 calories. Do you think her breakfast choice was a wise one? Do you agree with Alice's approach to losing weight? Why or why not?
2. Nutrition labels on food contain a great deal of information. What are some ways to use this information?
3. Compare these two child care lunches in terms of nutrition. Meal A: broiled chicken cutlet sandwich on a toasted whole wheat bun with a light covering of mayonnaise, lettuce, and tomato; a small fruit salad; a glass of orange juice. Meal B: breaded and fried chicken cutlet sandwich on a buttered bun; french fries; a soft drink.
4. When evaluating a child's diet, why is it more useful to consider what she eats over the course of a week rather than in one day alone?
5. Despite all the information available to the public on the importance of a low-fat diet, Americans still eat many foods that are high in fat. What are possible reasons for the public's resistance to change?

OBSERVATIONS AND APPLICATIONS

1. Go to a Head Start or other full-day child care program in which meals are prepared and served to children. Observe the preparations in the kitchen for a meal. How are the foods prepared? Are they broiled? Fried? Boiled? Are vegetables cut before cooking or after? Is salt added to the food being cooked? Are sanitary practices carefully followed? Do food preparers wear gloves? Do they wash their hands? Is the cutting board washed after meat is cut on it? Describe the preparation process and the apparent planning that went into it. What is served? What food groups are included in the menu for that meal?
2. Observe the children eating a meal you saw being prepared. Do the majority of the children eat the food served? What, if any, food is left over on the plates of the children? Note the comments the children make about the food during their meal. Note the age range of the children you observe.

3. Using Table 4.1 and Table 4.2 as your guides, prepare a day's worth of nutritious meals and snacks for a four-year-old.

4. Write down *everything* you ate and drank yesterday. (Be honest and complete.) Categorize the foods you ate into the six groups of the Food Guide Pyramid. (Remember that a slice of apple pie belongs in the tip of the pyramid, not in the fruits section.) How many servings did you eat from each category? Did any one category dominate your food choices? Was your diet for that day well balanced? Did you eat many foods that were nutrient dense? Did you eat an overabundance of food prepared in fat or foods that contained a lot of fat?

FOR FURTHER INFORMATION

Berman, C., & Fromer, J. (1991). *Meals without squeals*. Menlo Park, CA: Bull Publishing.

Brown, M. B. (1993). *Label facts for healthful eating: Educator's resource guide*. Washington, DC: Nabisco Foods Group and National Food Processors Association.

Edelstein, S. (1992). *Nutrition and meal planning in child-care programs: A practical guide*. Chicago: The American Dietetic Association.

U. S. Department of Agriculture. (1989). *Making bag lunches, snacks, and desserts*, Home and Garden Bulletin Number 232-9 (HG-232-9). Washington, DC: Human Nutrition Information Service.

U. S. Department of Agriculture. (1988). *Feeding infants: A guide for use in the child care food program*, Publication FNS-258. Washington, DC: Author, Food and Nutrition Service.

U. S. Department of Agriculture. (1989). *A planning guide for food service in child care centers*, Publication FNS-64. Washington, DC: Author, Food and Nutrition Service.

U. S. Department of Agriculture. (1992). *The food guide pyramid*, Home and Garden Bulletin Number 252 (HG-252). Washington, DC: Author, Human Nutrition Information Service.

U. S. Department of Agriculture and U. S. Department of Health and Human Services. (1990). *Nutrition and your health: Dietary guidelines for Americans* (3rd ed.), Home and Garden Bulletin Number 232 (HG-232). Washington, DC: Author.

PART 2

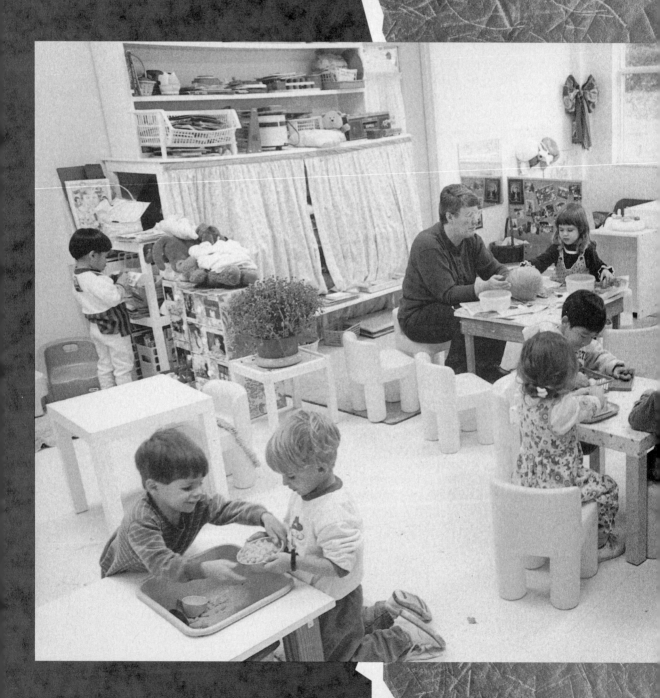

Different Needs at Different Ages

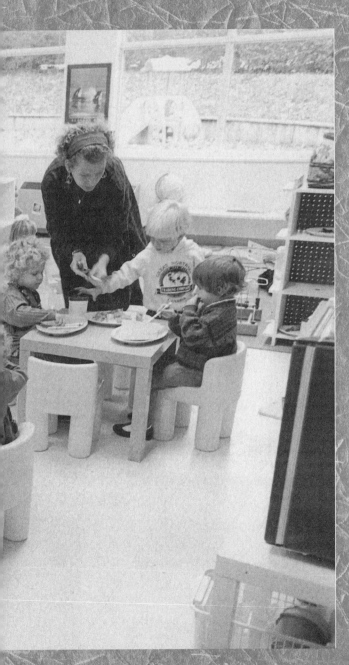

5 Growth and Development

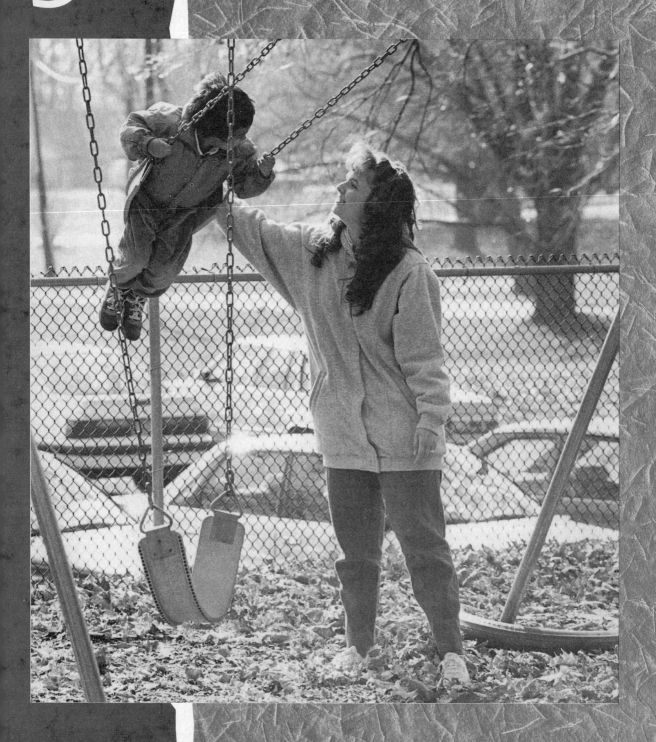

OBJECTIVES

Studying this chapter
will enable you to

- Describe the basic patterns of growth and development that occur in an embryo and fetus during pregnancy
- Summarize the physical, intellectual, social, and emotional changes that occur during the first five years
- Explain the role of food in growth and development
- List the major nutrients and explain why they are essential for growth and development
- Explain why and how a nutritional assessment is done

CHAPTER TERMS

deficiency disease
dehydration
development
enzymes
failure to thrive
fine motor skills
gross motor skills
growth
hormones
iron-deficiency anemia
nutritional status
rickets
tissue differentiation

THE children at the Green Valley Child Care Center were on the playground with Sandra, their teacher. The day was hot and humid, and the active children were sweating. Sandra set up cups and a pitcher of water on one of the picnic tables.

Marcie and Sasha stopped by for a drink, then raced off to the tricycles. Although Marcie and Sasha were born in the same month, Sasha was much more skilled at pedaling her tricycle. Marcie soon gave up and went to the climber. She climbed up the steps and slid down the small slide over and over.

Sandra felt especially close to this group of three-year-olds. She had begun caring for them when they were infants and moved along with them as they grew. It was Green Valley's policy to keep a teacher with the same children as long as possible to promote a sense of stability and security in the children.

Over by the fence, Richard played listlessly in the sandbox. He often seemed tired and irritable. Although there could be many reasons for his fatigue, Sandra wondered if Richard was getting all the nutrients his growing body needed. Richard and his family had recently become vegetarians, and Sandra knew that extra care is needed in planning vegetarian meals to ensure that they provide sufficient nutrients. Sandra made a mental note to suggest to Richard's mother that she mention that the family were vegetarians when she took Richard to the clinic for his checkup.

"Help me swing," called Tony insistently. Sandra pushed Tony for a few minutes. He had not yet learned how to pump for himself. When another child wanted water, Sandra left Tony swinging gently and went to pour the drink. Soon it would be time for the children to go in and listen to a story.

Major Milestones of Growth and Development

The children at the Green Valley Child Care Center had changed vastly in a few years. Their development mirrors that of children all over the world. A single fertilized cell becomes a walking, talking, thinking person. In an orderly sequence, growth and development begin before birth and continue well past legal adulthood. *Growth* occurs because cells increase in number and/or size. Various parts of the body grow at different rates and times. Immediately after birth, for example, the brain grows rapidly. The reproductive organs, on the other hand, grow very little until puberty.

Development refers to a change in function from simple to more complex. For example, babies at two months bat at objects with their hands. By nine months, they can pick up things and examine them because of the development of their nervous systems. Each stage of growth and development has characteristic events or milestones. The rate at which children reach these milestones depends on genetic and environmental factors.

Prenatal Growth and Development

During the prenatal period—the period before birth—a single cell grows and divides hundreds of times. Groups of cells become different from each other. Some form bone, muscle, and skin. Others become the heart, lungs, or other organs of the body. Pregnancy is often discussed in terms of three trimesters, or stages, each lasting three months.

Before birth, the developing baby, called an embryo from the second to the eighth weeks and then a fetus, depends on her mother for nourishment. Pregnant women need to eat a healthful, balanced diet that supplies additional calories and nutrients to support the developing fetus. Vitamin and mineral supplements are often prescribed by doctors to make sure that the nutritional needs of both mother and child are met. During pregnancy, a woman's personal habits, such as getting regular exercise, smoking cigarettes, or using alcohol, affect the growth and development of her baby (Milunsky, 1987).

Development, both prenatal and postnatal, progresses from head to foot. The term used to describe this is cephalocaudal. This means that the brain develops before the spinal column, and the spinal column develops before the nerves to the legs and feet.

Development is also proximodistal—it moves from the center of the body toward the extremities. Thus arms and legs form before fingers and toes. After birth, control of the arms comes before control of the fingers.

The First Trimester.   Eight to ten days after conception, the rapidly dividing fertilized egg attaches itself to the uterus of the mother. The placenta begins to form. The placenta allows the transfer of oxygen and nutrients from mother to child throughout pregnancy. It begins to function as early as the twelfth day after conception (Pillitteri, 1992).

Soon *tissue differentiation*, or the separation and specialization of groups of cells by function, occurs. The cells of the embryo separate into three different layers of tissue—the endoderm (inner layer), the mesoderm (middle layer), and the ectoderm (outer layer). Each layer develops into a different group of

---

FOCUS ON — Promoting Healthful Habits

Age-Appropriate Food Stations

The Katydid Child Care Center was one large multiuse room divided roughly in half by low shelves and further organized into several activity areas. One-half of the room was used by the two- and three-year-old group and the other half by the four- and five-year-old group.

In the reading corner, Vicky was just finishing a story with the twos and threes. She always read a quiet story just before snack time.

"Who's ready for a snack?" Vicky asked. The children responded enthusiastically. They headed for their very own "kitchen." This was a food station created with low tables and chairs. Low shelves, cupboards, and drawers were stocked with napkins and plastic plates and utensils. Even the sink was only 2 feet off the ground. The caregivers could help the children's small hands turn the faucets. The toddlers enjoyed filling cups with water or rinsing dishes—just like grown-ups.

Vicky knew it was important to give each child a responsibility. After having all the children wash their hands, she asked Martina to get plastic mugs and plates out of the low cupboard and place them around the table. Then Vicky handed Pierre a box of honey graham crackers. He reached in and filled a plate for each table. Vicky also helped Barry put apples in a colander and rinse them thoroughly. When the children were settled at the tables, Vicky poured milk in each child's mug and sliced the apples.

On the other side of the room, another small kitchen was sized appropriately for the fours and fives. It had slightly higher tables, chairs, and a sink, and more cooking utensils than the other food station. Liza, the older children's teacher, knew it was important to give them choices at snack time. She offered oranges, sliced bananas, or cheese and crackers. She let them peel the oranges and cut the bananas or cheese with blunt plastic knives. Yesterday, the children had enjoyed pummeling boiled potatoes with their own potato mashers. Next week, Liza planned to have them hand-squeeze their own fresh orange juice.

If the preschool where you worked didn't have the luxury of different food stations for each age group, how might you create your own? What different elements would you include for the younger and older preschoolers?

organs that performs special functions. The nervous system and skin come from the ectoderm. Bones, muscles, the heart, and the rest of the circulatory system come from the mesoderm cells. The endoderm forms part of the digestive system, the lungs, tonsils, and bladder.

All of the major organ systems have begun to develop by the end of eight weeks. During this time of rapid development, the embryo is especially susceptible to damage by viruses, drugs, and environmental toxins that may reach the embryo through the mother's body (Pillitteri, 1992). At the start of week nine, the embryo becomes known as a fetus.

By the end of the first trimester of pregnancy, the fetus is just over 3 inches (7.5 cm) long and weighs about 1 ounce (28 g). The brain is beginning to form and the heart is beating.

The Second Trimester.   Growth and development continue rapidly during the second trimester. The body grows rapidly in length. Flexible cartilage begins to turn to bone. The eyes, ears, and nose are formed. Hair appears. The heartbeat is strong enough to be heard with an ordinary stethoscope. By the middle of the second trimester of their pregnancies, most women are well aware of fetal movements.

The increase in fetal size is dramatic. By the end of the second trimester, the fetus is 11 to 14 inches (28 to 36 cm) long and weighs about 1½ pounds (680 g). At this point, it is possible, though unlikely, that a baby born prematurely could survive with intensive medical assistance.

The Third Trimester.   During the last trimester of pregnancy, many organs mature. The eyes open. The lungs complete their development, making it possible for babies to breathe air at birth. The brain continues developing rapidly. The fetus moves often and vigorously.

Over this period, the baby's body stores nutrients such as iron, fat, and calcium to use after birth. With each passing week, the chances of a baby surviving outside the uterus improve. The average baby born at the end of the third trimester weighs 7 to 7½ pounds (3.2 to 3.4 kg) and is about 19¾ inches (50 cm) long.

Growth and Development During the First Five Years

The pattern of growth and development in children is predictable and orderly. Physical development, including changes in height and weight, body proportions, and the function of organ systems, proceeds according to predictable patterns. Children develop physical, intellectual, social, and emotional skills in the same basic order. Growth and development are very interdependent. Skills such as walking, talking, drawing, and reasoning all depend on interactions among the maturing organ systems. A child needs adequate nutrition and rest and an emotionally supportive, caring environment to grow and develop these new capabilities and skills.

The rate at which each child moves through the developmental pattern varies from child to child. For every event, there is a range of times when

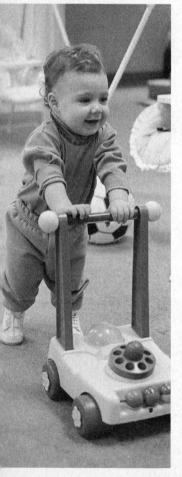

A child's ability to walk is one stage in a predictable pattern of growth and development.

normal children achieve that particular milestone. For example, Sasha could pedal a tricycle at age three, but Marcie could not; yet both children are normal. If a child's development falls far outside the normal range, evaluation by a health care professional is recommended.

Factors that affect the rate at which each child achieves certain developmental milestones include the child's genetic makeup, the home and community environment, nutrition, gender, birth order, and state of health. A child who reaches a developmental milestone early is not necessarily superior to one who achieves it later. Children may move ahead rapidly in one area of development, such as imitating speech, and lag in another, such as learning to walk.

Height and Weight. A steady gain in weight and height are usually signs of satisfactory growth. Babies grow rapidly during the first year, usually tripling their birth weight and increasing their birth length by 50 percent. The rate of growth is slightly slower during the toddler period, between ages one and three. Normally the height of toddlers at age two is approximately half their final adult height. By age 2½, toddlers weigh approximately four times their birth weight.

From age three until the growth spurt at the beginning of puberty (age 10 to 11 for girls and age 11 to 13 for boys), normal weight and height gains remain steady. Both boys and girls gain weight at a rate of 4½ to 6½ pounds (2 to 3 kg) each year. Their height increases by 2 to 3 inches (5 to 7.5 cm) yearly. Final adult height and weight depend on heredity, nutritional status throughout childhood, and general health. Final adult weight is also influenced by social and emotional factors.

If preschoolers and older children are poorly nourished, their growth will slow noticeably. If this condition is temporary, these children will grow at rapid rates once they receive adequate food until they catch up with children in their age group. Once they catch up, their rate of growth slows to average rates (Whaley & Wong, 1991). However, brief periods of malnutrition in infancy or continued severe malnutrition any time may result in permanent damage to the body.

Growth charts (see Appendix C) may be used to compare a child's height and weight to those of other children of the same age and sex. These charts are created using data from white and black American children. They may not provide appropriate comparisons for children from other backgrounds. Children tend to follow the general curve for growth. If a child's growth pattern shows major fluctuations from the curve, evaluation by a health care professional is recommended. Children at the extreme ends of the growth charts (below the fifth or above the ninety-fifth percentile) should be evaluated as well.

Changing Body Proportions. As children grow and develop, their body shape changes. Different parts of the body grow and mature at different rates. The brain develops early in life. The head of a newborn makes up almost 25 percent of her total body length. The circumference of her head is

FIGURE 5.1   Changing Body Proportions from Birth to Adulthood. The body proportions of an infant gradually shift to adult proportions over the years as different areas of the body grow at different rates.

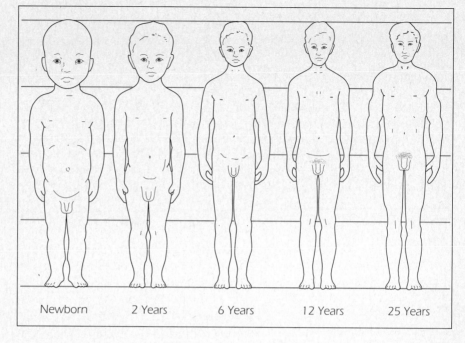

Newborn   2 Years   6 Years   12 Years   25 Years

larger than the circumference of her trunk. In adulthood, her head will be only 12 percent of total body length and its circumference will be less than that of her shoulders and hips (see Figure 5.1).

At birth, the legs are only about one-third of a newborn's total body length. Legs, however, continue growing rapidly until puberty, and eventually they make up about half an adult's height. Posture also changes with age. The spine of a newborn is curved, just as it was in the uterus. As children learn to walk, the curvature of their spines changes, as does their posture. Other external changes occur because of hormones produced during puberty. These hormones signal the body to develop typical male or female characteristics.

Growth changes the external shape of children and the relative proportions of some of their internal organs. The brain, for example, grows rapidly until a child is age two and will reach 90 percent of its adult size by the time a child is about age five. At birth, the lymph nodes, tonsils, adenoids, and spleen are large when compared to other organs. These organs grow rapidly until a child is age 6, then they grow more slowly until they reach twice their adult size at about the time a child is age 11. Their size then decreases until the end of adolescence (Whaley & Wong, 1991). There is very little growth of the reproductive organs during childhood, but their growth rate increases rapidly at the start of puberty.

Maturation of Organ Systems.   The central nervous system (CNS) is one of the earliest organ systems to mature. In fact, the CNS grows more rapidly during the three months before birth than at any other time. Development proceeds from the brain toward the hands and feet.

As the CNS develops, children's movements change from jerky, involuntary reflexes to controlled, voluntary movements. The amount of time children spend sleeping decreases gradually and the quality of their sleep (periods of active and quiet sleep) changes as the nervous system matures.

The newborn's digestive system is capable of digesting human milk (or baby formula) but is unable to process many other types of food. His stomach can hold about 3 ounces (90 ml) of milk, and his digestive system can break down human milk and baby formula and use the nutrients they provide. But the newborn's digestive system does not produce the substances that break down solid foods into usable nutrients. Within a year, however, the baby's intestines increase in length by 50 percent and begin producing the types and amounts of substances needed to digest most table foods (Mott, James, & Sperhac, 1990).

A baby's kidneys cannot remove water from the fluid that passes through them. A baby's urine is very dilute—mostly water—as a result. Until the kidneys can remove water from the urine, at the time a child is about the age of two, children are especially susceptible to serious water loss.

Major Motor Abilities.   There is a close relationship between the maturation of organ systems and the development of motor skills.

Gross motor skills are those that involve the use of large muscle groups. At birth, most gross motor movement occurs in response to primitive reflexes. As the nervous system matures and bones and muscles develop, actions become more smooth and voluntary. There is always a normal range of time during which particular skills are achieved by different children.

Within six months, children learn to control the movement of their heads and to sit up. By the end of the first year, babies will creep (pull themselves along with their arms), then crawl on their hands and knees. By 1½ years, they can toddle, holding onto something, and then walk unassisted. During the second year, toddlers learn to walk up stairs and kick a ball.

By age three, most preschoolers run and, like Sasha, pedal a tricycle. By age four, they can balance on one foot, catch a ball using their arms and bodies, and swing on a swing after being started by an adult. Younger children, like Tony, do not yet have the coordination to keep the swing in motion by themselves. A five-year-old can walk backwards, jump rope, and catch a ball using both hands.

Fine motor skills require control of the small muscles of the body. At birth, a newborn's fine motor behavior is reflexive. Within the first half year of life, however, babies learn to focus on and follow objects with their eyes and to grasp things using their whole hands. During the second half of infancy, babies are able to pick up objects with their thumbs and forefingers, and they develop an interest in feeding themselves.

Between ages two and three, toddlers develop enough fine motor control to build small block towers and put large pegs into holes. They also scribble on paper, but have little control over the marks they make.

Preschoolers have fairly advanced fine-motor control. Most can string beads, cut with scissors, draw, and paste.

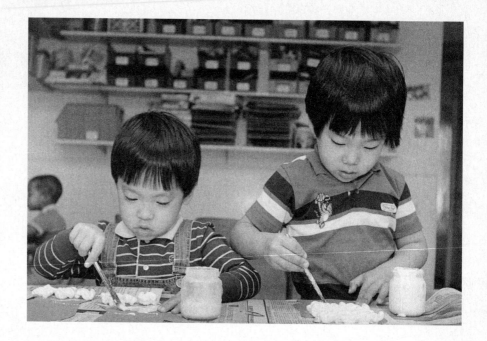

Preschoolers have better control over their hands. Between the ages of three and four, they learn to string beads, take apart and put together easy snap toys, and cut with safety scissors. By the time they are ready for kindergarten at age five, they can cut out and paste simple shapes and draw simple, recognizable pictures. Some begin writing their name in wavering, uneven letters.

Developing Language.   Babies cry from birth. Infants respond to sounds they hear, turning toward voices and later cooing in response to pleasant sounds. Crying, listening, and cooing in infancy help children develop more complex language skills later.

The ability to speak requires fine motor control of the small muscles of the tongue, mouth, and jaw, and maturation of the brain. Learning to talk requires a cycle of imitation, experimentation, and positive reinforcement from the caregiver. Children who are born profoundly deaf do not use oral speech without special training, even though their mouths and vocal cords are normal. This is because they hear no speech to imitate. Deaf children do, however, communicate through their own learned language—American Sign Language (ASL).

Children can understand spoken language before they can talk. Between nine months and one year of age, babies understand *no* and often respond to their names. During this same period—sometimes earlier—they begin babbling syllables such as "ba-ba" and "da-da." Gradually the babbling takes on the shape of the language being spoken, so that even though the child uses only nonsense syllables, these syllables sound like sentences.

FOCUS ON

Communicating with Parents

Serving Meat at the Child Care Center

It is the end of the day at the Foster Child Care Center, and parents are arriving to pick up their children. Five-year-old Sarah is helping Julie, one of the teachers, pick up toys.

Sarah's mother appears at the door. As Sarah gets her coat, Julie hands Sarah's mother a copy of the center's lunch menu for the following week.

SARAH'S MOTHER: (looking over the menu) Hmmm. Monday—red beans and rice. Tuesday—vegetable soup and peanut butter and jelly sandwiches. Except for the hamburgers on Wednesday and the sliced turkey on Thursday, I don't see much meat on this menu.

JULIE: We usually serve meat for lunch two or three times a week. Next week we're having chicken noodle soup on Wednesday and hamburgers on Thursday.

SARAH'S MOTHER: Well, I really don't think that's enough meat. Sarah never eats a big breakfast, and sometimes she's too tired to eat much at dinner. She gets her biggest meal here—not to mention snacks. Children need lots of protein every day to stay healthy.

JULIE: Sarah and all the other children get protein every day. But it's not always in the form of meat.

SARAH'S MOTHER: Everyone knows that meat is the best source of protein.

JULIE: Meat is a great source of protein, but it isn't the only one. Sarah will get the same quality of protein from the beans and rice on Monday's menu. The children are having yogurt jello fluff for a snack on Friday. The gelatin and yogurt in that provide protein too.

SARAH'S MOTHER: I don't know. It looks to me as if the center is trying to cut costs by serving less meat. I pay a lot to send my daughter to this center—it's one of the most expensive ones in town. I don't see why you can't afford meat every day.

JULIE: It's not really a matter of money. Our director, Mrs. Goodwin, likes to keep the menu fairly low in fat for the children over the age of two. Some other kinds of protein have less fat than meat.

SARAH'S MOTHER: Sarah is only five. It will be a long time before she has to worry about fat. Did you say that Mrs. Goodwin makes up the menus?

JULIE: Mrs. Goodwin and Arlene Benedict, a dietitian, make up the menus together. If you are concerned about the amount of meat on the menu, you should talk to them. Arlene has charts that show exactly how much protein children should have each day and which food combinations make complete proteins like those in meat.

SARAH'S MOTHER: I think I'll make an appointment with Mrs. Goodwin.

Do you think Julie handled the questions Sarah's mother asked effectively? Would you have added anything if you were talking with Sarah's mother?

A one-year-old may use a few words meaningfully. During the second year, that same child will become able to name a dozen things, make animal sounds, follow simple directions, and use two-word phrases. These great strides in language development often seem to happen quite suddenly.

Preschoolers start speaking in complete sentences that become more consistently structured as they approach school age. They are able to listen to and understand simple stories. By age five, their vocabulary is large enough to describe their wants, needs, and daily routines to people who do not know them.

Intellectual, Social, and Emotional Development. Newborns cannot distinguish between themselves and their environment. Between the fifth and eighth months of life, they begin to recognize this distinction. They start to learn that they can do things that change what's around them—they can make things happen. They can tip a cup and spill its contents; they can shake a rattle and make a noise. Much of the first year is spent experimenting with different ways to change the environment, imitating other people, and learning the effects of different actions.

Very early in life, infants learn to recognize their primary caregivers and respond with a smile. Forming an attachment to and a trusting relationship with the caregiver is an important part of infancy. The Green Valley Child Care Center's policy of keeping a caregiver with the same children for as long as possible is an acknowledgment of this need.

At about nine months, babies begin to respond negatively to strangers (stranger anxiety) and to separation from their parents or primary caregiver. This response confirms that the baby has formed a strong emotional attachment to the parent or caregiver. Although the baby's reaction may be difficult for those who care for the infant, it is a normal, healthy step in emotional development.

Active toddlers want to explore their world. They often resist adult control and have frequent temper tantrums, yet they are capable of showing genuine affection. Toddlers are unpredictable, moving rapidly from independent activities to shy or clinging behavior. At this stage, children often watch and try to imitate the actions of another child or an adult.

Preschoolers understand and can obey simple rules. However, they lack the ability to generalize. As a result, preschool children may learn and follow a rule that applies to one situation, but they are not able to make the mental comparison and connection to another situation in which the rule should clearly apply.

Preschoolers see events only from their own perspective (they are egocentric) and cannot interpret events from the viewpoint of any other person. This focus on themselves makes learning to share, take turns, and play with other children a slow process. The social skills preschoolers learn reflect what is considered valuable and socially appropriate in their own cultures.

The Role of Food in Growth and Development

Few aspects of a child's early life are as important as food. Food supplies the nutrients and energy children need to grow and thrive. It enhances their ability to interact with the environment and learn. Food also stimulates the development of identity and provides the opportunity for social interaction.

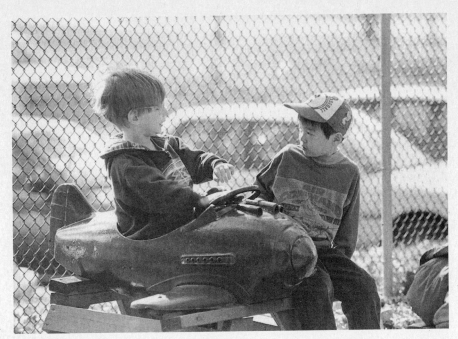

Preschoolers cannot interpret events from the viewpoint of another person. They need to learn how to take turns and share with other children.

Nutrition in Physical Development

What children eat has a far-reaching effect on their physical growth and development. It is important that children's diets provide the nutrients needed for each developmental stage. Children's *nutritional status*, which is the nutrients they take in compared with the nutrients they require, depends largely on diet.

A child's pattern of growth is partly influenced by heredity. Diet alone cannot override a child's genetic makeup. For example, a healthful diet will not make a short child grow into a tall adult. A healthful diet, however, will help children to grow and develop to their own potential.

While good nutrition maximizes a child's physical potential, inadequate nutrition limits physical development. *Failure to thrive*, or failure to grow at the expected rate over time, is caused by organic and environmental factors, including inadequate nutrient and caloric intake (Rallison, 1986).

Inadequate nutrient or caloric intake may result from neurological problems. It may also be caused by physical disabilities that interfere with a child's ability to suck, chew, swallow, or self-feed. Socioeconomic factors, such as child neglect, poor feeding practices, inadequate stimulation, or lack of food, may also be responsible for insufficient food intake. A family may not be able to buy enough food for the child because of poverty. However, some parents with adequate finances restrict a child's intake in an attempt to prevent obesity in the future by keeping children lean. The causes of failure to thrive are many.

Regular pediatric checkups evaluate incremental gains in growth. Children with delayed growth need professional evaluation to determine the cause(s). With appropriate intervention—including changes in feeding practices—most children can catch up with their growth curve, often growing at a faster rate than normal for a period of time.

Nutrition in Intellectual Development

A child's nutritional status and caloric intake are also related to intellectual, or cognitive, development. Intellectual development refers to the way children think and learn. It includes mental processes such as memory, comprehension, reasoning, problem solving, and attention.

Poor eating patterns can affect nutritional status and interfere with the learning process. Hunger pangs and hunger-induced headaches—often caused by skipping breakfast or by long intervals between meals and snacks—distract children from learning and exploring their environment. Studies of school-age children show that those who skip breakfast score lower on achievement tests; they have more school absenteeism and more behavior problems (McBean, 1993).

Healthful food patterns, on the other hand, enable children to learn. When children feel energetic and healthy, they relate better to their learning environment.

Nutrition in Psychosocial Development

Nutrition also promotes the emotional and social, or psychosocial, development of children. Psychosocial development refers to the development of attitudes, emotions, personality, identity, and social skills.

Many of a child's early life experiences relate to food—these range from the parent-child attachment that forms during feeding to the way caregivers respond to a child's cry of hunger, smile as a reward for appropriate eating behavior, or rebuke a child for spilling a glass of milk. These early food experiences affect lifelong food patterns and influence how children view themselves, others, and their world.

Careful management of a child's interaction with food and the food environment is important to the child's psychosocial development. A teacher or caregiver can make positive contributions to this process in many ways. Helping a child feel successful about eating builds self-esteem, and placing value on foods common to a child's culture reinforces the child's self-concept. By providing the opportunity to imitate and practice appropriate table behavior in a positive, supportive environment, the caregiver teaches a child valuable social skills.

The Role of Specific Nutrients in Growth and Development

Every cell in a child's body uses nutrients that come from the food she eats. Getting an adequate quantity of calories and a balance of nutrients is essential for the growth and development of tissues and organ systems and for the child's health as a whole. If a child does not get enough of a particular nutrient or group of nutrients, a *deficiency disease* may develop. With nutrients such as the B vitamin, folic acid, and the mineral zinc, deficiency directly interferes with growth. Other nutritional deficiencies disturb processes such as blood clotting (vitamin K) or water balance (potassium). As discussed in Chapter 3, six kinds of nutrients—carbohydrates, fats, proteins, vitamins, minerals, and water—are necessary for good health. Chapter 3 covered the main properties and sources of these nutrients. This chapter focuses on the roles these nutrients play in growth and development and how interdependent these roles are. These nutrients work together closely and must be provided to the body together. A balanced food intake is the best way to avoid deficiency diseases and provide all the nutrients needed for healthy growth and development in young children.

FOCUS ON Cultural Diversity

Staple Foods

Nutritionists agree that a low-fat, high-fiber diet is healthful for children and adults. As the number of children from diverse cultures increases in the preschool population, it is important for teachers to learn about low-fat, high-fiber foods from ethnic cuisines. Including these foods in snacks and lunches helps children from different backgrounds feel at home in the classroom. It also creates opportunities to introduce new foods that all the children may not get at home.

While some ethnic cuisines may seem exotic at first glance, many staple foods from these diets are naturally healthful and provide many essential nutrients.

- Mexican-Americans thrive on a diet rich in whole grains and beans. A bean burrito or taco for lunch provides fiber (from whole grains and beans), complex carbohydrates (whole grains), and vitamin B complex (beans).
- People from African nations and the Caribbean base many dishes on rice and beans. Again, beans provide fiber and B vitamins. Rice is a complex carbohydrate that's also rich in vitamins and high in fiber. Vegetables and lots of fruit round out the main ingredients in many African and Caribbean dishes.
- The Middle Eastern diet includes two delicious staple foods—sesame seeds and chick peas. Both are high in fiber, B vitamins, and all essential amino acids. Hummus, a spread made with mashed chick peas and crushed sesame seeds, on whole grain pita bread makes a great, nutritious snack.
- Asian cuisine is famous for its nutritional value. Rice, of course, is the foremost element. Fish and vegetables are two low-fat staples of the Asian diet. Food is often quickly stir-fried in vegetable oil. The food absorbs little of the oil, helping to keep the diet low in fat. Another low-fat, high-protein staple, tofu, is made from soybeans. Because tofu is bland, try serving it mixed in a salad for lunch. If possible, stir-fry it with vegetables.

Carbohydrates, Fats, and Proteins

Carbohydrates, fats, and proteins can all provide energy for the body. Carbohydrates are the main energy source in a balanced diet. Because only small amounts of carbohydrates are stored in the body (as glycogen), children need to eat carbohydrate-containing foods regularly. The amount of carbohydrates children need to consume to grow and stay healthy depends on how fast they are growing and how active they are.

Fats are a useful source of energy for the body, providing more calories per unit than any other nutrient. Fats are also essential for the proper growth and development of a child's nervous system and for maintaining healthy skin and hair. They are a source of essential fatty acids.

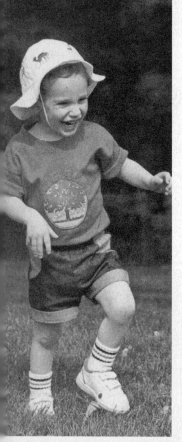

The eight B vitamins help to release energy from digested foods and build new body tissues. Growing toddlers require more folic acid, for example, for their size than do adults.

Essential fatty acids are needed to form myelin, a substance that surrounds nerves. Myelin must be present for the nerves to function properly. Infants are especially susceptible to deficiencies in essential fatty acids because their nervous systems are growing very rapidly.

Proteins are essential building materials in the body. This is their primary role in growth and development. The amino acids from digested proteins are used to build new protein in muscle, skin, hair, blood, internal organs, and other tissues. Amino acids also become part of *enzymes*, proteins that speed up chemical reactions in the body. *Hormones*, substances formed in one organ that are carried, often in the bloodstream, to another organ whose function they regulate, are generally made of protein as well. Proteins can be burned for energy when there is an inadequate supply of carbohydrates and fats in the diet, but this is not desirable, particularly for growing young children.

There are many protein sources, including meat, cheese, dried beans, and nuts. However, only animal products contain complete proteins. Foods that provide incomplete proteins should be served to children in combinations that provide all of the essential amino acids when eaten together (see Chapter 3). This is because a child's body must have an adequate supply of all nine essential amino acids from a meal's protein in order to use it for growing new tissues. Vegetarians like Richard's family need to be especially careful in planning meals that provide sufficient amounts of all nine essential amino acids.

Although protein deficiency is rare in the United States today, it is common in other parts of the world. Kwashiorkor is a disease that occurs when children receive enough calories but too little protein. Children with kwashiorkor lose weight and fail to grow. Their bodies retain water, making them look puffy and potbellied. Their skin becomes scaly and dry, and they almost always have other vitamin and mineral deficiencies.

Marasmus is a deficiency disease that results from too few calories and too little protein. Children with marasmus are simply not getting enough to eat. Often marasmus has an emotional as well as a dietary component, and it can be part of a general pattern of neglect. Children waste away. Their bodies appear old and wrinkled. Young children with kwashiorkor or marasmus also suffer mental retardation and have lowered resistance to infection. Complications from infection are often fatal.

Vitamin	Food Sources
TABLE 5.1 **Food Sources of Vitamins**	
Water-Soluble Vitamins	
B vitamins	
thiamin (B_1)	pork, liver, fish, eggs, legumes, whole grain breads and cereals, wheat germ, bran, brown rice, pasta, enriched grain products
riboflavin (B_2)	liver, eggs, milk, cheese, dark-green leafy vegetables, whole grain breads and cereals, brewer's yeast, enriched grain products
niacin	liver, lean meat, poultry, fish, nuts, dried beans, whole grains, enriched grain products
pyridoxine (B_6) pantothenic acid biotin	meats, fish, dried beans, vegetables, fruits, potatoes, whole grains, wheat germ
folic acid	liver, eggs, milk, dark-green leafy vegetables, enriched grain products
cobalamin (B_{12})	liver, eggs, milk, dark-green leafy vegetables
vitamin C	tomatoes, dark-green leafy vegetables, potatoes, green peppers, citrus fruits, strawberries, cantaloupe
Fat-Soluble Vitamins	
vitamin A	liver, fish-liver oils, egg yolk, milk and dairy products, margarine
(as beta carotene)	carrots, sweet potatoes, winter squash, kale, broccoli, spinach, apricots, peaches
vitamin D	liver, oily fish, egg yolks, fortified milk and other dairy products
vitamin E	meats, nuts, egg yolks, dark-green leafy vegetables, vegetable oils, cereals, wheat germ
vitamin K	pork, liver, egg yolks, cheese, dark-green leafy vegetables, cauliflower, vegetable oils

Vitamins and Minerals

Vitamins and minerals regulate the rate of many chemical reactions in the body. They are important throughout the lifetime. There are specific functions of vitamins and minerals that are crucial to growth and development.

Vitamins. Thirteen vitamins are essential to human health and need to be acquired through the diet (see Table 5.1 for specific sources). Vitamins play important roles in growth and development.

The eight B vitamins are required in reactions that release energy from digested foods. This is the energy that fuels the growth of young children. B vitamins also play a part in the manufacture of nonessential amino acids that are used in building new tissues. The B vitamin folic acid is especially important to growth because it is needed to make red blood cells and genetic material for all new cells. Growing infants need ten times more folic acid per pound of body weight than adults do. Deficiencies in folic acid or vitamin B_{12} (important for folic acid activity) can result in anemia, symptoms of which include fatigue, weakness, headaches, and irritability. Pregnant women also need increased amounts of folic acid; folic acid deficiencies are linked to birth defects.

Vitamin C is needed to form collagen, the most abundant protein in the body. Collagen is a strong connective tissue and is necessary for proper bone formation. Collagen forms tendons and ligaments, and is found in cartilage and blood vessels. Vitamin C also helps the body absorb iron, which is needed for making red blood cells. Scurvy is a disease resulting from insufficient vitamin C. The bones of a child with scurvy fail to grow. The gums bleed, teeth fall out, and joints become inflamed. Scurvy is rare in developed parts of the world.

Vitamin A is necessary for normal bone, tooth, and skin growth. It also plays a role in the formation of thyroxine, a hormone produced by the thyroid that regulates growth. Children who do not get enough vitamin A stop growing. Vitamin A is also used to make a light-sensing pigment in the eye.

Vitamin D helps the body absorb calcium. Calcium is the basic component of bone. Both vitamin D and calcium are necessary for skeletal bone growth. *Rickets* is a deficiency disease that occurs when there is too little vitamin D (see Chapter 9). The bones do not form properly, so that the legs of a toddler with rickets will not straighten normally but might become severely bowed. Breast-fed babies are often given vitamin D supplements, and commercial formulas routinely include vitamin D.

Vitamin E protects cell membranes from bursting and is especially important in preventing the rupture of red blood cells. It also helps protect vitamins A and C from being inactivated in the intestinal tract. All of these functions provide critical support to growth and development. Because vitamin E is found in many foods and is stored in body fat, deficiencies are limited to premature babies and people who do not absorb fats normally.

Vitamin K is needed for making proteins in bone, kidney, and blood plasma. It is also an essential factor for blood clotting. Newborns have no vitamin K stored in their bodies and do not yet have the bacteria that make vitamin K in their intestines. This makes them very vulnerable to internal bleeding that can result from minor bumps and handling that is part of their routine care. In hospitals, newborns are given an injection of vitamin K to prevent excessive bleeding.

Minerals.   There are 15 minerals that are essential for human nutrition. Chapter 3 discusses the general roles and food sources for all 15 of these minerals. The minerals discussed here play important roles in growth and development.

Calcium gives bones and teeth their strength. Without enough calcium, the bones become weak and fragile. Calcium deficiencies are fairly common, especially in women and young children. Pregnant women are often given calcium supplements to help their bodies meet the needs of the growing fetus. Growing children need more calcium for their size than do adults because children are making new bone and tooth tissue.

Phosphorus is the other major mineral in bones and teeth. Phosphorus deficiency is rare. Too much phosphorus, however, makes it difficult for the body to absorb calcium. This is one reason to encourage children to drink milk, which contains calcium and phosphorus, rather than soft drinks, which contain phosphorus but no calcium.

Sodium, chloride, and potassium help maintain the water balance of the body. Sodium excess is very common and probably plays a role in causing high blood pressure. Sodium deficiency causes muscle cramps and weakness. Chloride deficiency upsets the chemical balance in the body's fluids. These deficiencies usually result from prolonged, heavy sweating. Chronic potassium deficiencies are rare, but extended periods of diarrhea and vomiting can deplete the body's supply of potassium. This makes the water loss from diarrhea and vomiting more serious, since potassium is needed to restore the body's water balance. Since young children are especially susceptible to serious water loss, a potassium deficiency can be cause for concern. Electrolyte solutions, such as Pedialyte, may be used to help restore the chemical and water balance in infants when there is serious water loss.

As part of the cell's machinery for making protein and releasing energy, magnesium is essential to all growth and metabolism. Since it is also involved in muscle contraction and the transmission of nerve impulses, it is important to the development of gross and fine motor skills.

Iron is needed to form hemoglobin, the substance in red blood cells that transports oxygen from the lungs to all parts of the body. A good oxygen supply is essential to normal cell growth. Iron is also found in the muscle protein myoglobin. Children need more iron than adults because children are making new blood and muscle as they grow. Pregnant women need more iron for normal growth of the fetus. At birth, a baby's body has enough stored iron to last for about four months. After this period, children who are breast-fed should receive iron-fortified cereals. Bottle-fed babies should eat iron-fortified commercial formula.

People who do not get enough iron develop *iron-deficiency anemia* and may experience symptoms such as weakness, fatigue, headaches, and irritability. In children, iron-deficiency anemia can cause stunted growth and mental retardation. Iron-deficiency anemia is a common nutritional deficiency among preschool children in the United States today and will be further discussed in Chapter 9.

Iodine is needed only in tiny quantities, but it is essential for normal physical and mental growth. Iodine is a crucial element in the production of

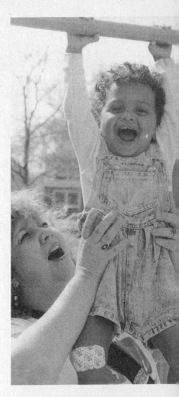

Minerals such as calcium and magnesium are important for normal muscle function and the development of gross motor skills.

the growth hormone thyroxine. Inadequate amounts of iodine in the diet can cause goiter, a swelling in the neck caused by enlargement of the thyroid gland, in people of any age. Iodine deficiency in a pregnant woman can result in mental retardation and severely stunted growth in the fetus. This condition, which is rare in the United States, is called cretinism. Once mental and physical growth have been retarded, the effects cannot be reversed.

Zinc is involved in making many proteins in the body and in producing the genetic material—the blueprint for inherited traits that is present in every cell. Therefore, zinc is important to growing children. The growth rate of children who do not have enough zinc in their diets slows down. This can result in dwarfism, in which children appear extremely small for their age.

Copper helps the body use iron in the production of hemoglobin. As previously discussed, iron deficiency can cause anemia. A deficiency of copper prevents proper use of iron and can, therefore, cause anemia as well.

Fluoride helps develop strong bones and teeth that are resistant to decay. Many communities add fluoride to their water. Infants who are breast-fed, and infants and children living in areas where the water is not fluoridated should take a fluoride supplement, available only by prescription. Recommended amounts vary according to age.

Water

Life without water is impossible. Water is found in all cells and tissues. It is part of most chemical reactions in the body. Water, as part of other body fluids, transports nutrients to and waste from all cells. Water also transports hormones that regulate growth and development.

Dehydration, or serious loss of water from the body, can be fatal. In infants and children, dehydration can occur rapidly. Vomiting and diarrhea are the chief causes of dehydration in infants and children. Both of these symptoms should be treated seriously. Medical help should be sought if caregivers suspect that children cannot take in enough liquids to replace what is lost through vomiting or diarrhea.

The amount of water people need varies with their level of activity and the outside temperature. Children lose more water due to evaporation from the skin than adults do. They should be encouraged to drink water often. It is particularly important to make water easily available to children during hot weather, as Sandra did when the children in her care played outside on a hot day. Sugary drinks and carbonated beverages should not be considered a substitute for water.

Nutrient Intake Assessments

To determine if a child is getting an adequate and balanced amount of nutrients, health care professionals sometimes conduct nutrient intake assessments. These involve recording everything that is consumed for a specific period of time.

Collecting Information

There are several ways to obtain information about nutrient intake. One method is the 24–hour recall. A health care professional interviews parents and asks them what and how much the child ate in the past 24 hours. The interviewer records this information for evaluation. However, it is often difficult to remember exactly what a child ate and estimate the quantities he consumed. Sometimes actual plastic or plaster models of food in different serving sizes are used to help people estimate portions. This method is used primarily to screen for nutrient intake problems.

More intensive methods of collecting information are used when detailed evaluation of a child's nutrient intake is needed. A commonly used tool that is considered to yield reliable information is the food diary. With this method, parents and caregivers measure or weigh every food that is provided to the child and any that is not finished and then record everything that the child eats. Usually food diaries are kept over a period of several days or a week to get an accurate picture of the child's diet. If caregivers are asked to keep a food diary for a child, they are provided with specific instructions and measuring devices.

Very detailed information about nutrient intake and eating patterns over time is sometimes collected through an interview or a questionnaire. In addition to questions about specific foods and amounts eaten, parents and caregivers are asked about the child's eating habits, whether the child skips meals, the frequency of snacks, how food is prepared, and when and where the child eats. They are asked other questions about the child's health history, appetite, and changes in eating patterns and exercise. If the child is an infant, parents and caregivers are asked about breast milk, including whether it is stored, how it is stored, and how it is later served. If the infant receives formula, it is equally important to know how the formula is prepared, stored, and served. Any vitamin or mineral supplements given to the child are also recorded.

Assessment

The information from a nutrient intake assessment is often supplemented with a physical examination and measurements of height, weight, head circumference, arm circumference, and body fat. In some cases, blood and urine tests are performed to obtain information about the levels of minerals and other substances and about general health.

To determine if eating patterns are balanced and adequate, a calculation is made of the total amounts of each nutrient in the foods consumed and the results are compared with a standard. In some cases, additional factors will be taken into account, for example when certain nutrients are not normally absorbed or metabolized by the child's body. Caregivers who suspect a child has a dietary deficiency should refer the child and family to a health care professional familiar with dietary assessments.

WHOLESOME SNACKS

Pineapple Cheese Spread

Ingredients:

8 ounces part-skim mozzarella cheese

½ cup crushed pineapple, packed in juice (undrained)

1 tablespoon additional pineapple juice

Directions:

1. Cut cheese into small pieces.

2. Let children help place all ingredients into a blender container. (Make sure the blender is unplugged or the container is removed from its stand.) Blend the ingredients, scraping the sides of the blender often. Blend until smooth and creamy.

3. Serve on whole wheat crackers.

Yield: 24 servings

Each serving contains:

Calories: 30
Protein: 3 g
Fat: 2 g
Carbohydrates: 1 g

Source: USDA. Making bag lunches, snacks, and desserts. HG-232-9. Washington, DC: Human Nutrition Information Service.

SUMMARY

- During the prenatal period and early years, growth occurs because cells increase in number and/or size. Various parts of the body grow at different rates and times in an orderly sequence.

- Development follows an orderly pattern. Most children go through the pattern in the same order, but the rate at which they develop varies.

- The nutritional status of the mother during pregnancy affects the growth and development of her baby before birth.

- By the end of the first trimester of pregnancy, all of the fetus's major organ systems have begun to develop and the heart is beating. During the second trimester, organ systems continue to develop and facial features form. In the third trimester, many organs mature, some nutrients are stored by the body, and the fetus steadily gains weight.

- Height and weight change during early childhood at fairly predictable rates. Growth charts can be used to compare a particular child's height and weight with those of other children of the same age and sex.

- A child's body proportions change as different parts of the child's body grow and mature. Organ systems also grow and mature at different rates and times.

- Children develop major motor abilities in the same basic sequence. The development of motor abilities is closely tied to the maturation of organ systems.

- Speaking requires fine motor control of the small muscles in the tongue, mouth, and jaw, and maturation of the brain.

- In the first year of life, babies learn that they are separate from their environment, that they can make things happen, and that different actions have different effects.

- Toddlers become active explorers who may shift quickly from independent activities to shy or clinging behavior.

- Preschoolers can obey simple rules but cannot make mental comparisons to related situations or see events from another person's perspective.

- Food provides the nutrients and energy children need for their physical, intellectual, and psychosocial development.

- The six basic nutrients children need to grow and develop are carbohydrates, fats, proteins, vitamins, minerals, and water.

- Carbohydrates, fats, and proteins can provide energy for the body.

- Fats are needed for the proper growth and development of a child's nervous system.

- Proteins are building materials in the body. All nine essential amino acids must be supplied from a meal's protein for that protein to be used in the growth of new tissues.

- Many functions of vitamins are essential to growth and development, including their roles in obtaining energy from digested food and in building various tissues.
- Minerals play many roles in growth and development as building materials, electrolytes, and important aids in chemical reactions that promote growth and development.
- Water performs so many functions that life cannot be maintained without it. Young children are especially susceptible to dehydration and should be encouraged to drink plenty of water.
- Health care professionals may conduct nutrient intake assessments to determine if a child is getting adequate and balanced amounts of nutrients. Different methods may be used to collect information and perform the assessment.

ACQUIRING KNOWLEDGE

1. Explain the difference between growth and development.
2. Why does a pregnant woman need to eat a healthful, balanced diet with additional calories?
3. Describe the two basic patterns of development.
4. Describe an aspect of fetal development that occurs during the second trimester.
5. During the third trimester, how does the baby's body prepare to function on its own after birth?
6. Describe the possible effects of a period of malnutrition on the rate of a child's development.
7. Describe three of the changes in body proportion that occur between infancy and adulthood.
8. Explain what type of food the newborn infant is able to digest and why this is so.
9. Define and give two examples each of gross motor skills and fine motor skills.
10. What aspect of emotional development causes a nine-month-old infant to become wary of strangers?
11. How does food contribute to a child's growth and development?
12. Will a short child who is given a healthful diet grow into a tall adult? Why or why not?
13. What does failure to thrive mean?
14. What impact do poor eating patterns have on a child's ability to learn?
15. What causes deficiency diseases?
16. How do carbohydrates contribute to a child's growth and development?
17. Where does the body obtain essential fatty acids? What role do they play in growth and development?
18. Why does a child need all of the essential amino acids?

19. Explain the role of vitamins in development.
20. Which minerals are especially important in the formation of bones and teeth?
21. Describe the role of sodium, chloride, and potassium in the body.
22. What is iron's role in development, and what are the results of iron deficiency?
23. Define dehydration and describe its chief causes in infants and children.
24. How can information about a child's nutrient intake be obtained?
25. What is involved in an assessment of nutrient intake?

THINKING CRITICALLY

1. A mother's responsibility for her child's nutrition begins long before birth. Explain what a woman can do during pregnancy to provide her child with adequate nutrition. Suggest ways in which a pregnant woman's nutritional habits might harm her baby.
2. What effect does the quality of a child's nutrition have on final adult height? Can good nutrition help a shorter-than-average child develop into a tall adult? Why or why not? Do any other factors affect height?
3. Children develop physical, intellectual, and social skills at their own pace. When do you think caregivers should become concerned about a child who fails to demonstrate a skill? What do you think a caregiver should do about a two-year-old who has not begun to walk, for example, or a three-year-old who does not talk?
4. Growth and development depend upon a wide variety of nutrients; yet, at some stages, young children may be choosy about the foods they are willing to eat. How might a caregiver cope with a child's food preferences and ensure that the child receives the nutrients needed during periods of rapid growth?
5. Give examples of some skills that children learn by imitating the people around them. What implications do you think this pattern of learning by imitation has on the development of a child's eating habits?

OBSERVATIONS AND APPLICATIONS

1. The rate at which children grow and develop varies widely. Observe two children in a preschool class that are close in age. Note similarities and differences in their physical development. Is one shorter and thinner than the other? Can one kick a ball while the other has not yet mastered that skill? Can one string beads while the other cannot? Observe the two children at snack time or mealtime. Does one finish everything and one hardly touch his food?
2. Children can understand language better than they themselves can express language. Observe this for yourself. Observe a child who is about 12 months old for 15 minutes. Write down what, if any, words the child says during that time. At the same time, note what the child understands. If her mother calls, "Come here," does the child go to her? When a caregiver

says, "It's time for juice and cookies," does the child get up and go over to the table? What examples do you observe?

3. Mrs. Calhoun tells you that while she knows sugar is bad for teeth and that eating too much of it contributes to weight problems, it is also a source of carbohydrates. Since children need a lot of carbohydrates, she does not limit her children's intake of commercially produced sugary products. Do you agree with Mrs. Calhoun's attitude toward sugar? Does its importance as a source of carbohydrates outweigh the problems it can cause? Why or why not?

4. Mr. Sanders tells you that his family has a history of high cholesterol levels and heart problems. He has read that diet can affect cholesterol level. He wants his son started on a diet that will not contribute to a high cholesterol level. What suggestions can you give him? At what age should his son start to follow these guidelines? Why is age a consideration?

FOR FURTHER INFORMATION

Berman, C., & Fromer, J. (1991). *Meals without squeals*. Menlo Park, CA: Bull Publishing.

Berman, C., & Fromer, J. (1991). *Teaching children about food*. Menlo Park, CA: Bull Publishing.

Dhopeshwarkar, G. (1983). *Nutrition and brain development*. New York: Plenum Press.

Frank, G. C. (1991). Taking a bite out of eating behavior: Food records and food recalls of children. *Journal of School Health, 61*, 198–200.

Hamilton, E., Whitney, E., & Sizer, F. (1991). *Nutrition concepts and controversies*. St. Paul, MN: West Publishing.

Insel, P. (1990). *Perspectives in nutrition*. St. Louis: Times Mirror/Mosby College Publishing.

Satter, E. (1987). *How to get your kid to eat, but not too much*. Menlo Park, CA: Bull Publishing.

U.S. Department of Agriculture. (1992). *Building for the future: Nutrition guidance for child nutrition programs*. Washington, DC: U.S. Government Printing Office.

Velazquez, A., & Bourges, H. (Eds.). (1984). *Genetic factors in nutrition*. Orlando, FL: Academic Press.

Nutritional Needs of the Developing Infant

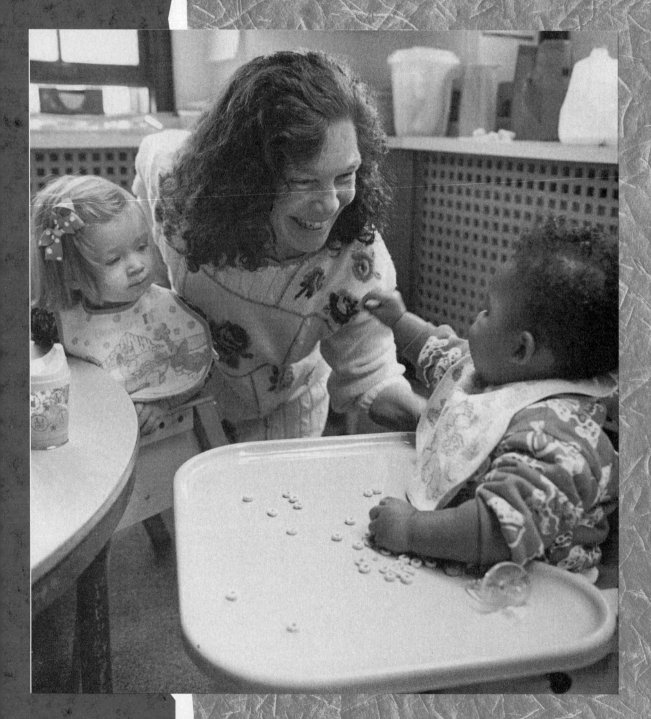

Studying this chapter
will enable you to

- Explain how changing growth rates during infancy affect an infant's nutritional needs
- Discuss how the changing mouth patterns of infants influence the foods they eat
- Identify which foods are unsafe or undesirable during the first year
- Explain why breast-feeding is the best way to feed an infant
- Discuss when solid food should be introduced and why
- Describe how new foods should be introduced to babies

CHAPTER TERMS

aspiration
bottle-feeding
breast-feeding
critical periods
infant botulism
mouth patterns
nursing bottle syndrome
palmar grasp
pincer grasp
teething
weaning

EDUARDO was ready to eat. Gloria, his caregiver at the Acorn Child Development Center, brought out the high chair and placed it next to Mary, who had just finished her lunch. The second Eduardo noticed the high chair, the eight-month-old began babbling excitedly.

"Hey Eduardo, just hang on a minute while I get ready," laughed Gloria as she tied a bib around his neck. Eduardo was an enthusiastic, but messy eater. Gloria lifted Eduardo into the high chair and secured the tray. She gave the hungry baby a few toasted oat rings to keep him occupied while she prepared his lunch.

Gloria washed her hands, then mixed some rice cereal with formula. She opened a jar of green peas and a jar of strained chicken and heated them up. Chicken was Eduardo's new food this week. So far, most of it had gone in his hair.

Across the room, Peter began to cry. Valerie, the other caregiver in the infant room, went to the refrigerator for a bottle.

Peter's mother provided breast milk she had frozen and stored in bottles, for Peter's feedings at the center. She felt strongly about Peter receiving breast milk, even though she was working.

This would be Peter's last bottle of the day. In an hour and a half, his mother would come for him. Valerie and Gloria tried to time Peter's last bottle so that he would be ready to eat again when she came to pick him up.

Cuddling Peter, Valerie listened to the satisfied sucking sounds Peter made as he drank. Occasionally she stopped to burp him.

Meanwhile, Gloria was feeding Eduardo as he stuck his hand into the rice cereal, then tried to put his whole fist in his mouth. Gloria offered Eduardo some apple juice in a cup, but most of it dribbled down his chin.

"I guess you're finished Peter," said Valerie, as he stopped sucking and turned away from the bottle. There was still an ounce of milk left, but Valerie discarded it. She knew it wasn't safe to save it and offer it to him later.

Growth During the First Year

Infants grow and develop more rapidly during the first year of life than at any other time during their lives. Over the span of 12 months, normal infants triple their birth weights, go from sucking at the breast or bottle to drinking from a cup, and develop the coordination and strength to support their weights while standing.

Good nutrition in the first year is a critical element in keeping children healthy and helping them reach their full developmental potential. But infants' nutritional needs change dramatically during the first year. Food that may be appropriate in early infancy may be inadequate to meet children's nutritional needs only a few months later.

Because of infants' rapidly changing needs, the caregiver plays an important role in monitoring nutritional status. This may involve educating parents about childrens' nutritional needs at different stages and coordinating feedings at the child care center with those at home.

The Newborn

The average newborn boy weighs 7½ pounds (3.4 kg) and is 20 inches (51 cm) long. Newborn girls are slightly smaller, averaging 7 pounds (3.2 kg) and 19¾ inches (50 cm). However, there is a normal range of variation in the birth weight of healthy babies of both sexes. Babies weighing between 5½ pounds (2.5 kg) and 9½ pounds (4.3 kg) are considered within the normal range. The average head circumference of a newborn is 13½ inches (34.3 cm).

A birth weight of less than 5½ pounds (2.5 kg) is considered low. Some low birth weights are the result of premature birth. However, full-term newborns may also have low birth weights if the mother's nutrient intake did not meet her nutritional needs during pregnancy, if she smokes tobacco, or if she uses alcohol or other drugs (Mott, James, & Sperhac, 1990).

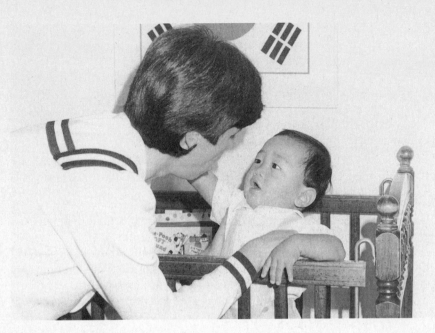

By the end of the first year, an infant will have tripled his birthweight.

The First Months

During the first six months of life, healthy infants double their birth weights, gaining approximately 1½ pounds (0.68 kg) each month. At the same time, infants grow in length by about 1 inch (2.5 cm) each month. The brain grows rapidly, resulting in an increase in head circumference of about ½ inch (1.5 cm) monthly.

During the second half of the first year, infant growth per month slows to about 1 pound (0.45 kg), ½ inch (1.3 cm) in length, and ¼ inch (0.6 cm) in head circumference. By the end of the first year, infants will have approximately tripled their birth weights, increased in height by 50 percent, and increased in head size by one-third.

Weight gain alone is not a reliable indication of normal growth. A baby should also show regular increases in height and head circumference. Growth charts indicate where a child's growth pattern falls relative to other normal infants of the same age (see growth charts in Appendix C). Growth is influenced by both the child's nutritional status and by hereditary factors. However, children who fall below the fifth percentile or above the ninety-fifth percentile may require evaluation by a health care professional.

The Infant's Changing Body

At birth, a baby's head makes up 25 percent of her body length as compared to 12 percent for an adult. The circumference of the head is larger than the circumference of the chest. A newborn's legs are only one-third of her body length compared to half the body length for an adult. These proportions give the newborn a very distinctive look.

HEALTH TIPS

**Infant Nasal
Congestion**

An infant's nasal
passages are very
narrow and are easily
blocked by nasal
congestion. Because
infants are primarily
nose breathers,
congestion can
seriously impede an
infant's breathing and
may even interfere with
feeding.

Caregivers can use a
specially designed
suction bulb to remove
excess mucus from the
nasal passages: press
the bulb, then gently
insert the rounded tip
into the open space in
the nasal passage. Be
extremely careful not to
touch the sensitive
membranes inside of
the nose. Release the
pressure on the bulb—
this sucks mucus into
the bulb. Use the
procedure only once.
The suction bulb
should be used for one
child only and must be
thoroughly cleaned
after each use.

Caregivers can also use
a cool mist humidifier
in a cool room (70 °F or
less) and raise the
upper half of an infant's
mattress to promote
nasal drainage.

During an infant's first year, her legs and trunk grow at approximately the same rate. In addition, her legs, which are bowed at birth, begin to straighten. Her chest circumference at the end of the first year is equal to her head circumference and will continue to increase in the following years. As an infant ends her first year, her body begins to take on the characteristic look of a toddler.

Along with overall growth, rapid development of the nervous system brings about great changes in a baby's ability to ingest and use nutrients during the first year. The baby's primitive reflexes, such as sucking, are replaced with voluntary movements, such as drinking from a cup. The digestive system of an infant, which is immature at birth, develops to the point where it can make use of a wide variety of solid foods. Likewise, the baby's immature kidneys become increasingly able to concentrate urine and adjust to varied amounts of liquids.

As the nervous system, digestive tract, kidneys, and other organ systems develop, the type of food an infant needs changes. Caregivers and parents who understand the physical changes an infant undergoes during the first year are better able to appreciate the changing nutritional requirements of the child.

Development and Feeding Behavior

The timing of certain developmental milestones, such as the eruption of teeth, varies from individual to individual. But the sequence of events, for example the order in which the teeth appear, remains constant for most infants. Both hereditary and environmental factors affect the timing of developmental events.

Mouth Patterns

During the first year of life, there are changes in the way babies manipulate food in their mouths. These changes in *mouth patterns* mark the transition from a liquid to a solid diet.

At birth, newborns display reflexes that help them obtain food. For example, the rooting reflex causes babies who are touched on the cheek to turn toward the touch and open their mouths. This helps them locate the breast and nipple. The suckling reflex is also present in newborns. Babies extend then pull back their tongues causing milk to flow from the nipple. The gag reflex helps to keep babies from inhaling breast milk or formula.

Within a short time, suckling gives way to sucking. The tongue movement in sucking differs in breast-fed and bottle-fed infants. In breast-fed infants, the tongue moves forward and back while the gums squeeze milk into the back of the mouth. This movement of the tongue helps babies suck, but discourages breast-fed babies from accepting food from a spoon.

In bottle-fed infants, the large, rigid nipple of the bottle interferes with the movement of the tongue. These babies thrust their tongues forward to control the flow of milk from the nipple and prevent choking. If continued beyond infancy, this tongue thrust behavior can deform the upper jaw and cause problems when speech begins to develop.

Around the fourth month, infants begin to develop a munching pattern, or up-and-down movement of the jaws. They continue to suck, but the munching pattern also allows babies to eat pureed food from a spoon. Later, in the seventh to ninth months, the facial muscles become strong enough for babies to drink from a cup without dribbling. Finally, as the first year comes to a close, babies begin to master rotary chewing or grinding and are then ready to eat soft table food.

Between the fourth and eighth months *teething* begins; teeth start to erupt through the gums into the mouth. When teething causes painful swelling of the gums, affected infants may find sucking on the breast or bottle uncomfortable and may lose interest in food. Teeth appear in a predictable pattern. The two lower front teeth usually come in first, followed by the two upper front teeth, the two upper side teeth, and the two lower side teeth. By age one, most infants have six to eight teeth.

Coordination and Feeding Behavior

At birth, babies can turn their heads from side to side and lift them briefly when lying on their stomachs. Their eyes focus on objects 8 to 10 inches (20 to 25 cm) away. Even with this limited ability to move, infants successfully nurse from the breast or bottle.

The vigorous growth of babies during the first half-year of life is accompanied by maturation of the central nervous system. And, as caregivers will notice, babies' range of movement increases with every month that passes. By the end of the fourth month, most infants can roll over.

Caregivers should not place babies in positions they are unable to achieve on their own. Putting them in positions, such as sitting unsupported, for which they are not physically ready can cause harm. Sometime during the fifth or sixth month, many infants can sit with support in a high chair.

In their first six months, babies become increasingly aware of their own hands and feet. Their first attempts at voluntary grasping result in a *palmar grasp*, where four fingers on the hand move simultaneously to grip an object against the palm (see Figure 6.1). Babies at this stage may want to hold their own bottles. They should never be left alone holding a bottle, however, nor should bottles ever be propped during feeding. Caregivers should hold infants while feeding them. All infants need continuous supervision while eating during the first year.

Around the eighth month, most infants are able to drink well from a cup. The fine motor coordination of the hands improves. Infants now begin using a *pincer grasp* to pick up small objects such as pieces of ground or chopped food between their thumb and forefinger (see Figure 6.1). At this age, many babies like Eduardo spend a large part of their mealtimes finger-feeding and exploring their food. Although it's a messy process, caregivers should encourage infants to explore the taste and textures of new foods. This exploration is a form of learning for infants.

FIGURE 6.1 Palmar Grasp and Pincer Grasp. An infant uses the palmar grasp to close his fingers around an object that touches his palm. As fine motor control develops, an infant can use his thumb and forefinger to pick up an object—an action referred to as the pincer grasp.

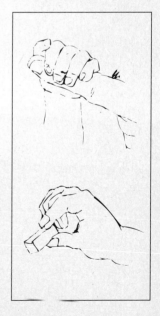

FOCUS ON — Communicating with Parents

Problem in an Infant's Diet

Monica was concerned about four-month-old Davy, the newest child at the center. When she changed his diaper earlier today, Davy's stool had an unmistakable tinge of green in it. Something was wrong. Monica had noticed that Davy seemed to be losing weight over the three weeks he'd been under her care. She was worried. When Mrs. Ellis came to pick Davy up, Monica approached her and described her concerns about Davy. Mrs. Ellis heard her out, but she was skeptical.

MRS. ELLIS: There's nothing wrong with Davy. My friend said it's natural for babies to lose some weight around this age.

MONICA: But Mrs. Ellis, Davy's stool is green. That shows that something's wrong. I think perhaps his formula is not agreeing with him.

MRS. ELLIS: That's nonsense. My pediatrician prescribed that formula herself. She said it's the best formula she knows of for infants. You must be mistaken. I think you're looking for problems where none exist.

MONICA: Please, Mrs. Ellis. Take Davy back to the pediatrician. And take a stool sample with you. I think the doctor may have to make only a simple change in the formula and then everything will be all right.

MRS. ELLIS: Do you expect me to tell my son's doctor that she doesn't know what she's talking about? To question her expertise and authority? I'd never do that!

MONICA: If it's easier, Mrs. Ellis, tell the doctor that Davy's caregiver is concerned. Then it won't seem as if you are personally questioning her judgment. I feel strongly that Davy's formula is causing him to lose weight. Wouldn't you rather be safe than sorry where Davy is concerned?

MRS. ELLIS: (sighing) Do you really think something may be wrong with Davy's formula? Something that's making him sick?

MONICA: Yes, Mrs. Ellis, I really think something may be wrong. But if it's caught right away—now—I'm sure it will be simple to correct.

MRS. ELLIS: But I never heard of such a thing before.

MONICA: It's actually a fairly common problem with infants. Many babies need small alterations in their formula if it doesn't agree with them. It's not serious. But it is something that must be taken care of right away.

MRS. ELLIS: Okay. I'll take Davy to the doctor. As you said, better safe than sorry. (pausing) You know, I really do appreciate your telling me about this. I see that Davy is in good hands and that makes me very happy.

Do you think Monica overreacted to the greenish color of Davy's stool? Do you think she handled Mrs. Ellis well? What might you have done differently?

By the time the first year comes to an end, voluntary muscle control has improved dramatically. Babies are interested in trying to feed themselves with a spoon. Although most of the food ends up on the babies or the floor, they eventually learn to control a spoon. Self-feeding is important in helping infants to develop a sense of independence.

Intellectual Development and Feeding Behavior

A newborn does not distinguish between himself and his environment. His actions are reflexive and not the product of conscious thought. During the first four months, sucking and grasping change increasingly from reflexive to deliberate acts. By six to eight weeks of age, a baby will smile in response to a smiling face. Sometime in the third month, he recognizes his primary caregiver and usually responds with smiles. Moreover, a baby begins to associate his caregiver with food and comfort.

Between the fifth and the eighth months, infants begin to distinguish themselves from their environment. They learn to perform deliberate acts that change their environment, such as shaking a rattle. Imitating the activities of others is deliberate and can be seen in babies' attempts to reproduce sounds that adults make. During these months, infants begin to understand some words. By this time, most infants also respond to their names.

By the ninth month, babies start showing stranger anxiety—a heightened wariness of strangers and distress when parents leave the room. This is because babies are beginning to understand that a thing or person continues to exist even when out of sight. (This idea is called object permanence.) Babies at this stage become unhappy when their reliable source of food and comfort goes elsewhere.

A little later, around 11 months, infants begin to combine the idea of object permanence with their new voluntary muscle skills by dropping objects and watching them fall. This can be especially frustrating for caregivers because it corresponds to the time when babies begin to feed themselves with a spoon. Many attempts at self-feeding become sidetracked by the game of dropping the spoon. Caregivers should keep in mind, however, that this game is one way that infants learn about their world.

Critical Periods of Development

There are specific times during development when children should have appropriate experiences if they are to continue to develop normally. These times are called *critical periods*. Sometime between the fourth and sixth months, babies begin to accept pureed foods from a spoon. The period between the sixth and the ninth months is best for developing the acceptance of foods with coarser textures. Babies are ready for these foods when they can sit up unaided, and when they develop the pincer grasp and chewing motion.

Caregivers should consult with parents about introducing minced, chopped, or mashed foods that have less water content and more texture than pureed foods during the sixth- to ninth-month period. Parents may supply food for their children. Children will have more difficulty accepting solid food introduced after this critical period. In some infants, however, such as those who were premature or of low birth weight, those who have experienced periods of illness, or those who are not thriving, the critical period may be delayed beyond the ninth month.

The Nutritional Requirements of Infants

Nutritional requirements of infants differ substantially from those of older children and adults. Infants require more of certain nutrients relative to their body weights than do older children. Meanwhile, their immature digestive systems and kidneys make it impossible to use some nutrients effectively. Some foods may, in fact, be harmful to babies during the first year. This will be discussed in more detail later in this chapter.

Physical Requirements

An individual's caloric requirements during the first six months of life are greater relative to the body weight than at any other time in the life cycle. This is because it is the period of most rapid growth. A newborn requires about 49 calories per pound (108 calories per kg) of body weight per day in order to grow and develop normally. In contrast, a young adult requires only about 18 calories per pound (40 calories per kg) daily. A newborn baby weighing 8 pounds needs about 400 calories per day.

After the first six months, growth slows. More calories are used in activity and fewer in growth and development. The caloric requirements for infants gradually decrease to about 44 calories per pound (98 calories per kg) toward the end of the first year.

Social and Emotional Requirements

Calories alone are not enough to make babies thrive. Babies also need to form close emotional bonds to their caregivers. Breast-feeding or cuddling babies during feeding, as Valerie did when she fed Peter at the center, helps promote a sense of security.

Feeding should be a pleasant, emotionally comforting time. A baby should be fed in a quiet, relaxed environment. The caregiver should be able to give the child her full attention and make eye contact during feeding.

Nonorganic failure to thrive, a failure of infants to grow and develop that is not caused by disease, sometimes occurs when infants receive an adequate number of calories but little emotional interaction with their caregivers. This can happen when parents are unable to adjust to the stresses of parenting or when they are unable to meet their children's emotional needs because of substance abuse or mental illness (Whaley & Wong, 1991).

Special Considerations of Infant Nutrition

Caregivers must be aware that many foods are not appropriate for infants. These foods can be presented either too early in development or in sizes or shapes that cause children to choke. Feeding inappropriate foods to infants can be fatal. Table 6.1 lists the most common of these foods.

Milk.   Human milk is the ideal food for infants. An acceptable alternative is commercially prepared iron-fortified infant formula (American Academy of

TABLE 6.1 Foods Not Appropriate for Infants	
Food	**Reaction**
cow's milk/goat's milk	lacks many substances necessary for growth; too much protein for baby's kidneys to process; more difficult to digest; may cause allergic reactions
high-nitrate vegetables (spinach, carrots, beets)	if given before four months, they can cause nitrate poisoning
honey	may cause infant botulism
flavorings/additives	may result in inappropriate food preferences later in life
eggs, wheat, soy, shellfish, nuts, chocolate, citrus fruits	may cause allergic reactions
raisins, nuts, small pieces of raw vegetables, popcorn, snack chips, whole grapes, circular hot dog pieces	may cause baby to choke

Pediatrics, 1989). While cow's milk is often among the ingredients in infant formulas, neither cow's milk nor goat's milk by itself is suitable for infant nutrition (Whaley & Wong, 1991).

Cow's milk is unacceptable for young infants for several reasons. It contains more protein than human milk, and processing this protein overworks babies' immature kidneys. In addition, cow's milk protein is much more difficult to digest than the protein in human milk. Cow's milk contains less vitamin C and vitamin E than human milk, and it lacks many factors present in human milk that are suited to human growth. Cow's milk may also cause allergic reactions. Goat's milk has similar limitations.

Many health care professionals recommend that infants should not be given cow's milk until age one. When cow's milk is introduced, whole milk, not low-fat or skim milk, should be used until age two. Low-fat and skim milk do not contain enough fat to allow the body to make myelin, a material essential to the rapidly growing central nervous system.

High-Nitrate Vegetables. Vegetables such as spinach, carrots, and beets contain large amounts of nitrates. Nitrates are chemical substances used by plants to make amino acids. If these vegetables are given to babies before they are four months old, their immature digestive systems cannot properly digest the nitrates. Nitrate poisoning can occur, causing a breakdown in hemoglobin that reduces the available oxygen in the blood and leaves babies' bodies with an inadequate oxygen supply.

Honey. Honey should not be given to children under one, either by itself or as a sweetener in baked goods, such as honey graham crackers (USDA,

1988). Honey may be contaminated with a bacterium called *Clostridium botulinum*, whose spores can grow in infants' bowels. As the spores become established, they release a toxin, or poison, that causes the sometimes fatal illness of *infant botulism*.

Flavorings and Additives.   Spices, salt, sugar, and fats should not be added to babies' food. Babies like bland foods and there are no nutritional reasons for adding seasonings to infants' food. In fact, early introduction of sugar or salt may result in an inappropriate preference for these additives later in life.

Food Allergies.   Allergic reactions to food are common during infancy because an infant's immature digestive system passes more unchanged proteins into the bloodstream. Among the common foods that can cause allergic reactions during the first year are cow's milk, eggs, wheat, soy, shellfish, nuts, chocolate, and citrus fruits (Whaley & Wong, 1991). The introduction of foods in this common allergen list in a child's diet is best delayed until after the first year. If these foods are introduced earlier, parents and caregivers should be alert for reactions to them.

Allergic reactions include diarrhea, vomiting, excessive gas, asthma, rashes, hives, and colic. Episodes of colic are characterized by irritability and excessive crying. Each of these symptoms can also be caused by other health problems, so it is important to work closely with parents and health care professionals when allergies are suspected.

Size and Shape of Food.   *Aspiration* is the inhaling of a foreign object into the airway. It is the leading cause of accidental death in infants (Pillitteri, 1992). Babies can aspirate liquids from a bottle if the nipple opening is too large or if a bottle is propped and they are unable to turn away or stop the flow of milk. Older children can aspirate solid food and small objects such as coins.

When babies begin to eat solid food, caregivers must pay special attention to the size and shape of the pieces of food that they are serving. Hot dogs must be cut so that the pieces are *not* circular. Grapes should be cut in quarters. Most child care centers avoid these foods completely for safety reasons. Raisins, nuts, small pieces of raw vegetables, popcorn, and snack chips are some of the foods that should never be given to young children because of the possibility of choking. The danger of aspiration is one reason why infants should never be left alone while eating.

Feeding During Early Infancy

Parents, often with guidance from health care professionals, make the first decisions about how to feed their babies before the children arrive at the child care center. They may choose *breast-feeding*, or nursing, in which the mother's breast milk provides nourishment, or *bottle-feeding*, usually with commercially prepared formula. Both are appropriate for a young infant, and both have advantages and disadvantages. Every family situation is unique, and caregivers should support the parents' decision about which method to use.

Breast-Feeding

Human milk is the preferred food for an infant. It is easily digested and rarely produces allergic reactions. The nutrients in breast milk depend somewhat on the diet of the mother. Women who are breast-feeding need to pay special attention to what they eat. The milk of a woman eating a healthful diet will contain the vitamins, minerals, and other nutrients her baby needs to grow and thrive during the first four to six months of life.

FOCUS ON ## Promoting Healthful Habits

Avoiding Nursing Bottle Syndrome

It was 5:30, and Mrs. Easton arrived to pick up her six-month-old daughter, Rosie. The infant began to cry as Louisa, the caregiver, lifted her out of her crib.

Mrs. Easton cradled her daughter in her arms and cooed softly to try to soothe her. She glanced up at Louisa. "Rosie's only been here a week," Mrs. Easton said. "Until she started here, she hardly ever cried. What's making her so cranky?"

Louisa, too, wanted to talk about Rosie's distress. She told Mrs. Easton that Rosie was not sleeping well. Rosie cried constantly when she was put in her crib to nap. Louisa asked Mrs. Easton how she prepared Rosie for her nap time at home.

"Well," said Mrs. Easton, "I usually have Rosie nap after she's eaten. I put her in the crib with a bottle so she can drink some more milk if she wants it. She usually sucks on the bottle a bit, then falls right to sleep."

Now Louisa knew why Rosie was so cranky. "I think Rosie misses her bottle in bed," Louisa told Mrs. Easton. "Here at the center, we never put infants to bed with their bottles because they can choke as they fall asleep. Drinking milk or juice in the crib also leads to what we

call 'nursing bottle syndrome.' Let me explain."

Louisa explained that milk or juice from the bottle remains in the sleeping infant's mouth. The liquids promote the growth of bacteria. These bacteria can eventually rot the infant's teeth.

Mrs. Easton thanked Louisa for the information. "I'll certainly stop giving Rosie a bottle at bedtime," she said.

"It will be hard at first to wean Rosie away from the bottle she's gotten used to when she's falling asleep," Louisa said. "She'll cry at first. But I'll help here. I hope it will only take a little while for her to get used to the new arrangement, and until she does we'll need to be very patient with her."

Mrs. Easton stroked Rosie's head. Then she shook Louisa's hand. "Thank you for telling me about this," she said. "I want to do the right thing for Rosie."

Do you think Louisa handled the problem well? Would you have told Mrs. Easton about nursing bottle syndrome? What if Mrs. Easton had refused to believe you?

Besides nutrients, human milk contains antibodies and other factors that help protect the baby from some bacterial and viral infections. Breast-fed babies seem to have fewer gastrointestinal disorders than bottle-fed babies (Eiger & Olds, 1987). In addition, when babies are breast-fed, there is no chance that their food will be incorrectly prepared or become contaminated during preparation. And the closeness and physical contact between mother and baby during nursing encourage a strong emotional attachment between mother and child. Many women who breast-feed find it convenient and rewarding.

Breast-fed babies need supplements of fluoride and iron. Fluoride helps build strong, decay-resistant teeth. It does not pass into the breast milk of nursing mothers, even when they drink fluoridated water. Iron supplements are needed from about the fourth month when the iron stores present in infants' bodies at birth begin to be depleted. Most doctors also recommend vitamin D supplements for breast-fed babies. There is some evidence, however, that these may be unnecessary (Greer & Marshall, 1989). Parents normally are responsible for giving these daily supplements to their babies, but caregivers should be aware that they are needed.

Women who breast-feed their babies must be extremely cautious about the use of any drug, including alcohol. Many drugs are passed to babies in breast milk and can cause serious damage to babies' developing organs and organ systems. Women need to be aware of all drug warnings and should consult a physician if in doubt about a particular drug. When certain drugs must be taken by nursing mothers for reasons relating to their own health, breast-feeding must be discontinued to protect children from drug damage. Some viruses, such as the human immunodeficiency virus (HIV), are also present in the breast milk of infected women (Whaley & Wong, 1991).

For some mothers, being the sole or main source of nourishment for a baby is a source of stress. They may be more comfortable combining breast-feeding with bottle-feeding. Others experience physical discomfort such as cracked or sore nipples while nursing. Special ointments can be used to relieve this problem if the mother continues breast-feeding. How long a mother breast-feeds is a matter of cultural and personal preference. Caregivers should respect the feeding decisions parents make.

Bottle-Feeding

Bottle-feeding allows other family members and caregivers to participate in and share the emotional closeness of feeding the baby. Some women feel more secure being able to measure how much formula their babies drink. Many women who return to work shortly after their babies are born find bottle-feeding the best choice for their family situation. Although it is possible for an adoptive mother to breast-feed, the process of stimulating milk production in a woman who has not been pregnant takes planning and determination. Most adoptive mothers bottle-feed their babies.

Commercial formulas contain a balance of nutrients similar to human milk but lack the infection-fighting factors of human milk. Caregivers

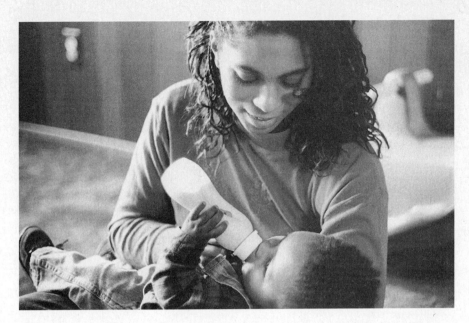

Bottle-feeding allows caregivers to share in the emotional closeness of feeding the baby.

should follow parents' instructions about the use of iron-fortified formula. Parents generally provide the formula to be fed to their children at the infant center. In rare cases in which an infant is unable to tolerate iron-fortified formula, caregivers should encourage parents to work closely with health care professionals to make sure that the baby's iron and other nutritional needs are met. Formulas are available in the form of powder, concentrated liquid, or ready-to-feed liquid. Care should be taken so that powdered and concentrated formulas are prepared properly.

Cleanliness is important in preparing bottles to protect them from contamination with bacteria and other microorganisms that cause illness. Before preparing bottles, hands and equipment should be washed and rinsed in hot water. Only water approved by the local health department should be used to dilute the formula—or for any other use in the child care environment. Formula-fed babies need fluoride supplements if unfluoridated water is used to prepare formula or if premixed formula is used.

Formulas provide 20 calories per ounce. An 8-pound (3.6 kg) baby needing about 400 calories per day will drink about 22 ounces (0.65 l) of formula usually spread out over six feedings. Formulas are available for infants with cow's milk or soy allergies, as well as fat or lactose intolerance. In addition, special formulas exist for children with metabolic disorders or other diseases.

Cereal or other solids should never be added to a bottle. This practice increases the chances of aspiration, adds unnecessary calories to babies' diets, and may result in an allergic reaction to the added food. Many parents believe that infants are more likely to sleep through the night if given solid food. This is not true. Babies begin sleeping through the night only when their nervous systems mature.

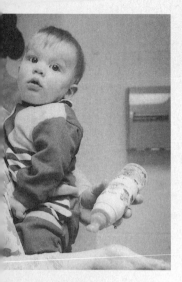

When feeding an infant with a bottle, caregivers should check the temperature of the milk by shaking the bottle and allowing a drop of milk to fall on the wrist.

Feeding at the Child Care Center

Many attitudes toward food are culturally based. Parents need to be supported in their feeding decisions as long as their choices result in a nutritionally balanced diet for their children. Mothers who place their babies in a center during infancy do not have to stop breast-feeding. Some mothers can visit the center during the day to breast-feed. Others provide breast milk in bottles, as Peter's mother did.

To encourage breast-feeding, child care centers should maintain a quiet place for mothers to nurse, and a refrigerator and freezer in which to store breast milk that mothers provide. Breast milk can be safely stored for up to 24 hours in the refrigerator or for several days if frozen. All bottles should be carefully labeled; they must be stored in the refrigerator and used within 24 hours. Once a baby is fed from a bottle, the remaining milk or formula will contain bacteria from the baby's mouth and should be discarded. Breast milk that has been thawed must never be refrozen. Caregivers should try to give the last bottle of the day 1 to 1½ hours before babies are picked up so they will be eager to nurse when their mothers arrive at the center.

Although there is no physiological reason why bottles need to be warmed, many parents and caregivers feel that warm bottles are more comforting. Caregivers should be sensitive to infant preferences and follow what is done at home. Bottles can be warmed in a pan of water. However, caregivers should check the temperature of all bottles before they are used. This is done by shaking the bottle, then allowing a drop of milk to fall on their wrists. The droplet should never feel hot.

Bottles should not be warmed in the microwave because the inner core of the bottle gets hot while the outside remains cool. There is a danger that caregivers will feel the outside of the bottle and believe that the milk is an acceptable temperature. Sensitive tissues in the infant's mouth and throat can be damaged by milk that is too hot.

Feeding provides a time for the caregiver to establish physical closeness and eye contact with the baby. Caregivers need to allow a minimum of 20 minutes for each child's feeding. Sit in a comfortable chair where the baby's head can be supported slightly above the rest of the body. Tip the nipple of the bottle so that it remains full of liquid and the baby does not swallow air.

The baby should be burped every few minutes. Pat the baby's back while holding her on your lap or resting her against your shoulder. Individual babies vary in how much air they take in during feeding. Some rarely burp. Others will spit up a small amount of milk as they burp. This is normal.

Babies who are full stop sucking, close their lips, or turn away from the bottle. Just as Valerie stopped feeding Peter when he refused more milk, caregivers should let babies' behavior signal the end of each feeding.

Bottle-fed infants can develop nursing bottle syndrome, also called nursing bottle caries. *Nursing bottle syndrome* is tooth decay that results when babies are permitted to fall asleep while drinking from bottles. Some of the bottle's contents remain in their mouths, promoting the growth of bacteria that cause tooth decay. Fruit juice is particularly damaging.

To prevent nursing bottle syndrome, bottles with formula, milk, or juice should be offered to infants only during their waking hours—never when it is time to sleep. If a parent requests that an infant have a bottle at nap time, fill it with plain water. An infant should never be left alone with a bottle, whether in a crib or elsewhere. Such a practice poses a choking hazard.

Feeding Older Infants

During the first year, infants graduate from drinking milk and formula to eating table foods (see Table 6.2). Introducing solid foods at the proper time is important in helping children make a successful change in diet. The choice

TABLE 6.2
Suggested Infant Meal Pattern

Age of Baby by Month	Breakfast	Lunch and Supper	Snack
Birth through 3 months	4–6 fluid ounces (fl. oz.) breast milk or formula[1]	4–6 fl. oz. breast milk or formula[1]	4–6 fl. oz. breast milk or formula[1]
4 months through 7 months	4–8 fl. oz. breast milk or formula[1] 0–3 tablespoons (tbsp.) infant cereal[2] (optional)	4–8 fl. oz. breast milk or formula[1] 0–3 tbsp. infant cereal[2] (optional) 0–3 tbsp. fruit and/or vegetable (optional)	4–6 fl. oz. breast milk or formula[1]
8 months through 11 months	6–8 fl. oz. breast milk, formula[1], or whole milk 2–4 tbsp. infant cereal[2] 1–4 tbsp. fruit and/or vegetable	6–8 fl. oz. breast milk, formula[1], or whole milk 2–4 tbsp. infant cereal[2] *and/or* 1–4 tbsp. meat, fish, poultry, egg yolk, or cooked dry beans or peas, *or* ½–2 oz. cheese, *or* 1–4 oz. cottage cheese, cheese food, or cheese spread 1–4 tbsp. fruit and/or vegetable	2–4 fl. oz. breast milk, formula[1], whole milk, or fruit juice[3] 0–½ slice bread or 0–2 crackers[4] (optional)

[1] Iron-fortified infant formula
[2] Iron-fortified dry infant cereal
[3] Full-strength fruit juice
[4] Made from whole grain or enriched meal or flour

Adapted from U. S. Department of Agriculture. (1988). *Feeding Infants: A Guide for Use in the Child Care Food Program.*

of food, the frequency with which new foods are introduced, and the atmosphere in which babies are fed all affect how well children adjust to changes in their diets.

When to Begin Semi-Solid Food

Developmental maturity is more important than chronological age in deciding when to introduce semi-solid food. Sometime between the fourth and sixth months, most babies are ready to eat pureed foods with a smooth consistency and high water content. Babies continue to need fluoride supplements and, if still nursing, supplemental iron and, possibly, vitamin D.

Bottle-fed babies who are ready for semi-solid food are usually drinking about a quart of formula a day. Babies who are ready for semi-solid food should be able to sit with support, draw their lips across a spoon, and keep the food in their mouths rather than using their tongues to thrust it back out. Premature babies, low birth weight babies, or infants who have been ill for extended periods may not be ready for semi-solid food even at six months.

Feeding Semi-Solid Foods

Good communication between the parent and child care provider is important during the introduction of semi-solid foods. New foods need to be introduced one at a time with a wait of about a week before the next new food is introduced. In this way, if the child shows an allergic reaction, the caregiver can inform the parent of the child's reaction to the food and encourage the parent to withdraw it from the baby's diet. Semi-solid food should be introduced in small quantities, initially at one meal a day. As the baby begins to accept these foods and becomes more skilled at eating them, the number of solid food meals can be increased.

Sequence of Solid Foods

Iron-fortified infant rice cereal is usually the first solid food offered to babies. It rarely causes an allergic reaction, is easily digested, and provides iron—an essential nutrient at this stage of a baby's life. Cereals made from other grains are more likely to cause allergic reactions and should not be served until a few months later.

After infant rice cereal, mild-tasting fruits and vegetables, such as bananas, peaches, apricots, green peas, and sweet potatoes, are good choices when properly prepared and introduced one at a time. Commercial baby food comes in jars or as dehydrated flakes. Either is acceptable. If using jarred foods, choose plain vegetables or fruits without added sugar, salt, or starch. There is no need to feed babies desserts. Baby food can also be made economically at home. Simmer or steam fresh fruits and vegetables, then puree them in a blender. Ripe bananas can be mashed without being cooked first. Homemade baby food can be frozen in ice cube trays and thawed as needed. Six to nine months is a critical period for the introduction of foods

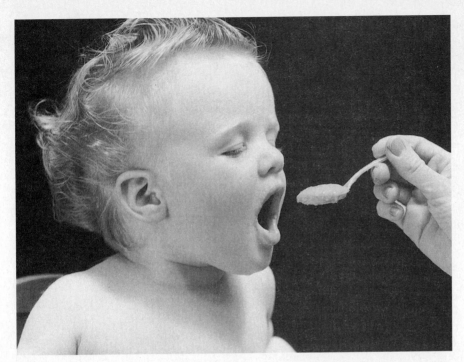

Most babies are ready to eat semi-solid foods between the ages of four and six months.

with more texture. As noted in the section on development, babies may refuse textured food if it is not introduced at this time. Examples of textured foods are mashed or minced vegetables, pureed meats, or banana slices.

Strained meats are usually served from the eighth month. Some babies do not like their consistency and will initially reject them unless they are mixed with vegetables. Avoid commercially prepared mixed dinners, however, because they often include added salt or starches. Parents who want to feed a vegetarian diet to their babies may need to consult a health care professional to make sure that their nutritional needs are met. It can be difficult to meet babies' nutritional needs with some very strict vegetarian diets (Whaley & Wong, 1991). Wheat products are not usually served until after the eighth month when they are less likely to cause allergies.

Using a Cup

Between the sixth and eighth months, babies can start drinking from a cup. Use a cup without a spout or "sippy lid" so they learn to drink rather than suck liquid. Apple juice is often the first drink served in a cup.

Introducing the cup marks the beginning of weaning. *Weaning* is the process of replacing the breast or bottle with drinking from a cup and eating table food. Gradually the number of bottle-feedings or nursings decreases. The number and size of solid food meals and the amount of liquids drunk from a cup increases so that by the middle of the second year weaning is usually complete.

FOCUS ON / **Cultural Diversity**

First Foods

Sometime during the first year of life, most children begin to eat "solid" food. At first, these solids are only a little thicker than breast milk or formula. As children get older and are better able to chew and swallow, the food they eat becomes less runny and closer in texture to adult food.

"Starter foods" vary depending on where children are raised. In general, children's first foods are made from the grains, fruits, and vegetables that are the staples of their culture.

In the United States, Canada, and western Europe, traditional baby foods have been replaced by prepackaged, dried cereals, which are mixed with breast milk or formula. Infants are introduced to cereals, then pureed fruits, vegetables, and meats. Eventually, the pureed foods give way to soft table food.

In other cultures, Western-style baby foods may not be available. If they are, they may be very expensive. Infants everywhere are weaned on foods based on local staples.

In India, a child's first solid food may be a mixture of steamed rice and beans. An Indian child may also eat mashed or shredded apples and bananas.

In parts of South America and Africa, children are fed a corn porridge, thinned with fresh or canned milk. African children may also eat a porridge made from dried beans that have been cooked and mashed with milk.

In Japan and parts of Africa where rice is a staple food, very young children eat rice that has been cooked with large amounts of water until it is very soft. Japanese mothers may add bits of ground vegetables or fish to the rice.

In many cultures, toddlers progress to soups made with finely chopped or diced ingredients. When this is part of the family's meal, the child's portion is taken out before spices and seasonings are added.

Feeding Techniques, Hunger, and Satiety

Feeding should be a pleasant time for children and caregivers. Put babies in high chairs where their feet are supported, and use bibs to keep their clothes clean. Start with very small amounts. One or two teaspoons of rice cereal once a day is enough to begin with. The cereal is mixed with formula or breast milk. Gradually increase the amount to several tablespoons at each feeding.

Babies who are hungry cry to be fed. When introducing solid food, it often works best to give babies a small bottle-feeding before trying to feed them solids. This gives them a chance to calm down and partially satisfy their hunger. Try to avoid letting them finish the bottle, however, because then they may be too full to have any interest in solid food.

A baby's mouth is sensitive to high temperatures so food should be served warm or at room temperature. If you do not expect the baby to consume the entire jar of food, transfer a portion into a clean dish. Choose a small spoon. When the baby opens his mouth, help him scrape the food off the spoon with his lips. Be patient. Some babies refuse solid food the first few times it is offered. If babies use their tongues to push all the food out of their mouths or continue to resist solid food after a few days, they may not be ready for solids.

Once babies have eaten their fill, or reached satiety, they will close their lips and turn their heads away. Older babies may try to push the spoon away. Do not try to force babies to continue eating, even if the amount eaten seems small. Infants can and should regulate their own appetites. Always discard any food that remains in the jar. Otherwise, harmful bacteria may grow.

Caregivers should follow parents' instructions about the quality and variety of foods to be offered to infants. The amount consumed must be left up to the children. Continually insisting that children "clean their plates" or eat more than they want may lead to poor eating habits and obesity later in life.

Self-Feeding

Learning to self-feed is an exciting activity for babies like Eduardo. It marks the beginning of increased independence. By about eight months, babies enjoy picking up small bits of food to eat with their fingers. Make sure the pieces are of a size and shape that will not be aspirated, or inhaled. Avoid hard foods, such as raw carrots, but gradually increase the texture of foods offered to babies during this period. Many babies of this age are teething

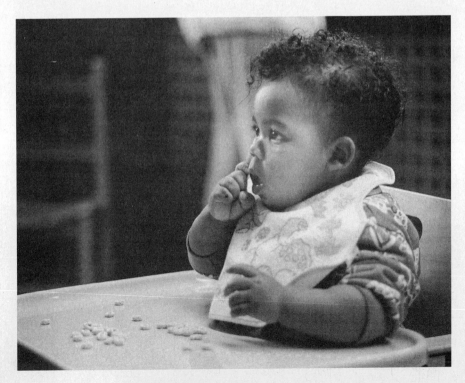

At about eight months old, babies learn to self-feed. They often enjoy picking up small pieces of food with their fingers.

and enjoy hard crackers and strips of dry toast as finger foods. Do not leave babies alone while they are feeding themselves because they can choke on almost any food, especially if they try to eat too much at one time.

Babies are naturally messy eaters. For them, food is something not only to be eaten but also to be touched, smelled, and played with. It is important that babies be allowed to learn about new foods in their own way. Parents can provide extra changes of clothes for messy eaters. For infants who habitually put food in their hair, caregivers can try covering the baby's hair with a shower cap while they are eating.

A plastic tablecloth under the high chair protects the floor and makes cleanup easier. Caregivers will still have to sponge off both the baby and the high chair after each meal. The baby's hands should be washed under running water before and after eating.

When babies want to use a spoon, give them one with a small bowl and a short handle. Offering small portions of food or a few tablespoons of juice in a cup will reduce the amount of cleanup required. Babies who self-feed still need supervision. By the end of the first year, children should be eating three or four meals of solid food a day and receiving substantially less from the breast or bottle.

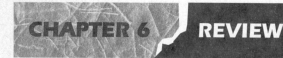

CHAPTER 6   REVIEW

SUMMARY

- Children grow more rapidly during their first year than at any other time during their lives. Although there is a wide range of variation in the rate of infant growth, good nutrition is critical to the healthy development of every infant.

- Changes in mouth patterns, coordination, and the maturation of the digestive and other organ systems determine when a child is ready for new foods.

- Infants who are not introduced to solid foods during the critical period of development may reject foods with increased textures that require chewing.

- Feeding should be a pleasant, emotionally comforting time for infants.

- Some foods are unsuitable or not recommended for babies during the first year. These include cow's milk, eggs, wheat, chocolate, and other foods likely to cause allergies as well as high-nitrate vegetables, which can cause nitrate poisoning, and honey, which may contain botulism spores.

- Aspiration is a leading cause of death in infants. Infants should never be left alone while eating and food should be of a size and shape that are unlikely to block a child's airway.

- Human milk is the best food for very young infants. It contains nutrients and protective factors that are suited to human growth. Breast-feeding mothers should be encouraged to continue breast-feeding even when their children are at child care centers.
- Iron-fortified infant formula is an acceptable substitute for breast milk. Cow's milk and goat's milk are not acceptable substitutes because they may produce allergic reactions and contain too much protein for an infant's immature digestive system to handle.
- Many food decisions are cultural. Caregivers should support parents' food choices as long as babies receive a nutritionally sound diet.
- Infants should not be permitted to fall asleep while drinking from a bottle because milk, formula, or juice remaining in a sleeping infant's mouth can cause tooth decay, or nursing bottle syndrome.
- Solids should be introduced when a child is developmentally ready, rather than at a specific chronological age.
- Caregivers should be sensitive to behavioral cues that babies have had enough to eat and should not urge them to eat more.
- Learning to self-feed is an important developmental step that should be encouraged by caregivers.

ACQUIRING KNOWLEDGE

1. What are two reasons why some full-term newborns have low birth weights?
2. Compare the rate of growth for height and weight during the first six months of life and the second six months.
3. How does the rapid development of the nervous system affect a baby's ability to use nutrients?
4. What is the rooting reflex and how does it help infants obtain food?
5. How does tongue movement differ in breast-fed and bottle-fed infants?
6. When are babies ready to eat soft table food?
7. What is a palmar grasp?
8. What is a pincer grasp?
9. Define object permanence.
10. What are critical periods?
11. Why should food with more texture be introduced during the sixth- to ninth-month period?
12. How do an infant's caloric requirements differ from the beginning to the end of the first year?
13. What is nonorganic failure to thrive?
14. Why is cow's milk unacceptable for infants?
15. What is the relationship between whole milk and the development of the nervous system?
16. Explain why honey should never be given to infants.
17. Why is the use of added salt or sugar not recommended for an infant's diet?

18. Name two common foods that can cause allergic reactions in a baby's first year.
19. What is aspiration? What are some guidelines to follow to lower the risk of aspiration?
20. Why is breast milk the preferred food for infants? What precautions do mothers who choose to breast-feed need to take?
21. What precautions should be taken when preparing baby bottles to protect them from contamination?
22. How can nursing bottle syndrome be prevented?
23. What are signs that a child is ready for semi-solid food?
24. What is the recommended sequence for introducing solid food? Why is the introduction of wheat products delayed?
25. What are signs that a baby has had enough to eat?

THINKING CRITICALLY

1. The practices of a child care center and the practices of parents may differ in some ways regarding the serving of food. How can potential problems be avoided when practices differ? Give examples of areas in which practices may differ.
2. When infants develop the pincer grasp, they are able to pick up small pieces of food and other objects by themselves. Although this is an exciting development, it is also worrisome because infants may pick up and try to swallow inappropriate food and objects. How can caregivers reduce the risk of choking once children develop the pincer grasp?
3. Why is the policy of insisting that children "clean their plates" a controversial one? How can caregivers reduce waste without forcing children to eat everything on their plates?
4. Weaning is no problem for some children but is met with resistance by others. Discuss how caregivers can help with the process of weaning.
5. Allowing one-year-olds to feed themselves may foster independence, but it can also be very messy. Caregivers often feel that it is easier to feed the children than to clean up the mess. What are some suggestions for reducing the amount of cleanup while allowing children to experiment with feeding themselves?

OBSERVATIONS AND APPLICATIONS

1. Observe an infant being fed from a bottle in a child care setting. Was the bottle warmed first? How? Do the caregiver and infant establish eye contact? Does the infant stop every now and then to smile at the caregiver? Does the caregiver talk or sing to the child? Does the caregiver burp the baby? How long does it take to feed the baby?
2. Observe infants between the ages of six months and one year being fed semi-solid and/or solid food in a child care setting. How many children are eating at one time? What are their ages? Do all the children eat the same food? What is served? Do any children try to feed themselves? Do the children themselves require a lot of cleanup when they finish?

3. A parent tells you that she is ready to start feeding her five-month-old semi-solid food. She wants to introduce a cereal, a vegetable, and a fruit each week. In the first week, she plans to introduce rice cereal, pureed peas, and pureed peaches. The next week she plans to introduce cream of wheat cereal, pureed carrots, and pureed bananas. She asks your opinion of her plan. What do you think of her plan? What changes would you suggest?

4. The mother of a three-month-old tells you that she plans to return to work soon. So far she has been breast-feeding her infant son. She plans to wean him before she returns to work. Explain what options she has instead of weaning her son.

FOR FURTHER INFORMATION

Cameron, M. E., & Hofvander, T. (1983). *Manual on feeding infants and young children* (3rd ed.). New York: Oxford University Press.

Dobbing, J. (Ed.). (1988). *Infant feeding*. New York: Springer-Verlag.

Kendrick, A. S., Kaufmann, R., & Messenger, K. P. (Eds.). (1991). *Healthy young children*. Washington, DC: National Association for the Education of Young Children.

Knight, K. (1992). *Baby cookbook: Tasty and nutritious meals for the whole family* (rev. ed.). New York: Morrow.

La Leche League International Staff. (1991). *The womanly art of breastfeeding*. New York: New American Library-Dutton.

Tsang, R. C., & Nichols, B. L. (Eds.). (1988). *Nutrition during infancy*. Philadelphia: Hanley & Belfus.

U.S. Department of Agriculture. (1988). *Feeding infants: A guide for use in the child care food program*. Publication ENS-258. Washington, DC: Author, Food and Nutrition Service.

Young, M. E., & Young, M. W. (1987). *The right start: Guidelines for your baby's nutrition and lifelong health*. New York: Walker & Company.

Nutritional Needs of the Developing Toddler

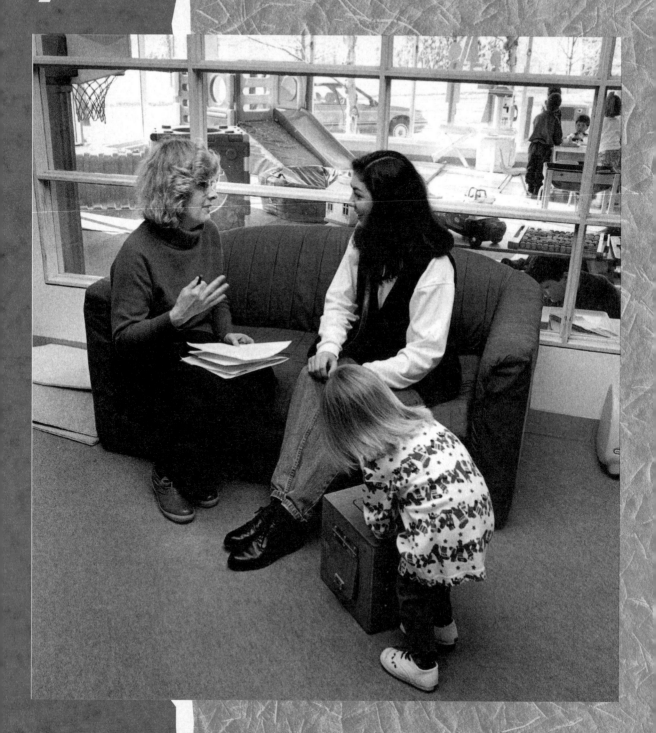

Studying this chapter
will enable you to

- Describe the changing growth rate and growth patterns that characterize the toddler years
- Summarize the motor, language, and psychosocial skills that toddlers develop
- Describe the energy needs of toddlers
- Discuss the changing needs of toddlers for particular nutrients
- Describe specific ways in which caregivers can meet the nutritional requirements of toddlers
- Identify diet-related issues that are of special concern to toddler care providers

CHAPTER TERMS

food jags
molars
rituals

BEFORE Kelly's daughter, Maya, began attending the New Horizons Learning Center, Kelly had a long talk with Maya's caregiver, Sharon, about Maya's eating habits. Kelly told Sharon that her two-year-old did not like to drink milk and that peanut butter and jelly sandwiches were all she would eat for lunch.

Sharon explained the way meals worked at the center. "Here at New Horizons," she told Kelly, "the children eat family style around the little tables you see in the main room. Every child is served a small amount of each food for that meal, including milk. If they want more of a particular food, they just need to ask. The children are encouraged to serve themselves as soon as they are interested and can handle the serving spoon. If they don't eat a particular food, that's fine too. In fact, we don't comment about which foods the children eat, but all of the choices are nutritious."

"What if they don't eat at all?" asked Kelly.

"Well," said Sharon, "that does happen occasionally, but it doesn't seem to last. With a little of each food on their plates at each meal and no pressure to eat, curiosity gets the best of them. Once they notice their peers and the adults eating, they start trying more foods and seem to eat quite well over time. We'll keep you posted on how Maya adjusts."

Kelly wasn't necessarily convinced by what Sharon said. She knew how strong-willed her daughter was. Nevertheless, within a couple of weeks, Maya was eating a wide variety of foods for lunch, and within a month, Maya was gulping down milk as if she had never disliked it. Kelly was impressed, and she soon began incorporating some of the center's ideas during mealtimes at home.

The Physical Growth of Toddlers

During the toddler years, between the ages of one and three, remarkable changes occur in a child's appearance. Toddlers do not simply become larger and larger babies. There are major shifts in their posture, body proportions, body fat, and muscle tone. Generally by the end of toddlerhood, the baby face and much of the baby fat of infancy have given way to the longer, leaner look of early childhood.

The Changing Growth Rate

One of the most striking differences between infancy and the toddler years is a change in the growth rate. Although toddlers continue to grow, their growth is at a steadier, slower pace. On average, toddlers gain between 4 and 6 pounds (1.8 and 2.7 kg) per year and add about 3 inches (7.5 cm) to their height each year.

During this period, the average boy continues to be heavier and taller than the average girl. However, the range of "normal" weights and heights is quite broad. The growth charts in Appendix C show just how wide-ranging a toddler's height and weight may be. It is only when heights and weights lie below the 5th or above the 95th percentile that there may be cause for concern.

Periodic measurement of the toddler's height and weight provides the most reliable means of documenting growth rate and detecting a possible growth problem. To measure a toddler's height, have the child stand with her back against a fixed measuring device. With her body centered, her feet together and touching the measuring tool, and her head erect, use the sliding bar to take the measurement. To measure weight, use a beam balance scale and make sure that the child is wearing similar clothing each time the measurement is taken.

Head circumference is another important measure of a child's growth. After infancy, a child's head increases in size more slowly. Between the ages of one and two, the head circumference grows about 1 inch (2.5 cm). At two years, the average toddler's head measures between 19.5 and 20 inches (49.5 and 51 cm). In subsequent years, a child's head typically grows less than 1 inch per year.

FOCUS ON **Communicating with Parents**

Food Jags

It is 8 A.M. on Monday at the Rock Ridge Child Care Center. Aaron, age three, is being dropped off by his father, who stops to talk to Liz, one of the teachers.

LIZ: (to Aaron) Good morning, Aaron. We're going to have lots of fun today—we're making fruit juice pops for snack time.

AARON'S FATHER: Good luck getting him to eat one!

LIZ: Why do you say that?

AARON'S FATHER: Because right now Aaron won't eat anything except carrots and potatoes. No meat, no fruit, no other vegetables—not even peanut butter!

LIZ: (laughing) Not even peanut butter? That *is* something!

AARON'S FATHER: You can say that again! (becoming more serious) His mother and I are worried that he isn't getting the foods he needs to stay healthy.

LIZ: Well, at least Aaron isn't the only one. A lot of the children go through food jags like this. For two weeks last month, my daughter Holly wouldn't touch green or yellow vegetables. One of Aaron's classmates wanted only bread and candy—and his mother didn't like the candy part! Usually the jag lasts only a short time.

AARON'S FATHER: This has been going on for three days now.

LIZ: Are you sure he isn't eating anything else? Is he drinking milk with his meals?

AARON'S FATHER: He isn't eating any other foods. He does drink milk with his meals though, and sometimes he has juice in between.

LIZ: Well, at least he's getting some protein from the milk and a few extra vitamins from the juice.

AARON'S FATHER: You said that some of the other children have done this. What did their parents do—make them take vitamins?

LIZ: No. The mother of the child who wanted bread and candy let him eat all the bread he wanted, but she kept offering him other foods too. After three days of nothing but bread, he finally ate a peanut butter and jelly sandwich. I didn't push Holly to eat green and yellow vegetables directly. Instead, I made a batch of pumpkin muffins, which Holly loves. And I used a few other "sneaky" tricks such as grating raw zucchini into her spaghetti sauce. Holly ate at least a few green and yellow vegetables without even knowing it!

AARON'S FATHER: I guess we'll have to keep trying and be patient until this thing blows over. I just hope Aaron doesn't end up getting sick.

LIZ: Aaron's classmate and Holly got through their food jags and are running around as fast as ever. Who knows, maybe if Aaron likes orange carrots, he'll eat an orange juice pop!

AARON'S FATHER: Let's hope so!

Would you have handled this situation in a similar way? Would you have done anything differently?

The Changing Growth Pattern

Some parts of a toddler's body grow more quickly than others. As a result, the toddler's body shape undergoes significant changes. During toddlerhood, the legs grow more rapidly than the trunk and the chest grows more rapidly than the abdominal areas, giving the young child a taller, thinner appearance. However, between the ages of one and two, the legs are still short relative to the trunk, and the weight of the trunk causes the legs to keep their bowed shape. As posture improves and the abdominal muscles grow stronger, the toddler begins to look more and more like a young child.

The brain cells, which are all present by the age of one, continue to grow in size. By two years of age, more than 70 percent of the brain's postnatal growth is complete. As head growth slows and other body parts grow more quickly, the relative size of the head decreases.

During the toddler years, children continue to cut teeth and their jaws grow larger. Between 12 and 24 months, toddlers get their first upper and lower molars (four teeth in all). *Molars* are the broad-surfaced teeth at the back of the mouth that are used for grinding food. By the time toddlers are 2½ to 3, most have a complete set of 20 teeth, including a second set of molars. The toddler face becomes less pudgy with the beginnings of a jawline and chin.

Proper nutrition is essential to normal toddler growth. As growth rates slow and activity levels increase, toddler appetites can fluctuate dramatically. And physical changes can prompt changes in what or how caregivers feed toddlers. For example, the eruption of molars can cause toddlers great discomfort. Toddlers find that they cannot comfort themselves by sucking because the action of the jaws against a bottle's nipple makes their gums hurt even more. Caregivers can put a toddler's drinks in a cup rather than a bottle to keep unnecessary pressure off the gums.

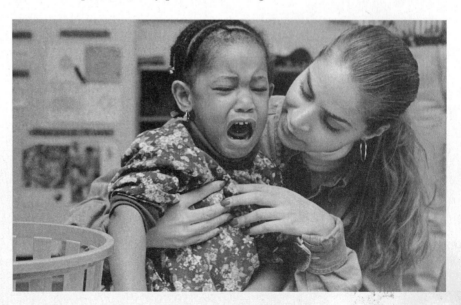

Children often throw temper tantrums and experience mood shifts during their toddler years.

The Development of Toddlers

Between the ages of one and three, young children go through an amazing developmental transformation. Although this transformation follows a predictable pattern, there are individual variations in timing. When toddlerhood begins, young children are still largely dependent on adults to meet their physical, social, and emotional needs. By the time they are three, young children have learned to take care of an increasing number of their own needs in a most independent and determined fashion. Although it is a welcome relief to parents and caregivers that toddlers are learning to do so much for themselves, the toddler years are often quite challenging. Temper tantrums, mood shifts, and negativism can make life in general and mealtimes in particular a test of adults' patience and creativity.

Gross Motor Skills

As toddlers gain control of the large muscles of their bodies, they develop a wide variety of gross motor skills. Walking is the most significant gross motor skill acquired during the toddler years. Most young children can walk alone by 15 months of age. By age three, walking is second nature to toddlers, and they no longer pay much attention to it.

As toddlers acquire greater control of their legs and feet, they begin to run, climb, and jump. By age two, they also learn to climb up and down stairs independently. Within the next six months, many toddlers learn to jump using both feet and to throw a ball using both hands.

Fine Motor Skills

While toddlers are learning to walk, they are also becoming more adept at using their hands. By age one, toddlers will have mastered the pincer grasp. Using the pincer grasp of forefinger and thumb, toddlers are able to pick up objects with some precision. The more they practice picking up objects with their fingers and hands, the smoother their movements become. Finger foods, such as banana chunks, small strips of tender meat, and even individual green peas, provide excellent practice and good nutrition for young toddlers.

As their manipulative skills and their eye-hand coordination improve, toddlers become very eager to do things for themselves, particularly in the area of self-feeding. By 18 months, most toddlers can use a spoon—although not without some spills—and they are drinking from a cup. At two, spoon-feeding is much improved, and most toddlers can handle a glass. By 2½, most toddlers have acquired good rotary chewing skills and are able to eat corn kernels and meat more easily than before (Mott, 1990).

The Development of Speech and Language

While toddlers are acquiring and refining gross and fine motor skills, they are also developing their language skills. Before young toddlers utter their first real words, they have gone through several stages of prelinguistic speech. One of the last stages of prelinguistic speech begins between 12 and

15 months, when the child uses jargoning, a kind of speech gibberish in which the young child strings together sounds so that they sound like sentences.

Between 15 months and 2 years, most toddlers make rapid progress in language development. By 18 months, most toddlers can say ten or more words. By the age of two, toddlers have a vocabulary of about 300 words, and they speak in sentences about 40 percent of the time. The rest of the time they use two- to three-word phrases. According to some experts, a two-year-old who does not talk in simple sentences should be examined to determine the cause (Pillitteri, 1992).

By the age of three, most toddlers talk all the time. Mealtimes and snack times are good opportunities for conversation that contributes to developing language skills, healthful eating habits, and good table manners. Listening to what children say and answering their questions encourage them to talk and express what they are thinking.

Psychosocial Development

Many of the skills that toddlers learn contribute to their growing sense of independence or autonomy. Toddlers need patience and understanding from caregivers as they acquire new skills. Caregivers should encourage toddlers to experiment with skills, such as feeding and dressing themselves, and then should praise their accomplishments. With the support they need to learn at their own pace and in their own time, toddlers develop a healthy independence.

As toddlers work to develop a sense of autonomy, they can experience great internal tension. They are torn between the security their relationships with parents and caregivers have given them and the need to explore independently the world around them and do things for themselves. Toddlers often express this tension in negativism—periods during which they refuse to do anything a parent or caregiver wants them to do. Child development experts agree that this is normal behavior for toddlers. In fact, experts consider this behavior a positive step in children's development because it shows that toddlers see themselves as individuals with their own needs (Pillitteri, 1992).

Toddler negativism can be limited so that parents and caregivers avoid constant confrontations. One method is to stop asking questions for which "no" is an answer and phrase questions so that the toddler can choose between two acceptable alternatives. For example, instead of asking a toddler if he is ready for his snack, you might ask him if he would like juice or milk with his snack.

In toddlers' determination to do things for themselves, they are often frustrated by their limited abilities. These frustrations can produce sudden mood shifts from enthusiastic involvement to temper tantrums or tears. For example, a perfectly happy toddler may sit down at the lunch table to feed herself with a spoon. Two minutes later, she may throw the spoon on the floor and start crying uncontrollably because she couldn't keep the spoon

FOCUS ON *Promoting Healthful Habits*

Avoiding the Clean Plate Trap

Lunch had been special today. Four-year-old Diane had brought in her mother's homemade spaghetti sauce. Alicia, the teacher, had helped the group prepare the spaghetti and sauce for lunch, along with a green salad and some toasted Italian bread.

As Alicia was finishing her meal, she heard Diane announce, "Joey has to clean his plate." Alicia walked over to the table where Diane and Joey and two other children sat. She noticed that Joey had eaten about half of the spaghetti on his plate, but that he was obviously done.

"Look," Diane said as she pointed to Joey's plate. "He didn't finish. He has to finish everything on his plate."

Alicia turned to Joey and asked if he had had enough to eat. He nodded. "Did you like the spaghetti and tomato sauce?" she asked.

"Yeah, I liked it," he said, "but I can't eat any more. I'm full."

Diane clearly expected Alicia to insist. Instead, Alicia explained to Diane that Joey was full and didn't have to clean his plate if he didn't want to.

"But my mother says I have to eat everything on my plate before I can leave the table," countered Diane. "Why doesn't Joey have to?"

This was tricky. How could Alicia explain the center's policy without contradicting Diane's mother? "I watch to make sure all of the children eat enough of the right food here at the center, and Joey did just fine," Alicia explained. "Sometimes the rules we have here are different from the ones you have at home."

Alicia made a mental note to talk to Diane's mother about the appetites of preschoolers. Alicia knew that young children eat as much as they want. Forcing them to 'clean their plates' can lead them to associate eating with a sense of being too full. That could lead to obesity. Alicia would be tactful with Diane's mother to try to convince her to trust her young daughter's appetite.

How well do you think Alicia dealt with Diane? With Joey? What do you think is the best way to approach Diane's mother? What might you have done differently?

---

level all the way to her mouth. Some adult comforting and encouragement will usually restore her to her former happy state.

In the midst of so many new experiences, toddlers often need something familiar and reassuring to cling to. *Rituals*—rigidly specific circumstances or requirements—become an important component of toddler behavior. At mealtime, for instance, a toddler may refuse to eat a sandwich until the crusts have been removed or the sandwich has been cut in half or in quarters. Some toddlers will not eat if the various foods on a plate are touching. Others demand that their dishes be placed on the table in a certain arrangement or that only certain dishes be used. Child development experts do not regard rituals such as these as a problem. Most ritualistic routines are given up as the child approaches three years of age. Children with an excessive number of rituals may be sending out a signal to adults that they need more structure or routine in their lives.

FOCUS ON / **Cultural Diversity**

First Utensils

Infants drink from the breast or the bottle until they are weaned. Then they are fed by an adult until they are old enough to feed themselves with hands or utensils—spoons, forks, knives, or chopsticks. A child who has learned to feed herself has made a developmental leap. Self-feeding brings both physical and emotional satisfaction to most toddlers.

Very young children often find that the most convenient eating utensils are at the end of their arms—their hands. African and Indian children are used to being fed from the hands of their mothers. These children are encouraged to use their own hands to feed themselves when they are ready. A spoon sometimes supplements hand-feeding in these cultures.

European and American children also start with a spoon, often one with a wide bowl and a short, easy-to-grasp handle. Some toddlers are given special child-sized versions of the full set of adult utensils. They are smaller and wider than their adult counterparts. The handle is thicker and easier to grip. In the case of forks and knives, these utensils are also blunter for safety reasons. In Asian cultures where chopsticks are important utensils, children use shorter "baby chopsticks" at mealtimes.

In almost every culture, children who are being taught to scoop or spear foods with the help of utensils may still rely on their fingers. They may do this when they are very focused on eating—or merely when their parents are not watching. It takes time and plenty of practice for children to adjust to adult eating behaviors.

The emphasis during the toddler years is on individual development. Toddlers are just beginning to develop social skills. They often engage in parallel play by imitating one another and playing side by side.

The Nutritional Requirements of Toddlers

When infants become toddlers, there are changes in growth rates and patterns and rapid increases in mobility as motor skills develop. These changes place new demands on a child's body. A toddler's body has specific needs for energy, basic building materials, and other nutrients.

The Energy Needs of Toddlers

Although toddlers are not growing as rapidly as infants, toddlers are still growing and their activity level is much greater than before. This translates into energy needs that are greater than those of a 6– to 12–month-old infant (see Table 3.1 in Chapter 3). Since there are broad differences in activity levels among children, the amount of energy needed will vary from one child to the next.

Nutritionists use several methods to determine the number of calories a toddler needs. One method is an age-related measure. The nutritionist starts with a base of 1,000 calories and adds 100 calories for each year of age. Using this method, a two-year-old would need 1,200 calories per day whereas a three-year-old would need 1,300.

Other approaches require the use of Recommended Dietary Allowances (RDAs) (National Research Council, 1989). The first of these methods is based on body weight. For children between one and three years of age, the RDA is approximately 46 calories per pound (102 calories per kg) of body weight. Thus, a toddler weighing 30 pounds (13.6 kg) would need about 1,380 calories per day. The other RDA method is based on height. For children between one and three, the RDA translates to about 37 calories per inch of height (about 15 calories per cm). A toddler who is 35 inches (88.9 cm) tall would need about 1,300 calories per day. With both the weight method and the height method, individual growth patterns are taken into account so that toddlers' diets can be altered to meet their caloric needs as they grow.

The Nutrient Needs of Toddlers

Toddlers have special nutrient needs that are different from the nutrient needs of babies, older children, and adults. Getting the recommended amounts of protein, minerals, and vitamins is of particular importance.

Although toddlers require less protein relative to their size than infants require, their protein needs exceed those of older age groups. Toddlers need protein for continuing tissue growth (National Research Council, 1989). The RDA for protein is about 0.54 grams per pound (1.2 grams per kg) of body weight. A 30-pound (13.6 kg) child would need about 16 grams of protein, which is the amount of protein found in 1 pint of milk, about 2 ounces of red meat or poultry, or about 1 cup of cooked dry beans.

Toddlers need more of most minerals—including calcium, phosphorus, magnesium, zinc, iodine, and selenium—than infants do (see Appendix A). If a toddler has dietary restrictions, some of his mineral needs may be hard to supply.

Calcium and phosphorus are needed in large amounts because of their structural role in the development of bones and teeth. Toddlers should have 800 milligrams each of calcium and phosphorus per day. Milk, cheese, and yogurt are good sources of both minerals. A cup (8 ounces) of milk or yogurt contains about 300 milligrams of calcium and about 240 milligrams of phosphorus. Thus, 3 cups of milk per day will meet the calcium requirement and about 90 percent of the RDA for phosphorus. Some children, however, cannot tolerate dairy products. It is a challenge to meet the RDAs for these minerals solely with other foods. Dark-green leafy vegetables are good sources of calcium with some phosphorus; cooked dry beans provide plenty of phosphorus and some calcium (see Appendix B). Tortillas and tofu that are processed with calcium contain significant amounts and some fruit juices and other foods are now fortified with calcium.

Another mineral that is vital to toddler growth is iron. Toddlers should have 10 milligrams of iron in their daily diets—the same amount that infants need. Once toddlers stop eating iron-fortified infant cereal and formula, it is important that other iron-rich foods be provided on a regular basis to meet daily needs. Virtually all breakfast cereals, sliced breads, and rolls are enriched with iron, so they are a good place to start. The body absorbs iron from animal and plant sources in different ways. More iron is absorbed from meat than from plant sources. When vegetables are eaten with meat, more of the iron in the vegetables is absorbed. Daily consumption of foods rich in vitamin C also enhances the absorption of iron.

Toddlers need more of most vitamins than infants need, but a balanced diet will most likely supply these. For example, the recommended allowance of vitamin C is 40 milligrams per day. This allowance can be met easily with ½ cup of orange juice or ½ cup of whole strawberries or cubed cantaloupe.

Nutritionists and health care professionals are not in total agreement over the need for vitamin or mineral supplements for toddlers. Most will agree that supplements are needed if a child is found to have a vitamin or mineral deficiency. Most also insist that a vitamin or mineral supplement is not an acceptable way to make up for poor eating habits. Vitamin and mineral supplements should be chosen carefully with the assistance of a health care professional because they can contain potentially harmful quantities of certain vitamins and minerals. Excessive amounts of vitamins such as A, D, E, and K, as well as calcium, iron, potassium, and other minerals, can be toxic.

Toddlers also need carbohydrates and fats in their diets. Carbohydrates are the main source of energy and should account for more than half of the calories provided by the toddler's diet. Most of the carbohydrates in a toddler's diet should be complex carbohydrates or starches from pasta, cereals, breads, rice, beans, and certain vegetables. Complex carbohydrates break down more slowly in the body than do sugars, providing energy over a longer period of time. They are generally a good source of other essential vitamins and minerals as well. If a toddler does not get sufficient carbohydrates, his body will begin to burn proteins for energy. Those proteins will no longer be available to assist in growth.

Fats also provide energy and serve many important functions in the body as discussed in Chapter 3. Low-fat milk and skim milk are not recommended for toddlers under the age of two because they do not contain enough fat for normal growth of the nervous system. For toddlers over the age of two, however, fats should constitute no more than 30 percent of total caloric intake.

Meeting the Nutritional Requirements of Toddlers

It takes careful planning, patience, and creativity to meet the nutritional requirements of toddlers. Although their need for many nutrients is on the increase, their appetite may be dwindling. Many toddlers get so busy exploring their world that mealtime becomes an unwelcome interruption of their activities. Putting together meals and snacks, creating a positive eating environment, and introducing new foods are challenging opportunities for parents and caregivers to provide toddlers with sound nutrition and a firm

TABLE 7.1 **Meal Pattern for Toddlers**	
Breakfast	**Children** **1 and 2 years**
Milk, fluid	½ cup
Juice or **fruit** or **vegetable**	¼ cup
Bread and/or **cereal,** enriched or whole grain	
Bread or	½ slice
Cereal: Cold dry or	¼ cup[1]
Hot cooked	¼ cup
Midmorning or midafternoon snack (supplement)	
(Select 2 of these 4 components)	
Milk, fluid	½ cup
Meat or **meat alternate**[2]	½ ounce
Juice or **fruit** or **vegetable**	½ cup
Bread and/or **cereal,** enriched or whole grain	
Bread or	½ slice
Cereal: Cold dry or	¼ cup[1]
Hot cooked	¼ cup
Lunch or supper	
Milk, fluid	½ cup
Meat or **meat alternate**	
Meat, poultry, or fish, cooked (lean meat without bone)	1 ounce
Cheese	1 ounce
Egg	1
Cooked dry beans and peas	¼ cup
Peanut butter or other nut or seed butters	2 tablespoons
Vegetable and/or **fruit** (two or more)	¼ cup
Bread or **bread alternate,** enriched or whole grain	½ slice

[1] ¼ cup (volume) or ⅓ ounce (weight), whichever is less.
[2] Yogurt may be used as a meat/meat alternate in the snack only. You may serve 2 ounces (weight) or ¼ cup (volume) of plain, or sweetened and flavored yogurt to fulfill the equivalent of ½ ounce of the meat/meat alternate component.
Adapted from U. S. Department of Agriculture. (1989). *A planning guide for food service in child care centers.*

foundation for healthful eating habits. The meal pattern shown in Table 7.1 can help keep a toddler's nutrition on track.

The Importance of Breakfast

Many nutritionists regard breakfast as the day's most important meal, especially for young children. Children are at their hungriest in the morning and are most likely to eat well if given appropriate choices and adequate time to eat. A good breakfast should provide the toddler with at least one-fifth of her energy requirements for the day.

Children who arrive at a child care center very early in the morning may not have had adequate time to eat a nutritious breakfast. Having breakfast foods available for these children is important. Many child care centers ask parents during the enrollment procedure whether they want their children to be given breakfast at the center. These centers usually give parents a description of the type of breakfast provided.

Meals and Snacks

Meals and snacks provided by child care centers for toddlers are generally designed around the meal pattern developed by the U. S. Department of Agriculture (USDA) Child Care Food Program (CCFP). As you can see in Table 7.1, the meal pattern gives serving sizes for general categories of food for each meal or snack. As toddlers approach the age of three, they may need larger serving sizes to support their continuing growth (see Table 8.1).

In addition to breakfast, most nutritionists agree that toddlers need two more meals and two to three snacks per day. Most toddlers cannot eat enough at mealtimes to provide them with their daily nutrient and caloric needs. And most toddlers are hungry within three hours of having a meal. Snacks are an important part of a well-balanced toddler diet. Foods eaten at snack time should provide nutrients that may be missing from other meals.

Meals for toddlers should contain foods from all five food groups. These are bread, cereal, rice, and pasta; fruits; vegetables; meat, poultry, fish, dry beans, eggs, and nuts; and milk, yogurt, and cheese. Snacks should contain foods from two of these groups. See Table 7.2 for a week of sample menus.

Bread, Cereal, Rice, and Pasta Group.   Enriched or whole grain breads and cereals provide toddlers with complex carbohydrates, B vitamins, minerals, and some protein. Whole grain breads and cereals are a better source of vitamins, minerals, and fiber than refined forms. Toddlers should have five or more servings per day of breads, cereals, or bread alternates. Bread alternates include taco shells, pancakes, chow mein noodles, crackers, grits, pasta, and rice.

Fruit Group.   Fruits are good sources of fiber, carbohydrates, vitamins, and minerals. Toddlers should have three or more servings of fruits each day. Variety is important since each fruit or vegetable supplies somewhat different nutrients. Consider fresh fruits, fruit juice, canned fruits in juice, and dried fruits when planning menus. Child care center menus should include fruits that are good sources of vitamin A, vitamin C, and iron (see Table 7.2). If fruits are served as part of a snack, individual portions should be larger than when they are served as part of a meal (see Table 7.1). One way to estimate toddler servings is 1 tablespoon for each year of age for cooked vegetables or cooked fruit. Thus, for example, a two-year-old should have 2 tablespoons of cooked apricots. If the fruit is raw, then toddlers

TABLE 7.2
Sample Menus for Toddlers

Day	Breakfast	A.M. Snack	Lunch or Supper	P.M. Snack
1	Orange juice ¼ cup Biscuit 1 biscuit Milk ½ cup Baked scrambled egg 2 tbsp.	Milk ½ cup Cinnamon toast ½ slice	Meat loaf 1 oz. meat Green beans ⅛ cup Pineapple cubes ⅛ cup Bread ½ slice Milk ½ cup	Mixed fruit juice ½ cup Celery sticks with peanut butter 1 tbsp.
2	Sliced banana ¼ cup Enriched cornflakes ¼ cup Milk ½ cup	Tomato juice ½ cup Cheese stick ½ oz.	Baked chicken 1 oz. meat Mashed potatoes ⅛ cup Peas ⅛ cup Carrot stick 1 stick Roll 1 small Milk ½ cup	Milk ½ cup Oatmeal cookie 1 cookie
3	Apricot halves ¼ cup Blueberry muffin ½ muffin Milk ½ cup	Milk ½ cup Enriched dry cereal ¼ cup	Chicken vegetable soup ½ cup Peanut butter and jelly sandwich ¼ sandwich Sliced peaches ¼ cup Milk ½ cup	Apple juice ½ cup Soft pretzel 1 pretzel
4	Fruit cup ¼ cup Hard-boiled egg ½ egg Toast ½ slice Milk ½ cup	Orange juice ½ cup Toasted raisin bread ½ slice	Spaghetti and meat sauce ½ cup Peas ⅛ cup Green salad ¼ cup French bread ½ slice Milk ½ cup	Milk ½ cup Peanut butter cookie 1 cookie Turnip stick 1 stick

(continued)

TABLE 7.2
Sample Menus for Toddlers *(continued)*

Day	Breakfast	A.M. Snack	Lunch or Supper	P.M. Snack
5	Grapefruit sections ¼ cup Rolled oats ¼ cup Milk ½ cup	Grape juice ½ cup Enriched soda crackers 2 crackers Peanut butter 1 tbsp.	Fish sticks 3 sticks (1 oz. fish) Spinach ⅛ cup Fresh pear half ⅛ cup Corn bread 1 square Milk ½ cup	Cottage cheese dip with zucchini sticks ¼ cup Melba toast 3 slices

Adapted from U. S. Department of Agriculture. (1989). *A planning guide for food service in child care centers.*

should receive twice this amount. However toddler portions are determined, they should be considered minimums.

Vegetable Group.   Like fruits, vegetables are good sources of fiber, carbohydrates, vitamins, and minerals. Each day, toddlers should have three or more servings of vegetables. A variety of vegetables is most likely to supply the toddler's needs for various nutrients. Dark-green leafy vegetables such as spinach are rich in iron, calcium, vitamin A, and vitamin C. Other dark green, yellow, and orange vegetables are especially good sources of vitamin A. Tomatoes, potatoes, broccoli, and cabbage are just a few of the vegetables rich in vitamin C. Toddler portions for the vegetables should be the same as for fruits. The alternate approach of 1 tablespoon for each year of age for cooked vegetables (2 tablespoons for raw) may also provide a useful estimate for minimum portion sizes.

Meat, Poultry, Fish, Dry Beans, Eggs, and Nuts Group.   Meat, poultry, fish, and meat alternates, such as eggs, beans, peas, and nut butters (peanut, almond, or cashew butter, for example), are good sources of protein, vitamins, iron, and other minerals. Meats, beans, and eggs should be cooked until tender and then offered to the child in pieces that are small enough to be picked up with the fingers or a spoon. Two or three servings of meat and meat alternates should be offered to the toddler daily. Nutritionists recommend 2 ounces of cooked meat each day along with one serving of a meat alternate. Examples of toddler servings might be ¼ cup of cooked dry beans or peas and 2 tablespoons of peanut butter. If a toddler is a vegetarian, you can substitute ¼ cup of cooked beans or peas for each ounce of meat called for in the daily diet.

Milk, Yogurt, and Cheese Group.   This group supplies calcium, phosphorus, riboflavin (vitamin B$_2$), protein, vitamin A, and other nutrients. Toddlers should consume 3 cups of milk or equivalent servings of yogurt or cheese each day. Food programs sponsored by the federal government require child care providers to serve milk at all meals. As mentioned above, only whole milk should be served to children under the age of two. Equivalent servings of yogurt and cheese vary according to which nutrients are of concern (see Appendix B). For example, 1 ounce of cheddar cheese, ⅔ cup of yogurt, or ¼ cup of ricotta cheese supplies as much protein as 1 cup of milk. To obtain amounts of calcium and phosphorus supplied by 1 cup of milk, however, requires 1½ ounces of cheddar cheese, ¾ cup of yogurt, or ½ cup of ricotta cheese. Chapter 9 discusses children with special nutritional needs.

Feeding at the Child Care Center

"She used to eat everything and now she's such a picky eater!" "I can't get him to sit down for a minute to eat his meals!" "Why did I ever give her peanut butter and jelly? Now it's the only thing she'll eat!" Feeding toddlers can be a challenging task. There are ways, however, to help toddlers make nutritious food choices.

Adjusting to the Toddler's Changing Needs.   Caregivers of toddlers must be prepared for a wide range of food-related patterns of behavior. Caregivers need to know when to reassure parents that a behavior is common and will pass in time. Caregivers must also be able to recognize when a

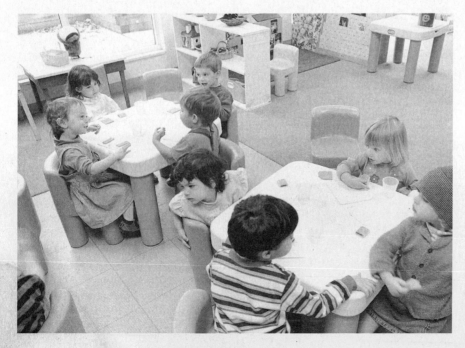

Some child care centers feed toddlers on demand, whereas others, such as this one, have specific schedules for meals and snacks.

child's eating pattern may be interfering with normal growth. In such a case, caregivers must share their concerns with the child's parents so that the parents can arrange for evaluation of their child by a health care professional.

Some child care centers feed toddlers on demand. Other centers have specific schedules for meals and snacks. Either approach can meet toddlers' nutritional needs. When a toddler who is accustomed to demand feeding enters a child care center that has specific snack and meal schedules, the situation may require extra patience and creativity on the caregiver's part. It may take considerable time for the child's appetite to adjust to the schedule. To ease the transition, some centers set aside a special table on which healthful snacks are made available in the morning or afternoon, allowing young children to help themselves when they are ready to eat.

Young children may have trouble settling down if they are brought in from active play and expected to sit down to a meal. They need some transition time and do well if quiet activities are scheduled before and after meals. This kind of break between active play and mealtime can improve appetites and make meals more pleasant.

Children also eat better when they are not too tired and have not had to wait too long since their last meal or snack. Tired, overly hungry toddlers often refuse the food that is offered. Children who are fed too frequently also lose their appetites. Toddlers should be fed five to six times a day at intervals of at least 2 to 2½ hours. Caregivers should set aside at least 30 minutes for each meal.

What kinds of foods appeal to toddlers? Most young children like foods that are seasoned simply and attractive to the eye. Casseroles and mixed foods are not always popular. Toddler meals should include cooked and raw foods that vary in size, shape, color, texture, and flavor. For instance, a meal of slender carrot sticks with mashed potatoes and small, tender cubes of cooked beef provides a variety of shapes, colors, textures, and flavors. The inclusion of a crunchy food, a soft food, and a chewy food helps toddlers improve their chewing skills. The more foods toddlers learn to eat, the more likely it is that they will get the nutrients they need now and later in life.

Because toddlers are just learning how to handle eating utensils, they should not be given too many foods that are hard to pick up with a spoon or fork. A mixture of finger foods and utensil foods will make meals less frustrating. To promote self-feeding and to make sure foods are easy to chew, meats and cheeses should be cut into cubes or strips, vegetables should be cut into sticks, and fruits should be cut into chunks or slices.

Toddlers' mouths are very sensitive to high and low temperatures. They prefer their food to be lukewarm. If food is too hot or too cold, toddlers may refuse to eat or may play with the food until it reaches the right temperature. When cooking food for toddlers, cook it properly, then allow it to cool off to an acceptable temperature before serving.

Creating a Positive Eating Environment.   The ideal environment for toddler meals is one that is developmentally appropriate. When children are eating together, toddler chairs and tables should be small and low. Toddlers should be able to touch their feet to the floor when sitting in their chairs.

Sitting family style around a table encourages toddlers to experiment with foods as they watch their caregivers and peers eat the foods being served. Maya, the toddler at the beginning of this chapter, became more adventurous with food after watching her playmates eat as they sat around the table. Family style eating also promotes independence. Toddlers can begin to help out with the food service by bringing things to the table and by picking up after the meal is finished. Since toddlers are prone to spills, caregivers can spread papers or plastic on the floor underneath the chairs to make cleanup easier.

Flatware should be toddler-sized and nonbreakable. Forks should have short, blunt tines with short, thick handles. Spoons should have similar handles and bowls that are shallow. Toddlers can be encouraged to use blunt, toddler-sized knives for spreading. Bowls and plates should have curved or upturned edges to make it easier for toddlers to get food onto their spoons. Cups should be small (4 to 6 ounces) and have broad bases for ease of handling and fewer spills.

A positive environment includes the atmosphere of the room and the attitude of caregivers at mealtimes. As toddlers prepare to sit down to a meal, the mood should be calm, pleasant, and encouraging. However, caregivers should be neutral about the foods once they have been served to the toddler. It is best not to comment on whether a toddler accepts or rejects a given

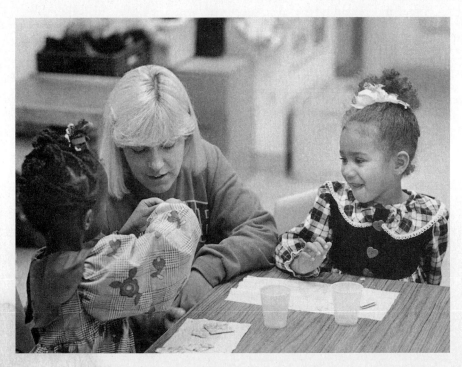

Caregivers should establish a calm, relaxed, and pleasant eating environment for the children.

Presenting new foods to toddlers can be a challenge, but frequently exposing them to a new item will encourage the toddlers to accept it.

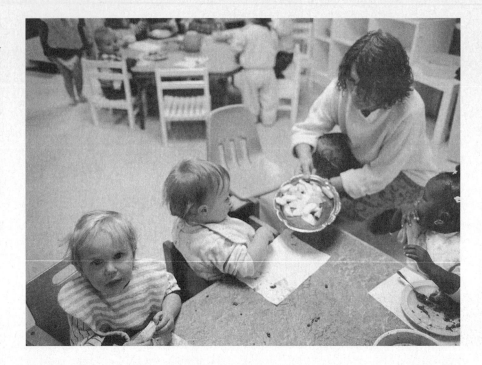

food. Maya's caregiver, Sharon, employed this technique, leaving the decision to Maya over what and how much to eat.

Toddlers should be given small portions so they can finish their meals and feel a sense of accomplishment. Small portions also give them the opportunity to assert their independence by asking for more. Cups should be partially filled for the same reason.

In child care centers that lack kitchen facilities, children must bring their lunches from home. Caregivers may notice that some toddlers come with lunches that are not nutritious or well balanced. In these cases, caregivers can send children home with information about the five food groups and with sample lunch menus that can be prepared easily at home. Child care centers should always keep food on hand to supplement children's meals as needed.

When children bring their own lunches to child care centers, they frequently feel that other children's food looks more appealing. In this situation, caregivers should encourage children to feel good about the food they have brought to eat. Caregivers might, for example, say a child's orange slices smell good or that her carrot sticks are very good for her.

Some children need to be on carefully controlled diets because of a medical condition. A child with phenylketonuria (PKU), for example, must avoid most foods that contain protein and the artificial sweetener aspartame. In situations such as these, it is best for the family to provide all the foods for the child's snacks and meals. The child's situation should be discussed with the entire group in a simple, direct manner so that the other children understand why it is important for the child with the medical condition to be on a special diet and why they should not share their food with this child.

Introducing New Foods. Although research shows that toddlers dislike unfamiliar foods (Burt & Hertzler, 1978), new foods can be presented in such a way that toddlers will eventually accept most of them. The key to making unfamiliar foods familiar is to give the child frequent exposure to them.

Child development experts and nutritionists suggest that no more than one new food be introduced each week. Caregivers should first serve the new food when the child is hungriest. If this is not possible, it should be served along with other, familiar foods. It is important to talk about the new food first. Comments might include its color, shape, and texture as well as where it comes from. The child should see caregivers enjoying the food. After the food has been presented or offered to the child, the caregiver's response should be a neutral one—whether the child chooses to try it or not. The new food should be served again eight to ten times during the next few weeks. This kind of frequency makes the food more familiar. Nutritionists advise that if more than a few days go by between tastings, it takes much longer for children to accept a food.

With new foods, it is also important to watch for signs of allergic reaction or intolerance to the food. Symptoms such as diarrhea, vomiting, abdominal pain, rash, irritability, and breathing problems are the most common signs of an allergic reaction. In some cases, the reaction may be immediate; in others, it may be delayed. The reaction can range from mild to severe. An allergic reaction to food should be treated as any other medical emergency. Parents should be consulted when their children have a reaction to a food, and caregivers should work with them to find acceptable substitutes. Some foods can be modified so that a child can tolerate them. For example, specially altered milks are available for people who have an intolerance to lactose, the sugar in milk.

Special Nutritional Concerns

The eating habits, physical development, and nutritional needs of children between the ages of one and three combine to pose special concerns for caregivers. Because toddlers are changing and learning so quickly, it is especially important that these concerns be carefully handled. Caregivers must protect the nutritional health of the toddlers under their care while promoting food attitudes and habits that will keep them healthy as they grow.

Aspiration or Choking Dangers

Children between the ages of one and four are more likely to choke on their food than any other age group. Their airways are still small and their feeding skills just developing. The foods most responsible for choking problems

---

WHOLESOME SNACKS

Frozen Bananas

Ingredients:

10 bananas
¾ cup peanut butter
10 graham crackers

Directions:

1. Peel bananas and cut in half lengthwise with a plastic knife.
2. Spread each half with a tablespoon of peanut butter and roll in graham cracker crumbs. (Children can crush graham crackers in a plastic bag using a child-sized rolling pin.)
3. Wrap in plastic wrap and freeze.

Yield: 20 servings

Each serving contains:

Calories: 177
Protein: 6 g
Fat: 9 g
Carbohydrates: 21 g

Source: University of Illinois at Urbana-Champaign Child Development Lab.

are firm, smooth, or slippery foods that can slide down the throat easily, such as circular pieces of hot dogs, hard candy, peanuts, and whole grapes. Other culprits include foods that are difficult to chew and easy to swallow whole, such as popcorn, snack chips, nuts and seeds, and small chunks of raw vegetables. Sticky or tough foods, such as peanut butter, tough meat, and raisins or other dried fruit, can clog the back of the throat or get stuck in the airway.

Most aspiration dangers from food can be avoided. Caregivers can cut hot dogs in short strips, grapes in quarters, and raw vegetables in slender sticks. Peanut butter can be spread thinly on bread or crackers. Although caregivers should avoid serving toddlers whole nuts or a handful of raisins, finely chopped nuts or a few raisins may be a fine addition to a 2½-year-old's yogurt or hot cereal. Foods such as hard candy, popcorn, snack chips, and tough meat should not be served to toddlers.

Caregivers need to help toddlers learn safe eating behaviors. Make sure all food is cut into bite-sized pieces and remind children to eat slowly and chew carefully. Teach children not to talk while their mouths are full and have them stay seated while they are eating. Choking is always a possibility, however, so be sure that all caregivers know how to handle a choking emergency. (See Chapter 13 for what to do if a child begins to choke.)

Milk Drinking and Dietary Balance

Drinking too much milk (or formula) is as bad for toddlers as drinking too little. Too much milk can keep toddlers' stomachs full, diminish their appetites, and lead to nutritional deficiencies as they choose milk over other foods. Toddlers who are still drinking from a bottle may be especially likely to have this problem.

Some toddlers, however, do not drink enough milk to supply the calcium, phosphorus, or other nutrients that their bodies need. For toddlers such as these, nutritionists recommend that meals begin with milk. As mentioned earlier, centers whose food programs are sponsored by the federal government are required to serve milk with meals. Milk should also be offered for snacks. If a toddler still is not getting enough milk, sufficient quantities of dairy products such as yogurt and cheeses should be offered.

Food Jags

Toddlers frequently go through *food jags*—periods of days or weeks when they are obsessive about certain foods. Maya, for example, would eat nothing but peanut butter and jelly for lunch before she came to the New Horizons Learning Center. During a food jag, a toddler may insist on eating the same food, the same color food, or foods of a particular shape at every meal for days at a time. Although toddlers are not getting a balanced diet when they are on food jags, the jags are usually brief. It is important to put other nutritious foods the toddler likes on her plate, even if she does not eat them. The jag will probably pass sooner if adults do not make an issue of it.

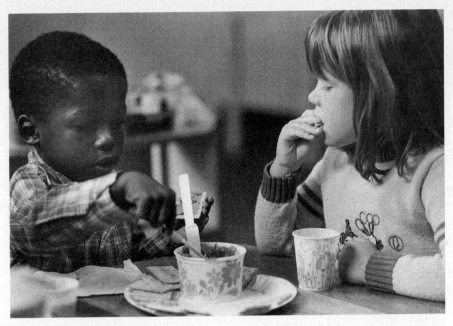

Many toddlers go through food jags. For example, a child may insist on eating nothing but peanut butter crackers for days on end.

In their efforts to get toddlers off a food jag or to modify other eating behaviors, adults are often tempted to use food as a reward. It is not uncommon to hear an adult say to a toddler, "If you eat something besides peanut butter for dinner, I will let you have dessert," or "If you eat all of your vegetables, you can have some candy." This kind of reinforcement transforms desserts and sweets into very desirable foods in the mind of the child. It is better to reward good eating behavior with words of praise or a hug. Caregivers should encourage children to see eating a variety of foods as a way to satisfy hunger and keep the body healthy.

Some adults use other kinds of rewards for good eating behavior. These are usually as ineffective as food rewards. They may increase the likelihood that a toddler will try a new food or eat all her vegetables, but they do not increase the toddler's acceptance of the food over time.

Excessive Sugar, Salt, and Fats

Nutritionists and health care professionals who work with young children have expressed increasing concern about excessive sugar, salt, and fats in the toddler diet. Foods that contain large amounts of added sugar, salt, and fats often provide calories but few essential nutrients. They can fill toddlers' stomachs without providing the vitamins, minerals, and protein children need. Naturally occurring sugars such as those found in milk and fruits provide a good energy source plus other nutrients a toddler's body requires for health and growth. A variety of fresh foods provides all the salt a toddler's body needs.

Whereas some dietary fat is necessary to maintain the proper balance of the body's fatty acids, too much fat in the diet can lead to heart disease.

Infants and toddlers require more dietary fat than older children because fatty acids are a major structural component in their rapidly growing brains and nervous systems. For this reason, whole milk should be served to toddlers until they reach two years of age. After two years, low-fat milk or skim milk may be served. For healthy people over the age of two, nutritionists suggest limiting foods that are high in fat, such as hot dogs, luncheon meats, butter, lard, and processed foods made with fats.

Much of the excess of sugar, salt, and fats in toddler diets comes from commercial snack foods and fast-food meals. Today, perhaps more than ever, caregivers need to provide toddlers with nutritious choices for snacks and meals. Caregivers can promote sound toddler nutrition and give toddlers a firm foundation for healthful eating as they continue to grow. Sharing nutritious food ideas with parents can help develop good eating practices at home as well.

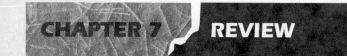

CHAPTER 7   REVIEW

SUMMARY

- Toddlers grow at a slower, steadier pace than infants. The best way to monitor toddlers' growth and detect possible growth problems is to have them measured periodically, usually by a health care professional.

- Physically, toddlers become longer and leaner in appearance. The brain cells continue to grow. Teeth continue to erupt until toddlers have a complete set, usually by the age of 2½ to 3.

- During the toddler years, young children master several gross motor skills including walking, climbing, running, and jumping.

- As the fine motor skills of toddlers develop, they become capable of picking up objects with some precision and using eating utensils. As their rotary chewing skills improve, the list of foods they can eat properly and safely expands.

- During the toddler years, young children learn how to speak. From a few real words toward the beginning of this period, the toddler vocabulary and phrase length increase steadily.

- The skills that toddlers learn contribute to their growing independence. Toddlers often feel torn between their need for security and their desire for independence.

- Toddlers' energy needs are greater than those of infants. There are several methods for determining the number of calories a toddler needs including an age-related measure, a weight-based measure, and a height-based measure.

- Although all nutrients are important to toddlers, it is particularly important that they get the recommended amounts of protein, minerals, and vitamins. Vitamin or mineral supplements should not be taken without the advice of a health care professional.

- Toddlers need three meals and two to three snacks each day. Meals should contain foods from all five groups in the recommended serving sizes.

- To promote healthful appetites, toddlers should have an opportunity to settle down before eating, intervals of at least two hours should separate meals and snacks, and at least 30 minutes should be set aside for eating each meal.

- Toddler meals should include cooked and raw foods in a variety of colors, textures, shapes, and flavors.

- A developmentally appropriate eating environment for toddlers contains toddler-sized tables, chairs, and eating utensils. A positive environment leads to greater food acceptance.

- In centers where children bring their own lunches, caregivers may need to send home information about the five food groups and sample lunch menus that can be prepared easily at home.

- Toddlers are more likely to accept new foods if they are given frequent exposure to them. After eating a new food, toddlers should be observed for possible allergic reactions or intolerances to the food.

- Caregivers should be familiar with the forms and types of food that pose choking hazards to toddlers so those foods can be avoided. Caregivers should also know how to handle a choking emergency.

- Excessive milk drinking can be as bad for toddlers as drinking too little milk because it may reduce their appetites for other important foods.

- Toddlers frequently go on food jags. These are usually brief and tend to pass more quickly if adults do not make an issue of them. Using food as a reward to change an eating pattern is not a wise nutritional practice.

- A toddler's intake of sugar, salt, and fats should be limited. However, whole milk should be served to toddlers until they reach two years of age.

- Toddlers need nutritious choices for snacks and meals. Caregivers can promote sound toddler nutrition and healthful eating habits that will help toddlers continue to grow and develop.

ACQUIRING KNOWLEDGE

1. Compare the growth rate of toddlers with that of infants.
2. List three differences in growth patterns between toddlers and infants.
3. What are four gross motor skills that are usually mastered during the toddler years?
4. Describe the development of two fine motor skills that promote self-feeding during the toddler years.
5. Describe the jargoning stage of language development.
6. Why does negativism appear in toddlers?
7. Why do many toddlers experience mood shifts?
8. What are toddler rituals?

9. Briefly describe three methods for determining the number of calories a toddler needs.

10. Compare the protein needs of toddlers with that of infants and older children.

11. Why do large amounts of calcium and phosphorus need to be supplied in the diet of a toddler?

12. What is the one nutrient type that should account for more than half of the calories in a toddler's diet? Why?

13. What are the advantages of whole grain breads and cereals over refined grain products?

14. What should a child care center consider when deciding which fruits to offer to a toddler?

15. List one vegetable that is a good source of each of the following nutrients: iron, vitamin A, vitamin C.

16. Identify two meat alternates.

17. List two circumstances that might interfere with toddlers' desire to eat at a child care center.

18. What are three general guidelines to follow when deciding what foods to serve toddlers?

19. How can caregivers create a positive eating environment for toddlers?

20. What are three general guidelines to follow when introducing a new food to a toddler?

21. What are two signs of allergic reaction or intolerance to food?

22. What are three foods that are potential choking hazards?

23. What problems can result from drinking too much milk?

24. What is a food jag?

25. List three reasons why added sugar, salt, and fats should be limited in the diet of a toddler.

THINKING CRITICALLY

1. Why is it useful for caregivers to be knowledgeable about the normal development of toddlers?

2. Toddlers often respond to "yes" and "no" type questions with "no." Sometimes when they are given a choice, they will respond negatively to both choices. What can you suggest to limit frustrating confrontations with toddlers?

3. Breads and cereals belong to one of the five food groups on the Food Guide Pyramid. Are all breads and cereals equal? For example, is a cereal whose second largest ingredient is sugar as good a choice as one with a small amount of added sugar? What guidelines should you keep in mind when choosing products from this category?

4. Food jags are common with young children. Can caregivers handle food jags in the same way that parents can? Explain your answer.

5. Limiting the amount of added sugar, salt, and fats in the diets of toddlers is important. Yet, the packaged foods that are marketed for this age often

contain large amounts of sugar, salt, or fats. How can caregivers limit the amounts of sugar, salt, and fats in the diets of the children in their care?

OBSERVATIONS AND APPLICATIONS

1. Observe toddlers being served a snack at a child care center. Is the snack served on demand or at a special time? Do you observe children asking for food? Do children and caregivers wash their hands before serving and eating the snack? What is served for the snack? Are utensils needed or are finger foods served?

2. Toddlers are in a very active stage of development. Observe three or four toddlers at a child care center for a period of 20 minutes. Note the age range of the children you observe. Describe the activities they are engaged in during that time period. How long do they stay with each activity? Do you note individual differences in activity level and attention span? Does one child sit and look through a book for a time while another child never sits still? Describe any interactions you observe between children.

3. Select six products at the grocery store aimed at children. These can include frozen dinners ("kids' meals"), granola bars, "fruit snacks," breakfast cereals, cookies, and so on. Read the food labels for each item. Then write down the answers to the following questions. How much sugar and salt are in each product? How much fat? How many calories are in each serving?

4. Using the food labels on packaged food as your guide, select four healthful snacks for toddlers. (For this exercise, choose packaged foods rather than fresh fruits or vegetables.) Check package claims carefully. Is the product really low-fat? Is it low in sugar but high in salt? Is it really "all natural"? (In other words, are sugar and salt artificial ingredients?)

FOR FURTHER INFORMATION

Baxter, K. M. (1989). *Come and get it: A natural foods cookbook for children* (rev. ed.). Ann Arbor, MI: Children First Press.

Castle, K. (1992). *The infant and toddler handbook: Invitations for optimum early development*. Atlanta: Humanics Ltd.

Cataldo, C. Z. (1983). *Infant and toddler programs: A guide to very early childhood education*. Reading, MA: Addison-Wesley.

Lansky, V. (1986). *Feed me, I'm yours* (rev. ed.). Deephaven, MN: Meadowbrook Press.

Leavitt, R. L., & Eheart, B. K. (1985). *Toddler day care: A guide to responsive caregiving*. Lexington, MA: D. C. Heath.

Wanamaker, N., Hearn, K., & Richarz, S. (1979). *More than graham crackers: Nutrition education and food preparation with young children*. Washington, DC: National Association for the Education of Young Children.

Wilson, L. C., & Headley, N. (1983). *Working with young children*. Wheaton, MD: Association for Childhood Education International.

Nutritional Needs of the Developing Preschooler

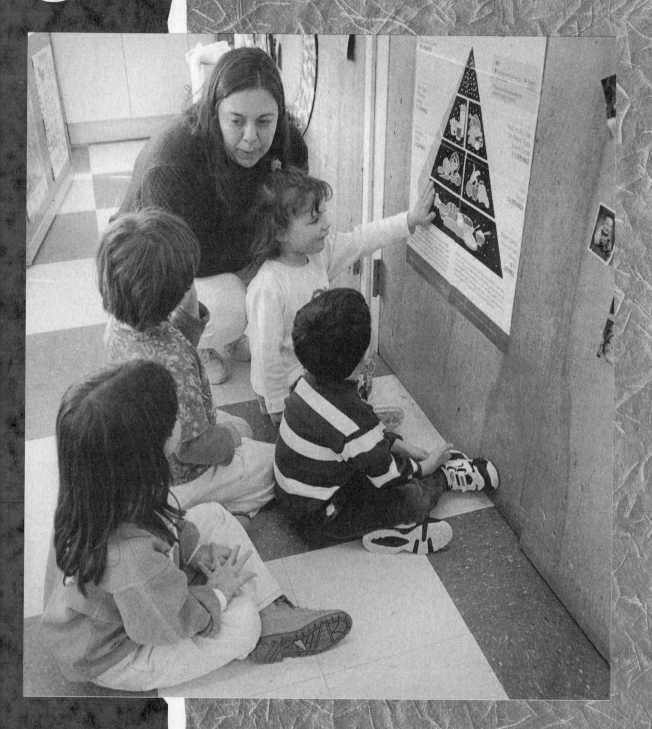

OBJECTIVES

Studying this chapter
will enable you to

- Describe the growth rate and growth patterns that characterize the preschool years
- Summarize the motor, language, and psychosocial skills that preschoolers develop
- Discuss the variations in the caloric and nutrient needs of preschoolers
- Describe specific ways in which teachers can help parents meet the nutritional requirements of preschoolers
- Identify diet-related issues that are of special concern to teachers

CHAPTER TERMS

food preferences
skinfold measurement

ELISA gathered her preschoolers into a circle. Today they were going to plan the menu for their "Super Breakfast." Elisa had explained to the children last week how important it was to eat a good breakfast. She told them it gave them energy to run and jump and play all morning. Elisa promised the group that they could eat breakfast together early the next week—their Super Breakfast. Elisa and the children studied the food pyramid chart on the wall. Last week the children had made a project of bringing in pictures of food and adding them to the chart.

"What should we have from the Fruit Group?" asked Elisa.

"Orange juice!" shouted Sam.

"Good idea, Sam," said Elisa. She noticed that Keshia looked a little sad. "What's wrong, Keshia?"

"I can't have orange juice," Keshia said. Elisa remembered that Keshia's mother said citrus juices gave Keshia a rash.

"We'll have apple juice, too, then," Elisa said. "And some banana slices."

Elisa offered to bring bran and blueberry muffins from home, as well as whole grain bread for toast. Bryan suggested serving milk with the meal.

"What about those other two groups?" Sam asked, pointing to the Vegetable Group and Meat, Poultry, Fish, Dry Beans, Eggs, and Nuts Group.

Elisa explained that it wasn't really necessary to include those two groups to have a complete breakfast. But then she remembered how much the children enjoyed a snack they'd tried last week.

"Maybe we *should* include those two groups, since you'll be eating a little later than usual," she said. "Why don't we have the celery sticks with peanut butter that you made last week? Then our Super Breakfast will include foods from all the groups."

The Super Breakfast was a hit with the preschoolers, and Elisa heard rave reviews from the parents afterward too.

"Sam never ate a blueberry muffin before, but now we've made them together twice," his mother marveled.

"Keshia used to insist on one type of cereal for breakfast. Now she is trying new cereals and she asks for banana or apple slices every morning," Keshia's mother said.

Elisa decided to write a short nutrition newsletter to send home with the children each month. It included basic nutrition information and ideas for child-friendly, nutritious meals and snacks. She asked parents to contribute their ideas and findings as well. Parents told Elisa that they looked forward to it each month.

"I don't have time to read nutrition books," said Bryan's mother. "But I always make time to read your newsletter and work those foods into our menu. We all eat better now."

The Physical Characteristics of Preschoolers

Photographs taken of the children in Elisa's class at age two and at age four would reveal definite physical changes. In the toddler photos, the children would more closely resemble infants with pudgy arms and legs and protruding bellies. As preschoolers, the children would look taller, slimmer, and more comfortable with their erect posture. The preschool years include the years from three to five when young children go through physical as well as developmental changes that mark the end of early childhood.

Height and Weight

During the preschool years, children continue to grow steadily. As children progress through the preschool years, teachers may notice differences in height and weight between individual children and between boys and girls. Whereas differences between male and female toddlers are quite small, by five years of age, the average boy is both heavier and taller than the average girl. Growth charts in Appendix C show height and weight ranges for average three- to five-year-olds.

As in other stages, the height and weight of individual children during the preschool years is a function of their genetic makeup and the state of their general health and nutrition. Children who are frequently or severely ill or who are poorly nourished may not experience normal growth. To detect possible growth problems among preschoolers, teachers can measure height and weight on a regular basis. (See Chapter 7 for information on measuring and weighing children.) These measurements should be recorded on a chart and compared with the normal range for the child's age. If the height or weight varies greatly from normal ranges for a significant period of time, teachers should report their findings to parents, who may want to consult the child's physician. Parents should be encouraged to take their children for regular health checkups during the preschool years.

As preschoolers grow, a smaller proportion of their weight gain is made up of fatty tissue. To gauge the percentage of body fat, health care providers sometimes perform a *skinfold measurement*, which uses an instrument known as a caliper to measure the fat under the skin at specific locations on the body. The most common sites for taking these measurements are on the back or arm. Skinfold measurements help health care providers distinguish between weight from muscle tissue and weight from fat. These measurements are generally used when children are underweight or overweight.

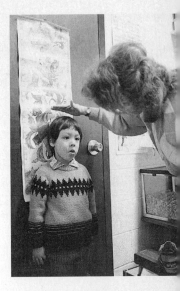

Preschoolers generally grow about 3 inches (7.6 cm) a year, and these height increases often come in spurts.

Growth Rates and Growth Patterns

The growth rate of children during the preschool years is slower than in earlier periods of development. Preschoolers generally gain an average of 4.5 pounds (2 kg) per year and grow about 3 inches (7.6 cm) per year. Increases in height often seem to come in spurts during the preschool years. These spurts are then followed by periods during which little or no growth occurs. Growth spurts are usually accompanied by increases in appetite, just as periods of little growth are accompanied by a decreased interest in food.

As preschoolers grow, their proportions change. The preschooler's head grows more slowly than the toddler's, but the face grows more rapidly and the jaw widens. Legs become longer in proportion to total body length. Whereas the legs make up about 34 percent of total body length at the age of two, by the age of five, this figure is 44 percent. During the preschool years, the spine straightens out and the abdomen protrudes less prominently. All of these changes make preschoolers look taller and more slender. At this age, girls and boys are still very similar in physical appearance.

Muscles and bones continue to grow and develop. Increasing muscle strength makes preschoolers more agile and coordinated than their toddler counterparts. Teachers may notice that some preschoolers look knock-kneed. This should not be cause for concern. As the skeletal system grows and develops, this condition will usually disappear.

Some preschoolers begin to get their permanent teeth while they are still five. This is frequently the case among children whose baby teeth erupted early. The first permanent teeth to appear are four molars. These teeth erupt behind the second molars.

The Development of Preschoolers

More than growth patterns and body proportions distinguish preschoolers from toddlers. Preschoolers acquire motor and language skills that enhance their abilities to learn about and understand the world around them. They want to know the "why" and "how" of everything and seem to talk constantly, using their rapidly growing vocabularies. Preschoolers are also whirlwinds of physical activity and love games that involve newly developed skills, rough-and-tumble play, and pretending. Although they still have difficulty seeing things from another person's point of view, preschoolers are learning to take turns and enjoy interactive play with other children.

Caring for preschoolers is quite different from caring for toddlers. Many of the children's personal care needs, from dressing to toileting to meal service, can be handled—to varying degrees—by the children themselves. Teachers should allow children to do as much as they can for themselves without becoming frustrated. This frees teachers so they can focus on creating an environment that is stimulating, safe, and enjoyable for children.

Gross Motor Skills

As with earlier stages of child development, the age at which preschoolers acquire specific skills will vary from one child to the next. The sequence of skill acquisition, however, is constant. For example, preschoolers learn to use alternate footing when going up stairs before they learn to do this when going down stairs. They become able to lace their shoes before they learn to tie laces in a bow.

During the preschool years, improving strength and muscular control of the arms and legs make it possible for preschoolers to take part in many meal-related activities. Teachers can encourage preschool children to carry serving dishes to the table, set the table, prepare certain foods (cereal with milk, for example), and clean the table. However, some states do not permit children in child care centers to take part in food preparation. They may also forbid family-style food service. It is important to be aware of state regulations before allowing children to help with meals.

Teachers should be prepared for occasional accidents when preschoolers are helping to serve food. A child may think she has safely placed a plate on a counter only to have it fall off. Another child may be briefly distracted while carrying food and spill some of it on the floor. Such mishaps are to be expected among children of this age group. A calm, nonjudgmental response to food accidents will help the children to develop a positive self-concept.

Fine Motor Skills

Improvements and refinements to fine motor skills continue during the preschool years. During this period, most children display a definite hand preference. Hand preference is the tendency to use one hand over the other to perform fine motor tasks. Approximately 90 percent of all people are right-handed (Whaley & Wong, 1991).

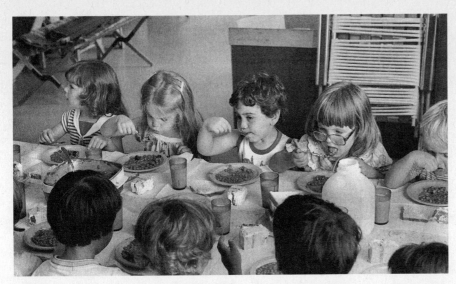

As their fine motor skills develop, preschoolers become more adept at handling eating utensils.

Many developing fine motor skills have important applications for mealtimes and nutrition. Preschoolers are more adept at handling their eating utensils and can serve themselves when bowls or platters of food are passed around. This enables children to make choices about what goes on their plates and how much of it they will eat. Preschoolers are able not only to handle dull-edged knives for peeling, slicing, or spreading foods on bread or sandwiches but also to crack eggs, stir, pour, measure, and beat. Thus, they can help with many aspects of meal and snack preparation. As mentioned earlier, always check state regulations regarding food preparation and service before planning such activities.

Language and Intellectual Development

One of the biggest differences between toddlers and preschoolers is the preschoolers' expanding use of language. Three-year-olds know their names and ages and typically speak in sentences that are three to four words long. Most have a vocabulary of about 900 words (Pillitteri, 1992) and use language all the time and for many purposes.

By the age of four, most preschoolers have expanded their vocabularies to 1,500 words. Between ages four and five, preschoolers' sentences become longer, typically four to five words in length. They also begin to use various parts of speech, such as prepositions and adjectives, to make the meaning of their conversations clearer (Pillitteri, 1992; Whaley & Wong, 1991).

By the age of five, most young children have a vocabulary of more than 2,100 words and can use different parts of speech properly. Sentences tend to be six to eight words long (Pillitteri, 1992; Whaley & Wong, 1991).

During the preschool years, young children begin the slow shift from egocentric thinking to an awareness of and a consideration for other points of view. They still, however, use appearance rather than logic to make decisions and draw conclusions. For example, a preschooler will look at the

FOCUS ON Promoting Healthful Habits

Field Trip to an Orchard

The buzz of excited four-year-old voices got louder as the bus approached the apple orchard. Elaine, the teacher, had planned this field trip so the children could see how apples grow and have the chance to pick their own fruit. She knew that children this age would learn a lot from a hands-on experience.

Elaine had her hands full trying to keep order as the children got out of the bus in front of the visitor's center. Mr. Bradley, an orchard employee, greeted the visitors and announced that they should follow him to pick their own apples off of the dwarf apple trees.

The class moved off toward the orchard. Elaine asked the children what they already knew about apples.

"They're round and red," said George.

"And green and yellow too," added Sally.

"Apples are my favorite fruit," said Josie.

The children grew excited as they neared the dwarf trees. Daniel jumped up and down and clapped his hands.

"Okay, children," said Mr. Bradley. "Now you're going to pick some apples. Please be sure to pick ripe apples—when they are ripe, they are red."

The children were delighted as they pulled apples from the branches. "There sure are a lot of apples on this tree!" exclaimed Josie. "Can I eat one now?"

Elaine explained that as soon as each child had picked some apples, they would go into the orchard store where they would wash the apples and their hands. Then they would all taste the fruit together.

"But I already took a bite of this one," said George.

"Well, George, just don't eat any more until we've had a chance to wash up," Elaine responded.

Fifteen minutes later, the children were sampling their apples. By the time they were heading back to the bus, apples were everyone's favorite fruit. And Elaine was already planning some special apple snacks for later in the week.

Do you think Elaine prepared for the field trip well? Did she handle the situation well once she and the children got to the orchard? What would you have done differently?

same quantity of liquid in a short, wide cup and in a tall, narrow cup and conclude that there is more liquid in the tall cup. Cheese that is cut into small pieces seems smaller than a broad slab of the same quantity of cheese. By understanding how a preschooler thinks, teachers can avoid many mealtime conflicts. In general, preschoolers will feel more comfortable if liquids are placed in child-sized cups and food is served in small pieces.

During this phase of intellectual development, preschoolers can recognize similarities and differences between objects. They know, for example, that corn and zucchini are vegetables and that grapes and apples are fruits. Thus, teachers can begin teaching young children about nutrition. Preschoolers can also follow simple directions, and learn the concepts of solid and liquid measurement terms and comparisons. Basic cooking projects, if permitted by state regulations, can become part of a center's daily activities.

Psychosocial Development

The physical and intellectual skills that preschoolers acquire give them a sense of autonomy about their lives. They can eat without assistance, dress themselves, and go to the bathroom independently. They can get a snack for themselves, clean up their toys, and decide what or who to play with next. These accomplishments make preschoolers proud of all the "big" things they can do. Parents and teachers can encourage preschoolers' initiative by allowing them to choose what and how much they want to eat from a nutritious selection of foods.

Preschoolers also show a willingness to participate in new experiences. Their developing sense of self allows them to focus their attention and curiosity on the world around them. Teachers can channel some of this curiosity toward the food the children eat. Snacks and mealtimes are good opportunities for discussing concepts such as shape, color, texture, and size. "Hands-on" learning experiences, where children can touch and manipulate the materials that illustrate a concept, are particularly meaningful for preschoolers. The food on a child's plate can be a starting point for a discussion on where the food comes from and how it is grown, processed, packaged, and prepared. Field trips to a dairy, a food processing plant, a farm, a supermarket, or a restaurant kitchen can be stimulating for children in this age group. Creating learning centers based on these places in your school extends the experience.

Curiosity also helps preschoolers to enjoy tasting new foods. Have the children sample foods from various cultures represented at the center. Then encourage them to talk about the food by discussing its tastes and textures and by comparing it with foods they are familiar with. Involve parents at the center by having them contribute favorite family dishes or recipes. Check state regulations to make sure that food from home is allowed to be served in class.

The Nutritional Requirements of Preschoolers

Encouraging preschoolers to try new foods not only promotes their psychosocial development but also helps them meet their daily nutritional needs. Because preschoolers are still growing, it is extremely important that they eat adequate amounts of nutritious foods.

The Energy Needs of Preschoolers

The same methods used to determine the energy needs of toddlers can be used to determine the energy needs of preschoolers. The age-related measure starts with a base of 1,000 calories and adds 100 calories for each year of age. Thus, a three-year-old would need 1,300 calories per day, whereas a five-year-old would need 1,500.

As explained in Chapter 7, the two other methods require the use of Recommended Dietary Allowances (RDAs) (National Research Council, 1989).

The first method is based on weight. For children between one and three years of age, the RDA is about 46 calories per pound (102 calories per kg) of body weight. Thus, a three-year-old weighing 32 pounds (14.5 kg) would need about 1,470 calories per day. According to the weight method, the energy needs of four- to six-year-olds are a bit lower. They require about 41 calories per pound (90 calories per kg) of body weight. A five-year-old who weighs 40 pounds (18 kg) would need about 1,640 calories per day.

If height is used as the basis, for children between one and three, the RDA translates to about 37 calories per inch of height (about 15 calories per cm). A three-year-old who is 38 inches (96.5 cm) tall would need about 1,410 calories per day. For children between four and six years, the RDA translates to about 41 calories per inch (about 16 calories per cm). A five-year-old who is 43 inches (109 cm) tall would need approximately 1,760 calories per day. Both the weight method and the height method take individual growth patterns into account, allowing parents and teachers to alter children's diets as they grow. There are also computer programs that help teachers to calculate the daily caloric needs for each child.

Whichever method is used, it is important to remember that energy needs vary from child to child and should be linked to the child's level of activity. Preschoolers need energy as much for their level of activity as for growth. The more active a child is, the greater the child's energy needs will be.

The Nutrient Needs of Preschoolers

As with daily caloric requirements, the specific nutrient needs of preschoolers are different for three-year-olds than for four- and five-year-olds. Older preschoolers need more protein, more vitamins A, C, and K, and more magnesium and iodine than their three-year-old companions. The most recent Recommended Dietary Allowances for major nutrients for these age groups can be found in Appendix A.

Preschoolers need protein for the growth and maintenance of body tissues. They can meet this requirement by drinking two or three 8–ounce cups of milk and eating 2 ounces of meat daily. Young children can get additional protein from dairy foods, eggs, nuts, seeds, legumes, and grains.

Carbohydrates provide the body with energy and are essential to a healthful diet. More than half (55 to 60 percent) of the preschooler's caloric needs should be supplied by carbohydrates, primarily complex carbohydrates such as starches. All plant sources of food and some animal products, such as milk, contain carbohydrates. Grain products, vegetables, and legumes are good sources of complex carbohydrates.

Fats also provide the body with energy and are important in growth and development. Most Americans, including preschoolers, have plenty of fat in their diets. Fats should make up no more than 30 percent of the total caloric intake of preschoolers. It is important to remember that each gram of fat yields 9 calories—more than twice the 4-calorie yield of a gram of protein or carbohydrate. Dietary fats can be found in margarine, vegetable oils, meat, fish, poultry, nuts, and dairy products.

FOCUS ON Cultural Diversity

Holiday and Birthday Foods

Most children love birthdays and holidays. Families get together to share special songs, to play games, and—most of all—to eat special foods. The dishes may vary from culture to culture, but they almost always contain ingredients that are not eaten every day.

In many cultures, birthdays are the sweetest days of the year. American and western European children celebrate with decorated birthday cakes. In England, special charms or favors are baked into the cake and the children who find them in their portions get to keep them. Fancy pastries with fruit filling and whipped cream are sometimes served to guests at Spanish and Dutch birthday parties. Indian children are treated to a favorite sweet dish in honor of the day.

Other foods also make birthdays special. In Ghana, the birthday child's mother may prepare a special dish containing yams, eggs, and palm oil. Other dishes, made with larger-than-normal portions of expensive ingredients such as meat, may also be served.

Danish children eat sweet, round white breads call boller on their birthdays. In Iceland, thin pancakes called ponnukokur are served with strawberry jam and whipped cream for a treat. In Japan, osekihan, a dish of red beans and rice, is a favorite birthday food.

Holiday foods sometimes symbolize the theme or idea behind the celebration. Mexicans and Filipinos celebrate All Saints' Day in early November by eating Pan De Muerto (Bread of the Dead), which is shaped like a skull and crossbones. During the celebration of the Chinese New Year, guests are offered a variety of fresh and preserved fruits as a way of wishing a sweet new year.

Some holiday foods are special because certain ingredients are not used. Jews do not eat food containing yeast during the Passover season, and many Christians do not eat meat on Fridays during all or part of Lent. To make up for the food not eaten, these seasons sometimes begin or end with a feast.

Satisfying the RDAs for most vitamins is not difficult because the amount of vitamins required is small, and each vitamin can be found in many different foods. Vegetables, fruits, and grain products are good sources of vitamins.

Some minerals such as calcium, phosphorus, and magnesium are needed by the body in significant amounts. Others, such as zinc, are needed in much smaller amounts. Preschoolers should consume 800 milligrams of calcium per day. Three cups of milk will meet this requirement. Other dairy products such as cheese and yogurt can also help to satisfy the requirement. Meeting the dietary allowances for most other minerals is not difficult for preschoolers. Iron, however, is often the exception. (For more detailed information about meeting iron needs and iron deficiency, see chapters 7 and 9, respectively.) Young children sometimes become iron deficient because they drink large amounts of milk and have no appetite left for foods that are richer in iron. Good sources of iron include whole grain breads, dark-green leafy vegetables, meat, egg yolks, and legumes.

Recommendations about vitamin and mineral supplements for preschoolers are similar to those for toddlers (see Chapter 7). The only supplements a child should take are those prescribed or recommended by his physician. Over-the-counter supplements may contain more of certain vitamins and minerals than the child needs and can be toxic in large doses. Supplement bottles should have child safety caps and should be kept out of the reach of children. Many children's vitamin and mineral supplements look and taste like candy and children might be tempted to consume too many of them.

Supplements may be needed by children with vitamin or mineral deficiencies. They may also be recommended for preschoolers who follow a vegetarian diet that includes no animal products. Children who do not eat milk, eggs, meat, or fish may need a vitamin B_{12} supplement, for example. Again, this supplement should only be prescribed by the child's physician.

Meeting the Nutritional Requirements of Preschoolers

Knowing what preschoolers need to eat to have a healthful diet and making sure they are offered those foods are the two sides of the nutrition coin. To meet the nutritional requirements of preschoolers, teachers must know what and how much to serve, when to serve it, and how to promote the formation of good eating habits in young children. Elisa's Super Breakfast, described at the opening of this chapter, shows one way to accomplish this task. The preschooler's job is to decide how much of which foods to eat.

Meals and Snacks

When child care centers provide meals and snacks to children, they usually use the meal pattern developed by the U. S. Department of Agriculture (USDA) Child Care Food Program (CCFP) as a guide. The requirements for children three through five are shown in Table 8.1. The plan includes foods from the five major food groups as outlined in the USDA's Food Guide Pyramid. (See Chapter 4 for more on the pyramid.) The food groups are the Bread, Cereal, Rice, and Pasta Group; the Fruit Group; the Vegetable Group; the Meat, Poultry, Fish, Dry Beans, Eggs, and Nuts Group; and the Milk, Yogurt, and Cheese Group. Table 8.2 provides a week of sample menus that meet the CCFP requirements.

Bread, Cereal, Rice, and Pasta Group.   Breads and cereals are a good source of carbohydrates, B vitamins, and iron (if the breads and cereals are enriched or fortified). Preschoolers should have a minimum of four servings from this food group. Nutritious breads and cereals include whole wheat bread, enriched white bread, macaroni or spaghetti, rice, and unsweetened cereals. Wheat germ is also a part of this food group and can be sprinkled on yogurt, cereal, and other foods. Teachers should note that wheat germ is a good source of iron and, when toasted, is well accepted by children.

TABLE 8.1 **Meal Pattern for Preschoolers**	
Breakfast	**Children 3 through 5 years**
Milk, fluid	¾ cup
Juice or **fruit** or **vegetable**	½ cup
Bread and/or **cereal,** enriched or whole grain	
Bread or	½ slice
Cereal: Cold dry or	⅓ cup[1]
Hot cooked	¼ cup
Midmorning or midafternoon snack (supplement)	
(Select 2 of these 4 components)	
Milk, fluid	½ cup
Meat or **meat alternate**[2]	½ ounce
Juice or **fruit** or **vegetable**	½ cup
Bread and/or **cereal,** enriched or whole grain	
Bread or	½ slice
Cereal: Cold dry or	⅓ cup[1]
Hot cooked	¼ cup
Lunch or supper	
Milk, fluid	¾ cup
Meat or **meat alternate**	
Meat, poultry, or fish, cooked (lean meat without bone)	1½ ounces
Cheese	1½ ounces
Egg	1
Cooked dry beans and peas	⅜ cup
Peanut butter or other nut or seed butters	3 tablespoons
Nuts and/or seeds	¾ ounce[3]
Vegetable and/or **fruit** (two or more)	½ cup
Bread or **bread alternate,** enriched or whole grain	½ slice

[1] ⅓ cup (volume) or ½ ounce (weight), whichever is less.

[2] Yogurt may be used as a meat/meat alternate in the snack only. You may serve 2 ounces (weight) or ¼ cup (volume) of plain, or sweetened and flavored yogurt to fulfill the equivalent of ½ ounce of the meat/meat alternate requirement.

[3] This portion can meet only one-half of the total serving of the meat/meat alternate requirement for lunch or supper. Nuts or seeds must be combined with another meat/meat alternate to fulfill the requirement. For determining combinations, 1 ounce of nuts or seeds is equal to 1 ounce of cooked lean meat, poultry, or fish.

CAUTION: Children under 5 are at the highest risk of choking. USDA recommends that any nuts and/or seeds be served to them in a prepared food and be ground or finely chopped.

Adapted from U. S. Department of Agriculture. (1989). *A planning guide for food service in child care centers.*

TABLE 8.2
Sample Menus for Preschoolers

Day	Breakfast	A.M. Snack	Lunch or Supper	P.M. SNACK
1	Purple plums ½ cup Cheese toast ½ slice Milk ¾ cup	Grapefruit juice ⅜ cup Carrot sticks 3 sticks Whole grain rye wafers 2 wafers	Swiss steak cubes 1½ oz. meat Mixed vegetables ¼ cup Orange sections ¼ cup Rice ¼ cup Milk ¾ cup	Milk ½ cup Granola bar 1 small
2	Orange juice ½ cup Enriched English muffin ½ muffin Milk ¾ cup	Dry Cereal ⅓ cup, with banana slices Milk ½ cup	Macaroni, cheese, and ham casserole ⅓ cup Green beans ¼ cup Fresh fruit cup ¼ cup Pita bread ½ round Milk ¾ cup	Milk ½ cup Tortilla with refried beans ½ tortilla
3	Sliced peaches ½ cup Corn grits ¼ cup Milk ¾ cup	Apple juice ½ cup Bagel ½ bagel	Pizza 1 slice Green salad ¼ cup Tomato wedge ¼ cup Milk ¾ cup	Pineapple chunks ¼ cup with cottage cheese Bread sticks 2 sticks
4	Applesauce ½ cup Scrambled egg 2 tbsp. Whole wheat toast ½ slice Cocoa ¾ cup	Orange juice ¼ cup Muffin ½ muffin Raisins ¼ cup	Lean beef patty 1½ oz. Whole wheat bun ½ bun Carrots ⅜ cup Apple wedge ⅛ cup Milk ¾ cup Chocolate pudding 2 tbsp.	Milk ½ cup Saltines 4 with cheese
5	Tomato juice	Milk	Salmon loaf	Fresh fruit cup *(continued)*

TABLE 8.2
Sample Menus for Preschoolers *(continued)*

Day Breakfast	A.M. Snack	Lunch or Supper	P.M. SNACK
½ cup **Farina** ¼ cup **Milk** ¾ cup	½ cup **Enriched soda crackers** 2 crackers **Peanut butter**	1½ oz. fish **Boiled potatoes** ¼ cup **Broccoli** ¼ cup **Milk** ¾ cup **Roll** 1 roll	½ cup **Bran muffin** ½ muffin

Adapted from U. S. Department of Agriculture. (1989). *A planning guide for food service in child care centers.*

Fruit Group.   Preschoolers should have two or more servings of fruits daily. A serving of fruits, as specified in Table 8.1, may be offered at lunch or supper and other servings can be provided at snack times or at other meals. Servings can also be estimated at 1 tablespoon of cooked fruit or 2 tablespoons of raw fruit for each year of age. Thus, a four-year-old should have 4 tablespoons of cooked applesauce or 8 tablespoons of raw fruit.

Include a variety of fruits that are good sources of vitamin A, vitamin C, and other vitamins and minerals. One serving of cantaloupe can satisfy a preschooler's requirement for vitamin A. To meet their vitamin C needs, they should have at least one serving per day of oranges, grapefruit, orange juice, grapefruit juice, tangerines, or strawberries. Other fruits that are good sources of vitamins and minerals include apples, bananas, grapes, plums, and peaches.

Fresh fruits are the best choice, but frozen fruits are preferable to the canned variety. When canned fruits are served, use those packed in water or fruit juice rather than in syrup.

Vegetable Group.   Preschoolers should have a minimum of three servings of vegetables per day. One serving per day of carrots, sweet potatoes, collard or turnip greens, winter squash, or broccoli will meet a preschooler's vitamin A requirements. Vitamin C needs can be satisfied through one serving per day of green pepper, broccoli, or brussels sprouts. Other vegetables that are good sources of vitamins and minerals include potatoes, corn, green beans, peas, lettuce, cucumbers, and spinach.

Nutritionists recommend at least one serving of vegetables at lunch or dinner. Vegetables are more likely to be eaten if they are not overcooked. Steaming vegetables leaves them with a crunchy texture and allows them to retain more of their nutritional value. Raw vegetables such as carrot sticks and cucumber wedges are enjoyable and nutritious snacks. Serving sizes for vegetables are the same as for fruits, and as with fruits, fresh or frozen varieties are preferable to canned.

Meat, Poultry, Fish, Dry Beans, Eggs, and Nuts Group. Preschoolers should have a minimum of two servings of meat or meat alternates each day. For preschoolers, a meal serving of meat, fish, or poultry is 1½ ounces. One egg, ⅜ cup of cooked dry beans or peas, or 3 tablespoons of peanut butter are equivalent servings (see Table 8.1).

The foods in this group should be cooked until tender so that preschoolers can easily cut them with a dull knife or eat them with their fingers. Meat and meat alternates that are high in salt and fat such as hot dogs or luncheon meats should be limited.

Milk, Yogurt, and Cheese Group. Milk and milk products are good sources of calcium and protein. Teachers should use low-fat milk, cheese, and yogurt to supply the nutrients in this food group to preschoolers.

Preschoolers should have three servings of milk and milk products each day. Alternatives should be provided for children who have difficulty digesting milk and milk products.

Other Considerations. It is important that teachers be familiar with the dietary needs of all the children in their care and plan meals and snacks accordingly. Teachers should invite parents to explain any dietary restrictions they would like their children to follow at the center. For example, some children may be vegetarians, whereas others may not be able to eat foods such as pork because of religious restrictions. Teachers should accept a child's family values and understand that children can get all of the nutrients they need even when their diets are limited in some way. Find out from parents exactly what each child can and cannot eat. Then discuss ways in which you can provide substitutes for restricted foods for the child. Center staff should be aware of children's food allergies and any restricted foods; for example, this information could be posted in the children's classrooms and in the center kitchen.

Be sure to offer children a variety of foods. This is essential to good nutrition since each food provides different nutrients. The greater the variety of foods eaten, the more likely it is that all nutrient needs will be met. Variety also makes mealtimes and snacks more interesting. Children will look forward to meals and snacks when a variety of foods are offered.

Preschool children are sensitive to the way foods look; they enjoy variety in the texture, shape, and color of their food. Foods that appeal to children visually can help to encourage good eating habits. Although a plate with corn, rice, apple slices, and chicken provides variety, it isn't as visually appealing as one with green beans, sweet potatoes, kiwi, and chicken.

Finally, variety in the diet can teach children about foods that are associated with other cultures. When you serve foods from different cultures, you expand children's experiences and let the children of that particular culture know that you accept and respect their ways and practices.

Importance of Snacks. Preschoolers need snacks because they have small stomachs and they cannot eat large enough portions to keep them

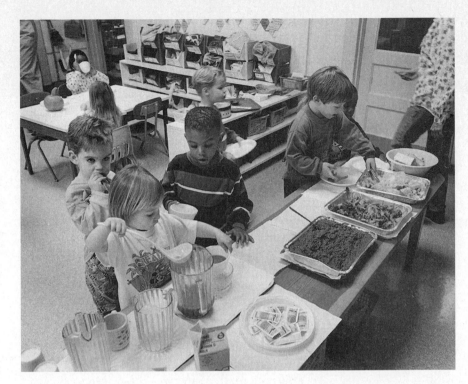

If children are offered a variety of foods, their nutrient needs are more likely to be met. This center is providing a choice of main dishes at lunch.

going from one meal to the next. Snacks also provide an important opportunity to fill in any nutritional gaps in their diets. Thus, morning and afternoon snacks should be a part of the child care center's activities and food plan.

Serving Food at the Child Care Center

State regulations generally govern such things as the types of food served, the frequency of food service, and the way food is prepared and served in child care centers. These regulations have been developed in conjunction with nutrition and child development professionals to ensure that children receive nutritious food in a sanitary environment. Although the regulations of many states may be identical to the recommendations presented here, be sure you are familiar with your state's rules.

Scheduling and Frequency of Meals.   Most nutrition and child development professionals recommend that children in care for six to eight hours be fed at least one meal and two snacks, or two meals and one snack. Children in care for nine hours or more should be offered at least two meals and two snacks, or three snacks and one meal. Meals and snacks should be served at two- to three-hour intervals. Snacks are best served at midmorning and midafternoon (American Public Health Association & the American Academy of Pediatrics, 1992). Breakfast should be provided for children who arrive at the child care center without having eaten.

Encouraging Good Eating Habits.   Teachers should keep in mind that preschoolers have fluctuating appetites that often increase and decrease in conjunction with periods of growth. Appetites may vary from one day to the next and even from one meal to the next. This kind of irregularity is not unusual. As long as children are offered a nutritious selection of foods at snack times and mealtimes, they will get the nutrients they need. If a change in a child's appetite lasts for more than a few days, however, teachers should share their observations with the child's parents.

If state regulations permit, allow children to take part in all phases of meal activity. When children can help in these ways, they learn about such things as the importance of handwashing, food safety, and the many ways foods can be prepared nutritiously. Letting them help—whether it involves setting the table or cleaning up after a meal—adds to their sense of accomplishment and responsibility.

Whenever possible, include both children and adults in the mealtime environment. This helps to make meals a social experience. With adults at the table, preschoolers can observe good table manners and watch adults eating and enjoying their food. Preschoolers love to imitate the adults around them. When they see adults reacting positively to nutritious foods, they will mimic these behaviors.

Introducing New Foods

Most preschoolers are reluctant to eat foods they have never tried before. Despite such resistance, it is important for teachers and parents to continue exposing children to new foods. When this is done consistently, in a positive atmosphere, children can become more adventurous about food choice. The more variety there is in a preschooler's diet, the more well balanced that diet is likely to be.

Methods and Timing.   Many of the methods for introducing new foods to preschoolers are similar to those for introducing new foods to toddlers (see Chapter 7). New foods can be introduced slightly more often, leaving a few days between each new food. Follow the guidelines of serving the new food with familiar foods, talking about the food with the children, enjoying it yourself, and presenting a neutral response to the child's acceptance or refusal. Continue to offer the new food to children.

Another way of encouraging children to try new foods is to take the children along on a trip to the grocery store. Children can be encouraged to select a new vegetable or fruit that they would like to try. Where there is room to do so, starting a vegetable garden at the child care center can be an excellent method for introducing new foods.

When introducing new foods, teachers should keep in mind the cultural and religious diversity of their groups. Group differences can provide avenues for finding new food choices. Teachers should, however, avoid offering foods that a particular child cannot eat for cultural or religious reasons.

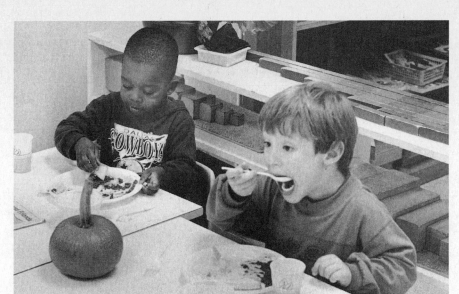

Preschoolers' appetites do fluctuate. A child who has an excellent appetite one day may be relatively uninterested in food a day or two later.

Allergies or Food Intolerances.   When serving new foods to preschoolers, it is still important to watch children for signs of a reaction or intolerance (see Chapter 7). Foods most likely to cause an allergic reaction are nuts, peanuts, eggs, cow's milk, wheat, fish, shellfish, and citrus fruits (Kendrick, Kaufman, & Messenger, 1991). Fewer food allergies are likely to appear in this age group, however, because preschoolers have a more mature digestive system than toddlers. Also, parents are likely to know about their children's allergies by this stage and will probably have told teachers about them ahead of time. Teachers should, however, be familiar with signs of allergic reactions and intolerances and know the steps to take should a child have a severe allergic reaction. Teachers also need to make sure that they advise parents of any food allergies or intolerances that they notice.

Special Nutritional Concerns

The very qualities that make preschoolers so exciting and interesting to work with—their curiosity, independence, and awareness of the world around them—can create special nutritional concerns for teachers of this age group. Preschoolers usually have definite opinions about food, and they are likely to be influenced in their choices by advertising and the choices of their peers. Teachers can help preschoolers by consistently providing nutritious, well-balanced meals and snacks at the child care facility.

Food Preferences

Most preschoolers have strong *food preferences*, meaning they are partial to certain groups of foods or certain types of food preparation. At snack time,

WHOLESOME SNACKS

Pasta Alfredo

Ingredients:

1 pound uncooked spaghetti

8 ounces parmesan cheese

4 cups skim milk

Directions:

1. Cook and drain the pasta before bringing it into the classroom.
2. Have the children help you grate the cheese and pour the milk into small pitchers.
3. Give the children bowls of pasta and allow them to sprinkle on their own cheese, add milk, and stir.

Yield: 20 servings

Each serving contains:

Calories: 135
Protein: 7.2 g
Fat: 2 g
Carbohydrates: 22 g

Source: University of Illinois at Urbana-Champaign Child Development Lab.

preschoolers will frequently ask for cookies, crackers, or cereal. They may like potatoes—but only when they are mashed, not baked. They may insist on chocolate milk at every meal. When one of these foods is an appropriate item on the menu, teachers should make no comment on a child's choice. This does not mean that preferred foods should be specially prepared for a child or that cookies, for example, should be available for breakfast.

Although some children's food preferences become extreme, most of these disappear over time. Teachers and parents can ease the process by not making an issue of the preferences but continuing to offer a variety of nutritious foods. It is helpful to remember that choice is an important element in getting young children to eat. Offering two kinds of fruit, for example, and allowing the child to help himself gives the child control.

Restricting Certain Foods

Although variety is essential in the preschooler's diet, some foods should be served only in restricted quantities. These include foods high in added sugar, salt, and fats. It is important to read food labels carefully for hidden sugar, sodium, and fat. This information can be found under "Nutrition Facts" and in the list of ingredients.

Sugar. Processed sugar should be limited not only because it is a nutritionally empty source of calories but also because it is a major factor in causing dental caries, or tooth decay. Bacteria in the mouth feed on sugars as well as starches, forming a substance that destroys the tooth enamel and creates a cavity. Teachers should not add sugar or sweeteners to vegetables, fruits, or cereal. They should not serve candy; sweetened beverages; or refined, sweetened baked goods. For birthdays, suggest that parents consider more nutritious snacks than cake or cookies. Treats such as a hollowed-out watermelon filled with fruit, fruit with a yogurt dip, or whole grain muffins could satisfy both children's desire for sweets and adults' nutritional concerns.

Salt. The connection between too much salt in the diet and high blood pressure, or hypertension, has already been discussed in Chapter 4. Teachers can limit salt intake by keeping saltshakers off the table, reducing the amount of salt used in cooking, and making sure that the prepared foods served are low in sodium.

Fats. Fats are a dietary concern because a diet too high in fats has been linked to obesity, cardiovascular disease, and some cancers. Saturated fats should be restricted because they are linked to heart disease. Thus, foods that have a high saturated fat content, such as hot dogs, luncheon meats, and ice cream, should be served sparingly to children.

FOCUS ON Communicating with Children

Healthful Meals and Snacks

All the preschoolers at the Linden Day Nursery School gather together for circle time every day. Paul, one of the teachers, is talking with the children about the letter *C*, which is the sound theme for the week.

PAUL: Who can tell me some words that start with the letter *C*?

LEAH: Cat and crib. My baby sister has a crib!

PAUL: Right, Leah. Cat and crib both start with the letter *C*. Does anyone else know a *C* word?

ROBERT: Candy. That starts with *C*. I wish I could eat candy all the time, but my mom won't let me! (The children begin to talk among themselves about candy.)

PAUL: Wait a minute. Let's not all talk at once. You're right Robert. Candy is a *C* word. Let's talk about candy for a minute. Robert, you said that your mom won't let you eat candy all the time. Has she told you why?

ROBERT: She says it's bad for my tummy and my teeth. But I like candy!

PAUL: Candy does taste good and it's okay to have it once in a while, but you have to eat other foods too. Your body needs growing foods like fruits, vegetables, meat, and cereals to keep you healthy. And growing foods don't have to taste bad. Does anyone here ever eat bananas?

KATHY: I do. Yesterday, I had a banana for a snack. I like bananas.

PAUL: Bananas are a good-tasting growing food. So are other fruits like apples, oranges, and grapes. You can eat them for snacks or for breakfast or even for supper.

LEAH: Bananas for supper?

PAUL: Sure. I bet I know another growing food that most of you like—pizza.

ROBERT: Pizza is a growing food?

PAUL: Yes, it is. The crust is made from flour, so it's sort of like bread. It's covered with sauce made from tomatoes—a vegetable—and cheese, which is made from milk. All of those foods are growing foods.

ROBERT: Do you know what growing food I hate? Vegetables! I hate vegetables!

PAUL: How many of you hate vegetables? (All of the children raise their hands.) That's too bad, because there are lots of really good vegetables. Do you remember the bread we had for snack yesterday that Sally's mother brought in? (Several of the children nod their heads.) Well, that was zucchini bread. And it had the vegetable zucchini in it.

LEAH: Sally's mom played a trick on us!

PAUL: Not really. She just found a way to make a vegetable into something tasty. I bet I know a vegetable that most of you like—carrot sticks. How many of you like carrot sticks? (About half of the children raise their hands.) In fact, carrots would be a perfect snack to have today because carrots start with the letter *C*.

Did Paul do a good job of talking to the children about healthful foods? What other examples of good-tasting growing foods would you have used?

Snacks and Fast Foods

In many families, snack foods and fast foods are replacing home-cooked meals with growing frequency. Parents may feel they are fighting a losing battle in their struggle to give their children nutritious diets. Many fast-food restaurants offer fresh vegetable salads, milk, and fruit juices in addition to foods high in fat, salt, and added sugar. Processed snack foods seldom provide the vitamins, minerals, protein, and complex carbohydrates important for growing young bodies, although they may have a high caloric content because of added sugar and fats used in processing. Applying the key principles of variety, balance, and moderation over time (not necessarily to each and every meal and snack) will ensure a healthful diet.

Teachers can help both parents and children by making nutrition education a part of the child care program. Talking with children about the commercials they see on television can help to correct some of the misinformation these advertisements provide. Providing parents with written nutrition information, as Elisa did with her newsletter, helps them to make wise choices when they eat out with their children or purchase foods at the grocery store.

Nutritional Concerns for After-School Programs

Some child care centers look after older children in the afternoons after school lets out. These centers are required to provide the school-age children with at least one snack if the children are there for two or more hours. Snacks are just as important to school-age children as they are to preschoolers. These children need to eat after school to maintain their high energy level and to support their continued growth. Thus, snacks for school-age children should be nutritious and should help to meet their nutritional requirements for the day.

Teachers can encourage school-age children to eat the right kinds of snacks by involving the children in planning and preparing what they will eat. Teachers should avoid offering foods that are high in fat. Fruits and vegetables; whole grain muffins, crackers, and bagels; and low-fat cheese and yogurt products make satisfying snacks that school-age children like to eat. Such snacks are high in complex carbohydrates and are excellent sources of energy, vitamins, and protein.

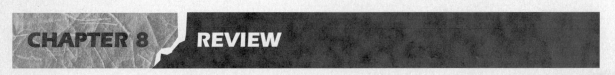

CHAPTER 8   REVIEW

SUMMARY

- As preschoolers grow, they look taller, slimmer, and more comfortable with their erect posture. Their legs get longer, their spines straighten out, and their abdomens protrude less prominently.

- Preschoolers acquire new gross and fine motor skills and refine others. These abilities enable them to take a more active role during mealtime, setting the table, preparing food, and even serving themselves.

- The level of intellectual development of preschoolers means they are ready and able to learn about nutrition. In serving foods, however, teachers must take into account the ways preschoolers perceive amounts.

- Teachers can direct the preschooler's curiosity about the outside world and new experiences toward food and nutrition-related activities.

- Age-, weight-, and height-related measures can be used to determine a preschooler's daily caloric needs. A child's energy needs are also linked to his level of activity.

- Meals and snacks for preschoolers should contain a variety of foods. Preschoolers should have at least four servings each day of bread, cereal, rice, and pasta. They should have two servings a day of fruits and meats or meat alternates; and three servings a day of vegetables and milk or milk products.

- Variety in the diet exposes preschoolers to new foods, makes meals more interesting, and teaches children about cultural diversity.

- Meals and snacks should be served at two- to three-hour intervals. If state regulations permit, preschoolers should be encouraged to take part in all phases of meal activity.

- New foods should be introduced one at a time and served with familiar foods. Teachers should react neutrally whether children try the new food or not. Teachers should continue to serve the new food so that it becomes familiar, and they should let the children see adults eating and enjoying it.

- Sugar, salt, and fats, particularly saturated fats, should be offered sparingly to preschoolers.

- Nutrition education can help parents and preschoolers. Teachers should explain what makes up a healthful diet and help children and parents cope with the influences of advertisers on food-buying habits.

- Child care centers that care for school-age children in the afternoons need to provide these children with snacks. Teachers should make sure that the foods offered are nutritious.

ACQUIRING KNOWLEDGE

1. How does the height and weight of the average five-year-old boy compare with that of the average five-year-old girl?
2. What is the relationship between growth spurts and the appetite of preschoolers?
3. Describe the way body proportions change as a preschooler grows.
4. What are two meal-related activities that preschoolers can be expected to handle?
5. Compare the language skills of a typical three-year-old with those of a typical five-year-old.

6. What are two tasks preschoolers can accomplish without assistance as a result of their psychosocial development?
7. Why is it important to take into account a child's activity level when deciding how much food he or she should be encouraged to eat?
8. What percentage of the total caloric intake of preschoolers should be eaten in the form of fats?
9. Name two of the minerals that are needed by preschoolers' bodies in significant amounts.
10. What are three sources of iron?
11. Why are vitamin and mineral supplements generally not needed? Who should take supplements?
12. Why is it preferable to serve breads and cereals that have been enriched or fortified?
13. How many servings of fruits should preschoolers eat each day?
14. How many servings of vegetables should preschoolers eat each day?
15. How many servings from the Meat, Poultry, Fish, Dry Beans, Eggs, and Nuts Group should preschoolers eat each day?
16. How many servings from the Milk, Yogurt, and Cheese Group should preschoolers receive each day?
17. Why should preschoolers be served snacks?
18. What are three aspects of food service in child care centers that are generally covered by state regulations? What is the purpose of these state regulations? Are regulations the same in all states?
19. How many meals and snacks should children in care for six to eight hours be fed? How often should children in child care be fed?
20. Why should adults eat with children?
21. Why are food allergies less of a problem with this age group than with toddlers?
22. How should teachers respond when a child shows a strong like or dislike for a particular food?
23. Explain how sugar contributes to tooth decay.
24. What are two ways to limit salt intake?
25. Why should intake of saturated fats be restricted?

THINKING CRITICALLY

1. The chapter mentions that physicians sometimes measure a child's percentage of body fat. Why would this measurement be taken? How do you think the results of the test would be used?
2. The chapter mentions three methods for determining the caloric needs of preschoolers. Which is the easiest method for teachers to use? Why? What are advantages of the other two methods? Of what use is the information about caloric needs to teachers?
3. Fats should take up no more than 30 percent of a child's daily caloric intake. How can you plan meals and snacks for children that fall within these guidelines; especially since, in some cases, you will not know exactly how much fat is in a particular food?

4. Home-cooked meals are often a series of prepackaged foods heated up in a microwave oven. Many of these foods are high in fats, sugar, and salt. What can teachers do to help limit the amount of these foods in the diets of preschoolers in their care?

5. A common attitude toward serving food to preschoolers is that serving them a wide variety of foods is wasteful. Preschoolers are picky eaters whose general likes and dislikes are predictable. Serving milk or juice and cookies for snack, with an occasional piece of cut-up fruit, reduces waste. Children can be counted on to eat these foods. What do you think?

OBSERVATIONS AND APPLICATIONS

1. Observe three-year-old children playing on a playground. What gross motor skills do you observe them using? What equipment do they use? Can they use the swings by themselves? Observe four-year-old children playing on a playground. What gross motor skills do you observe them using? What equipment do they use? Can they use the swings by themselves? What similarities and differences do you observe between the gross motor skill development of the three- and four-year-olds?

2. Observe children helping to prepare food at a preschool. What are they preparing? What jobs do the children do? How are jobs divided? How much can they do on their own? How many children are involved in the preparations?

3. A mother tells you that she is concerned about her son. He is a picky eater. Lately, this problem has worsened. He only wants to eat macaroni and cheese. She thinks that macaroni and cheese is fine occasionally, but not for lunch and dinner every day of the week. She is worried that his diet isn't varied enough and that his nutritional needs are not being met. Even though she has tried, she has not been able to get him to eat anything else. What advice would you give this mother?

4. Suppose you work in a child care center where a midmorning snack, lunch, and a midafternoon snack are served. Plan snacks and meals for the preschoolers for three days. What alternatives would you make available to children who do not want to eat a food you offer?

FOR FURTHER INFORMATION

Berman, C., & Fromer, J. (1991). *Teaching children about food: A teaching and activities guide.* Menlo Park, CA: Bull Publishing.

Brazelton, T. B. (1992). *Touchpoints: Your child's emotional and behavioral development, the essential reference.* Reading, MA: Addison-Wesley.

Galinsky, E., & David, J. (1991). *The preschool years: Family strategies that work—from experts and parents.* New York: Ballantine Books.

Lansky, V. (1986). *Feed me, I'm yours* (rev. ed.). Deephaven, MN: Meadowbrook Press.

Satter, E. (1987). *How to get your kid to eat . . . but not too much.* Menlo Park, CA: Bull Publishing.

9

Children with Special Nutritional Needs

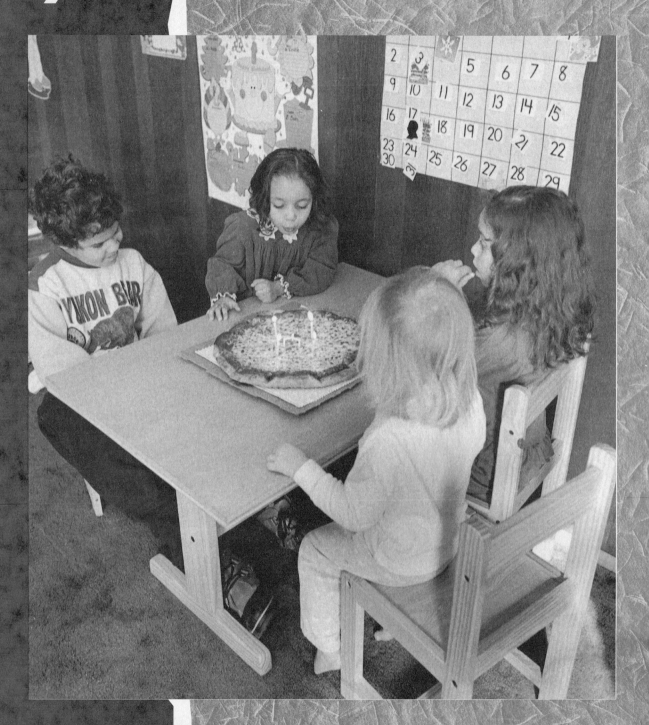

OBJECTIVES

Studying this chapter
will enable you to

- Describe the causes and remedies
  for iron-deficiency anemia and
  other nutritional deficiencies
- Explain why obesity is a major
  nutritional problem and identify
  ways that teachers can help obese
  children achieve normal weights
- Describe the difference between
  food allergies and food
  intolerances and suggest how
  these conditions might be handled
  in a child care setting
- Discuss how developmental delays
  can affect nutritional status
- Summarize the effects of low birth
  weight on the nutritional needs of
  infants and young children

CHAPTER TERMS

allergen
anemia
cystic fibrosis
diabetes mellitus
eczema
food allergy
food intolerances
hyperlipidemia
lactose intolerance
malabsorption
obesity
phenylketonuria

IT was a beautiful fall day and the preschool class at Mountainview Children's Center was enjoying the last few minutes of its outdoor play period. Sonia, the teacher, called them indoors. Today was Marcella's birthday, and her grandmother had brought pizza as a snack. At the beginning of the year, Mountainview handed out guidelines for birthday celebrations that encouraged families to provide nutritious snacks rather than cake or candy.

Fortunately, Marcella's grandmother understood why the center wanted to limit sweets, and she had consulted Sonia a few days earlier about what foods would be appropriate. Not all families were as cooperative as Marcella's. A few felt that their children were being deprived of enjoyment on their special days if they didn't celebrate with cake.

Marcella blew out the candles on her pizza while the class sang "Happy Birthday." Suddenly Alyssa started to cry.

"It's not fair. You know I can't eat pizza," sobbed Alyssa. Alyssa was allergic to milk proteins. The cheese on the pizza would make her break out in hives.

"Look, Alyssa," said Sonia. "I have a special treat for you." From the refrigerator, she brought Alyssa a fruit plate. The pieces of fruit had been cut and arranged to look like a smiling face. Realizing that she wasn't going to be overlooked, Alyssa brightened.

"Wow!" said Ari, looking at the fruit plate. "Can we make those for snack sometime?"

Nutritional Deficiencies

Although food is generally abundant in North America, caregivers may work with children who suffer from nutritional deficiencies. Some children have nutritional deficiencies because of inadequate diets. Their families may not be able to afford a variety of foods or may make poor choices about which foods to serve. A few children may have nutritional deficiencies because strongly held cultural beliefs limit the variety of foods they are served. Occasionally children with behavioral problems such as attention deficit-hyperactivity disorder (ADHD) find it difficult to focus on eating long enough to consume adequate amounts of food. These children need to eat in an environment as free of distractions as possible. They may also benefit from being offered smaller amounts more frequently than other children. Some children with emotional disturbances may exhibit peculiar eating patterns that lead to unbalanced diets. Intervention by a trained therapist is often needed to change their eating patterns.

Homelessness is a social condition that may lead to nutritional deficiencies. Because homeless people have little money and usually lack the opportunity to cook for themselves, their food choices are limited. One study found that single mothers and their children in temporary housing were getting less than 50 percent of the Recommended Dietary Allowances for iron, magnesium, zinc, and folic acid (Drake, 1992). Another study found that the rate of iron-deficiency anemia was twice as high in homeless children as it was in children with permanent homes (Wiecha, Dwyer, & Dunn-Stroheckerr, 1991).

Nutritional deficiencies also can occur for other reasons. Children may have an illness or physical condition that prevents their bodies from utilizing certain nutrients. Others may be taking medication that interferes with the use or storage of nutrients. Still other children may have physical disabilities that make eating challenging. Recent immigrants from politically troubled or poverty-stricken parts of the world may have diseases or disorders uncommon in the United States, including deficiency diseases.

Anemia

Some conditions can have a variety of causes, including nutritional deficiencies. *Anemia* is such a condition. People with anemia do not have enough hemoglobin or red blood cells to carry oxygen from the lungs to all parts of the body. Hemoglobin is the substance that actually carries the oxygen throughout the body.

It can be difficult to detect anemia. Some children who have anemia appear pale and tired and are more susceptible to infection. Others show few outward signs of the problem. A simple blood test can measure the volume of red blood cells in the blood to detect anemia. This test is performed by a health care professional when anemia is suspected.

Causes of Anemia.   Anemia can have several different causes. The most common cause for anemia in childhood is insufficient iron in the diet. Iron is an essential mineral for the formation of hemoglobin and red blood cells. Children who do not receive enough iron from their food will develop iron-deficiency anemia. Deficiencies in either of the B vitamins—folic acid or cobalamin (B_{12})—or copper can also cause anemia.

Excessive external or internal bleeding also causes anemia. After heavy bleeding, the fluid volume of the blood is usually replaced within a few days, but the number of red blood cells remains low. In healthy people, it takes about a month to replace the red blood cells lost during a serious bleeding episode (Whaley & Wong, 1991).

Another cause of anemia involves red blood cell destruction. Red blood cells can be destroyed faster than the body can replace them. This happens with inherited diseases such as sickle cell disease and infections such as malaria. Lead poisoning, burns, and some drugs also destroy red blood cells.

Decreased production of red blood cells can be caused either by damage to the bone marrow, where red blood cells are made, or by insufficient supplies of nutrients to make new cells. Diseases such as leukemia reduce the functioning of the bone marrow. Exposure to radiation, certain chemicals, and some drugs also reduce the number of red blood cells the bone marrow makes. If the body makes too little of the growth-regulating hormone thyroxine, an insufficient number of red blood cells is produced.

Iron-Deficiency Anemia.   Caregivers of preschool children may be responsible for a child with iron-deficiency anemia. This type of anemia is most common in children between the ages of six months and three years (Lanzkowsky, 1985). While reports vary on the percentage of children affected, iron-deficiency anemia remains common in the United States today.

Iron-deficiency anemia is generally the result of insufficient iron in the diet. Children need a greater amount of iron per pound of body weight than do adults. This is because children must both replace red blood cells that are destroyed through normal processes and make additional red blood cells to increase the volume of blood their bodies need as they grow. Children are most vulnerable to iron-deficiency anemia during periods of rapid growth.

Full-term infants have about a four-month supply of iron stored in their bodies; premature infants have far less. Formula-fed babies should be given iron-fortified commercial formula to prevent an iron deficiency. Breast-fed babies need iron supplements starting around the fourth month, when their iron stores become depleted. Premature breast-fed babies need supplements starting at around two months. Babies who do not receive iron from food or supplements by the time their iron stores are used up become iron deficient.

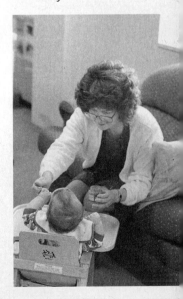

Children need a greater amount of iron per pound of body weight than do adults. Giving babies iron-fortified infant cereal can help to prevent iron deficiency.

WHOLESOME SNACKS

Fruit Juice Cubes

Ingredients:

1½ envelopes
unflavored gelatin

¾ cup water

6-ounce can frozen
grape or apple juice
concentrate

Directions:

1. Very lightly grease a
9" x 5" loaf pan or
plastic ice cube trays.
2. Dissolve gelatin in
water in saucepan over
low heat.
3. Mix in fruit juice
concentrate, and pour
into pan or trays.
4. Cover. Refrigerate
until set.
5. Cut into 1-inch cubes
and serve.

Yield: 45 cubes

Each cube contains:

Calories: 10
Protein: trace
Fat: trace
Carbohydrates: 1 g

*Source: USDA. Making bag lunches,
snacks, and desserts. HG-232-9.
Washington, DC: Human Nutrition
Information Service.*

Older babies who drink cow's milk may suffer from iron deficiency as well, since milk is not a good source of iron. Babies who drink too much milk don't eat enough of other foods, such as iron-fortified infant cereal, mashed dark-green leafy vegetables, and strained meats, all of which provide iron.

Children on strict vegetarian (vegan) diets have particular difficulty getting enough iron. The foods in their diets provide little of this mineral. To get enough iron without eating any meat, these children may have to eat larger quantities of food than they can comfortably consume. (Vegetarian diets are discussed in Chapter 4.)

Access to a wide variety of foods, especially iron-rich foods such as meats, is closely tied to economic status. Children from lower socioeconomic groups tend to have a higher rate of iron-deficiency anemia than do children of higher economic status.

Sometimes iron-deficiency anemia is caused by *malabsorption*, or poor absorption, of iron into the body. Malabsorption can occur because of the presence of iron-inhibiting compounds, certain diseases, or long-term diarrhea. Generally, the absorption of iron from foods can be increased by combining foods high in vitamin C with iron-rich foods. For example, eating a hamburger along with a sliced tomato salad will increase the absorption of iron from the meat. Iron in vegetables is better absorbed when they are eaten with meat.

Children who have iron-deficiency anemia need an increase in the amount of iron in their diets. Depending on the cause and severity of the condition, they may need iron supplements.

Other Nutritional Deficiencies

There are several classic nutritional deficiencies. Scurvy, marasmus, and kwashiorkor are discussed in Chapter 5. Beriberi results from a thiamin deficiency and pellagra is caused by a deficiency of niacin. Both of these B vitamins are added to enriched grain products in this country. All of these nutritional deficiencies are rare in the United States. They are still found, however, in many other parts of the world, and caregivers may see some of these diseases in children who have recently immigrated to this country. Caregivers may also see a child who has grown up in this country and has a nutritional deficiency caused by limited food choices, disease, or medication.

Vitamin D-Deficiency Rickets.   The body needs vitamin D in order to absorb calcium and phosphorous, two minerals essential for creating and maintaining bones and teeth. Vitamin D-deficiency rickets occurs when there is inadequate vitamin D to allow the body to absorb all the calcium and phosphorus it needs. Children with rickets have bowed legs, present a "pigeon chest" appearance because the breast bone protrudes, and are late to get teeth. The head bones in infants may remain soft, and the spine takes on an abnormal shape.

When skin is exposed to direct sunlight, the body normally makes its own vitamin D. Some children, however, do not get enough sunlight. A child who is hospitalized would probably not be exposed directly to the sun. In recent years, there has been an increase in rickets among urban children who are kept indoors much of the time or who live in high pollution areas. Children with dark skin are more at risk than children with light skin (Whaley & Wong, 1991). Breast-fed babies of vitamin D-deficient mothers may also develop rickets. Many doctors recommend vitamin D supplements for all breast-fed babies. Children on vegan diets are also likely to be vitamin D-deficient. These children need vitamin D supplements.

Vitamin D is normally added to commercially produced formula, milk, cream, and butter. Children who drink unprocessed, unsupplemented milk might be at risk for vitamin D deficiency.

Malabsorption Conditions.   Some diseases reduce the amount of nutrients the body can absorb as food passes through the intestines. Cystic fibrosis is the most common of these malabsorption disorders.

Cystic fibrosis is an inherited disease that affects the mucus-producing glands of both the lungs and the digestive system. It is estimated to occur in 1 out of every 1,600 white children, and much less often in blacks and Asians (Nora & Fraser, 1989). The severity of symptoms varies widely from child to child. Often the first sign of cystic fibrosis is failure to thrive—these children do not grow as expected over time.

Children with cystic fibrosis need respiratory therapy to keep their lungs clear. They also have special nutritional needs. For example, they may need up to 50 percent more calories than other children their age. Children with cystic fibrosis have difficulty digesting fats. Health care providers must, therefore, monitor the children's intake of the fat-soluble vitamins A, D, E, and K. Enzymes to help fat digestion are also given. To ensure that children with cystic fibrosis get adequate nutrition, they need to follow diets planned by health care professionals.

Drug-Induced Deficiencies.   Certain medications interfere with the body's use of nutrients. High levels of salicylates, compounds found in aspirin, can reduce the body's ability to store vitamin C. Anticonvulsant drugs increase the need for vitamin D and interfere with the body's use of calcium and folic acid. Health care professionals treating children who use these drugs can provide guidance about appropriate diets.

Obesity

Obesity is the excessive storing of fat in the body. It is another common nutritional problem in the United States today. Obesity results from consuming more calories than are used for growth and activity over a prolonged period. The number of obese children has increased steadily over the past 20 years.

Children who appear to be obese should be evaluated by a health care professional. Evaluation usually involves assessment of body fat content,

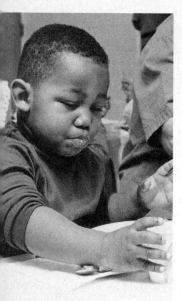

since an overweight child may merely have more muscle tissue than average. A child is not considered obese unless there is excessive body fat. Although obesity is generally easy to recognize, its causes are complex.

The cost of obesity is high. Children who are obese have significantly lower self-esteem and less satisfying social lives than normal weight children (Whaley & Wong, 1991). They are also susceptible to various physical problems, including skeletal-muscular disorders, hypertension, respiratory problems, and diabetes.

Causes of Obesity

There is no single reason why some people are obese and others are not. Many different factors can play a role. Because there are many different reasons for obesity, the problem is difficult to correct.

Physical Causes of Obesity.   There is good evidence that both weight and body shape are influenced by genetic factors. Less than 10 percent of children born to normal weight parents are obese. A very high percentage of obese children and adolescents have at least one obese parent. Although it is difficult to separate genetic and life-style causes for obesity, studies show that identical twins raised in separate households tend to have similar weights (Strunkard, Harris, Pedersen, & McClearn, 1990). Adopted children have body weights closer to those of their biological parents than to those of their adoptive parents (Strunkard, Sorensen, Hanis, Teasdale, Chakraborty, Schull, & Schulsinger, 1986). These facts and findings strongly suggest that there is a genetic role in determining body weight. This does not mean that obese parents are certain to have obese children, but it means that these children are at higher risk for obesity.

Some people are obese because their bodies store fat too efficiently or the mechanism for retrieving fat for use by the body functions poorly. These fat storage problems are among genetic factors that contribute to obesity.

A very small percentage of children are obese as a result of a disease or endocrine disorder. In hypothyroidism, for example, the thyroid gland makes too little of the growth-regulating hormone thyroxine, and obesity can result. Obesity is sometimes a complication of muscular dystrophy and some fairly rare inherited diseases. Children with these disorders should be under the supervision of a health care professional who can advise the children's caregivers about the children's diets.

Life-Style Causes of Obesity.   Perhaps no other human activity is influenced as much by social and cultural values as is eating. One's culture heavily influences which foods are considered appropriate and desirable, how they are prepared, and when and where they are eaten. Cultures that emphasize large family meals with many high-fat foods tend to promote obesity more than those that value spare meals with little red meat.

Societal attitudes toward exercise and physical activity also influence whether or not children become obese. Obese children tend to be less active

Although obesity is strongly linked to heredity, overeating and consuming high-fat foods can contribute to this problem.

FOCUS ON Cultural Diversity

Perceptions About Weight

Like adults, children come in a wide variety of shapes and sizes. Ideas about what are normal or desirable body types vary from group to group. The same child might be called "fat," "thin," or "average" depending on the surrounding culture. In some upper-middle-class American communities, for example, a desire for thinness among adults may lead parents to limit the amount of food that their children eat, resulting in slender youngsters. In this culture, even a child whose bone and muscle structure give him a large appearance may be seen as overweight.

In cultures where food is less plentiful, a plump or stocky child may be considered more healthy and attractive than his thinner friends. This has to do with survival. Where medical care is less adequate, infants and children with more body fat stand a better chance than oth-ers of surviving childhood illnesses. Plumpness, therefore, becomes a desired trait.

Such attitudes can be hard to change even when conditions change. People who leave an area where food is scarce to settle in one where food is easy to get may still cling to the idea that a healthy child should have some extra fat on his body.

Unless a child's weight is endangering her health, it is best to accept it without comment. The child's appearance may be related to many factors, including the rate at which she is growing, the body types of her parents, and how her culture views attractiveness. Even when a child is obese, other children should never be allowed to tease her. Ideas about "ideal weight" may change from time to time and place to place, but childhood hurts can be painful for a lifetime.

than other children, but whether this is a cause or effect of obesity is not clear. Many societies consider plumpness a sign of well-being, and many parents still believe that a fat baby is a healthy baby.

There is some question about whether television watching causes obesity. Without a doubt, time spent watching television is time not spent in more vigorous physical activities. Also, children who watch television tend to snack more. Many advertisements promote high-calorie, low-nutrient foods. However, a direct link between television watching and obesity has not been clearly established (Mitchell, 1993).

Psychological Causes of Obesity. Eating is a pleasurable social activity. Babies associate eating with the security and comfort provided by those who care for them. Older children may continue to associate food with social situations in which they receive attention from adults.

Adults often believe subconsciously that food is an expression of love. They may try to show their love for their children by providing extra helpings or food treats. Some parents overestimate the amount of food children need and insist that children eat all the food on their plates, even if the children are full.

Sometimes children overeat in response to stress in their lives. Changes in eating patterns often occur after separation, divorce, or other traumatic events in children's lives. Children who eat for emotional reasons eat even when they are not hungry. Patterns of overeating in response to stress or for comfort tend to perpetuate themselves and are difficult to change.

Controlling Obesity

Child care professionals, along with center directors and the parents themselves, share responsibility for the quality and quantity of food served to preschool children in their care. The food habits young children develop tend to influence their eating patterns for a lifetime. Teachers should work actively to promote good food habits in children. The teacher's own eating and exercise habits should also provide a positive example.

Diet.   In children, obesity is controlled by reducing the rate of weight gain rather than by weight reduction. If the rate of weight gain is slowed, children will arrive at a normal weight as they grow taller. Child care providers need to work with parents to balance food eaten at the child care center with food eaten at home. In some cases, teachers can play an important role in educating parents about controlling obesity.

Caregivers need to provide plenty of high-nutrient, low-calorie snacks. Healthful, nutritious food should be offered to all children, not just to children with weight control problems. Singling out an overweight child for a special diet can make the child self-conscious or uncooperative. It is the responsibility of the teacher to help obese children find foods they can eat rather than to simply eliminate foods they should not eat.

Exercise.   Children who are obese tend to exercise less than children of normal weight. As obese children become older, they often become self-conscious about their physical skills and reluctant to join in sports and games. Teachers need to encourage obese children to participate in all physical activities. Activities that stress individual abilities instead of competition allow all children to succeed.

Preschool programs should provide ample time for active outdoor play. Parents who live in apartments or in neighborhoods where they feel it is unsafe to let their children play outdoors can be encouraged to find other recreational opportunities for their children. Some communities offer organized activities for children of various ages. Parents can make regular trips to local parks a special opportunity to share active play with their young children.

Behavior Modification and Psychological Support.   Obese people often eat in response to cues other than hunger. They may eat or overeat only at certain times of the day or in specific social settings. Making parents and children aware of these eating patterns is the first step in changing them. Caregivers can offer children alternative activities when overeating

FOCUS ON / **Promoting Healthful Habits**

Encouraging Exercise for an Obese Child

Suzanne stood in the middle of the child care center playground supervising the children in her group. It was a fine spring day and most of the children were involved in lively games. Deena, however, was sitting quietly on a bench, observing the others. Suzanne was concerned about Deena because she was overweight, and Suzanne wondered if lack of exercise was contributing to Deena's problem.

"It's a beautiful day," Suzanne said as she sat down beside Deena. "Why don't you go and play with the others?"

"Oh," Deena said, "Do I have to? I'm too tired."

"We're going to play tag later," Suzanne said. "That's a lot of fun. You'll play, won't you?"

Deena thought a moment, her face clouding briefly. "Maybe," Deena said slowly. "I don't like tag. I'm *always* it."

"Deena," she said, "I bet if you played more, you'd get better at tag. You would be able to move more quickly and you wouldn't get so tired. But you wouldn't have to play just tag. You could jump rope and play lots of games. You don't really like getting tired so easily, do you?"

"No," Deena answered sadly. "I hate being tired and I hate being slow."

That gave Suzanne an idea. She began to describe some simple games she and Deena could play together. "If you like," she said, "we can be a special team. We'll play together. It will be fun. And pretty soon you'll be playing games all day without getting tired. What do you say?"

Deena smiled at Suzanne. "Can I really be on your team?" Deena asked.

"You sure can," replied Suzanne. "Let's play right now!"

Did Suzanne present this delicate subject well? Is being Deena's partner in exercise a good idea? What might you have done in Suzanne's place?

occurs in response to situations that arise at the child care center. A hug and a chat about how they are feeling can help start the process of learning constructive, rather than destructive, ways of dealing with stress.

Controlling obesity is a difficult proposition. Caregivers need to offer families that are working to control obesity as much support as possible, especially in cases where the parents themselves are obese. Parents need help in planning special events such as birthday celebrations so that they include attractive foods that their obese children can eat. Teachers can also encourage all parents to send nutritious snacks rather than high-calorie, low-nutrient foods for special occasions.

Food should never be used as a reward for any child. Obese children may need a great deal of help separating food from feeling loved and appreciated. Child care providers need to be patient and persistent as they offer encouragement and nonfood rewards to obese children who are learning new, healthier associations. Understanding some of the social and cultural factors that play a role in a child's weight problems can be crucial to finding acceptable strategies for weight control.

Obesity and Certain Medical Conditions

Obesity can predispose people to, if not actually cause, some serious medical conditions. Once these conditions are present, obesity aggravates them. Although a person who is not obese can develop hypertension, hyperlipidemia, or diabetes, careful weight control is essential in treating all three conditions. When these conditions exist, guidance from a health care professional concerning diet is essential.

Hypertension.   Hypertension, or high blood pressure, is usually thought of as a problem of middle age. Some children, however, also have high blood pressure. Most children exhibit hypertension as a complication of other medical disorders, such as kidney or cardiovascular disease. However, one study found that 1 to 2 percent of children under age 20 with no other apparent health problems had high blood pressure (Cranwell, 1984).

Obesity and hypertension are closely related. In children with no other medical problems, control of hypertension involves maintaining a normal weight and reducing salt (sodium) intake, getting regular exercise, and reducing stress. Blood pressure screening for hypertension is part of every routine medical examination.

Hyperlipidemia.   *Hyperlipidemia* means having excess lipids, including cholesterol, in the blood. High lipid and cholesterol levels are believed to increase the risk of developing heart disease. People who have high cholesterol levels as children are likely to continue to have high cholesterol levels as adults (Newburger, 1990).

Children whose family medical history suggests the possibility of hyperlipidemia should be screened for this condition. Some pediatricians prefer to screen all children rather than only those obviously at risk. Controlling hyperlipidemia in children involves substantially reducing the amount of fat in the diet, developing a regular aerobic exercise program, and weight loss if the child is obese.

Diabetes.   In *diabetes*, or more correctly diabetes mellitus, the body produces an inadequate amount of the hormone insulin. This interferes with the metabolism of sugars. Early signs of diabetes include irritability, unusual thirst or fatigue, and abdominal discomfort. Children with diabetes must take insulin several times a day, usually by injection, and the timing and content of their meals and snacks must be controlled.

Successful control of diabetes requires strict monitoring of a diet in which sources of carbohydrates are controlled, especially concentrated sweets. Activity is not restricted. In fact, children with diabetes have grown up to become professional athletes. What is required for successful management of diabetes is the coordination of diet, exercise, and insulin intake.

Teachers of diabetic children must work closely with parents and health care professionals to ensure that the children's consumption of food is timed

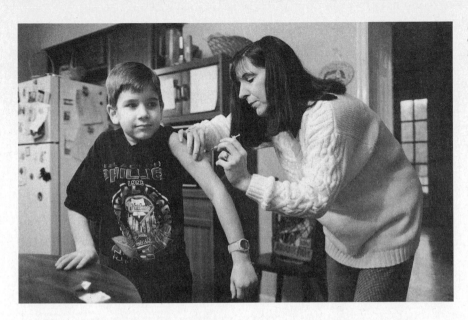

Most children who have diabetes take insulin by injection.

to coincide with the actual availability of insulin in the child's system. Consideration of activity levels, emotional states, and general health are also important to proper control of diabetes.

Food Sensitivities

Caregivers of preschool children are fairly likely to deal with food sensitivities on a day-to-day basis. Reactions to a particular food can range in severity from irritating, such as a mild itch or upset stomach, to fatal, for example hives or swelling that close off the airway. Helping children avoid foods to which they are sensitive means reading food labels for hidden sources of food irritants as well as avoiding obvious sources of the problem food.

When food sensitivities eliminate large numbers of food categories from a child's diet, special foods from home or specific diets prepared by heath care professionals may be needed. Dietary supplements for nutrients that are not available in adequate amounts may be prescribed as well.

Food Allergies

In a true *food allergy*, the body's immune system reacts to a food substance as if it were an attacking organism. This is known as an immune response. The food is an *allergen*, which is any substance that causes an allergic reaction. Allergic reactions are most common during infancy, because the immature intestines allow more proteins to pass into the bloodstream (Whaley & Wong, 1991). Many children "outgrow" their allergies as they mature. Others develop food allergies only during certain stages of development. Food allergies tend to be inherited. The best way to control a food allergy is to avoid the food that causes it.

Symptoms of Food Allergies.   Food allergies can be difficult to pinpoint. The symptoms of food allergies are diverse and range widely in their seriousness. Symptoms can be immediate or delayed for several days. Common digestive system responses to food allergies include vomiting, diarrhea, excessive gas, and abdominal pain. Other symptoms include asthma, runny nose, hives, rashes, and *eczema*—a condition characterized by skin inflammation. Although food allergies may aggravate hyperactive behavior, they do not necessarily cause hyperactivity (Whaley & Wong, 1991).

Because many medical problems have similar symptoms, it is often difficult to say for sure that the problem is a food allergy. Food allergy is suspected when removing the food from a child's diet causes the symptoms to disappear. It is confirmed if reintroduction of the same food causes the symptoms to reappear. Coordination between the home and the child care facility is important during this process.

Common Food Allergens.   Cow's milk is one of the foods that most commonly causes an allergic reaction in infants and young children. Children who are allergic to milk cannot eat milk proteins in any form. This is why Alyssa could not eat the pizza Marcella's grandmother brought to celebrate Marcella's birthday. When a child is allergic to milk, teachers must read nutrition labels closely to eliminate from the diet any foods made with milk or dried milk solids.

Infant allergies to cow's milk can be avoided by breast-feeding. Food allergens rarely pass from mother to child in breast milk. In cases where this does happen, the mother can eliminate milk and milk products from her diet. Milk-free commercial formulas are also available. Fortunately, many children outgrow their allergic reactions to milk by age five.

Eggs, wheat, corn, soy, peanuts, chocolate, citrus fruits, strawberries, fish, and shellfish are all common allergens in young children. Many allergic reactions to these foods disappear by the time children reach school age.

Handling Food Allergies in Child Care Settings.   Because allergic reactions to foods can be severe, caregivers must be serious about removing known allergens from a child's diet. Wheat, usually in the form of flour, is found in many foods, especially baked goods. It is also added to sauces and gravies and is used in coating foods such as fried chicken. Eggs and corn are also difficult to avoid, especially in prepared foods. Soy proteins are added to many foods and condiments.

Caregivers need to work with the parents of a child with a food allergy to find an appropriate diet. Since many child care centers allow children to bring food from home to share with the class for birthdays or other celebrations, caregivers may want to alert all parents to any special dietary needs of children in their classes. Caregivers should request ingredient lists for foods prepared outside the center in order to determine whether a child with a food allergy can safely eat them. Even so, permission from the allergic child's parent should be obtained before serving the child any special foods not prepared at the center.

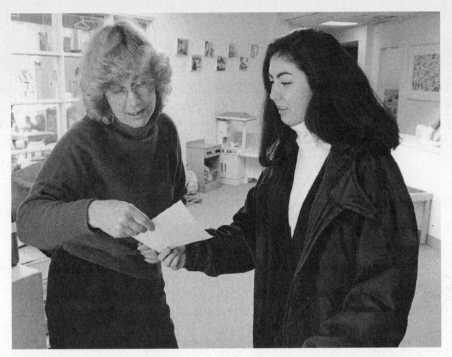

To prevent allergic reactions to foods, caregivers should request ingredient lists from parents for snacks and meals prepared outside the center.

When a child in the class is allergic to a common food such as wheat, it is helpful to keep on hand a supply of appealing allergen-free foods. This allows the child with the food allergy to be included in special celebrations even if she cannot eat the treat provided. When Sonia prepared a special fruit plate for Alyssa, she was responding to the reality that Alyssa's allergy meant she could not eat the pizza and to Alyssa's need to join in the celebration.

Food Intolerances

Food intolerances do not involve an immune response; they are the result of inherited or inborn errors of metabolism. The body lacks the enzyme(s) needed to make use of a particular food. The symptoms of food intolerances are similar to those of food allergies and, from the caregiver's viewpoint, these situations are handled the same way. Each problem food is eliminated from the child's diet.

Lactose Intolerance.   Children with *lactose intolerance* are unable to digest lactose, the sugar found in milk. Children with lactose intolerance may complain of abdominal pain, excessive gas, or diarrhea soon after drinking milk. In contrast to a milk allergy, lactose intolerance may not be an all-or-nothing phenomenon. Some children tolerate small amounts of milk at a sitting, but react unfavorably to larger amounts. Children with lactose intolerance may be able to eat yogurt, cheese, and buttermilk because the

FOCUS ON   Communicating with Children

Special Nutritional Needs of a Classmate

It is morning at the University Child Care Center. Sandhya, one of the teachers, has just finished playing a lotto game with a group of four-year-olds. She steps away for a moment to talk to Mrs. Lee, the center's director.

SANDHYA: (returning to the group): Jimmy's mother just called. He isn't feeling well, so he won't be with us today.

KIM: What's wrong with him?

SANDHYA: His stomach is upset, that's all.

CHRISTOPHER: Well I think he's sick because he doesn't drink his milk! My mom says milk helps me to be healthy. Jimmy never drinks milk, so now he's sick!

SANDHYA: It's true that Jimmy doesn't drink milk, but that doesn't have anything to do with his stomachache.

KIM: But why doesn't he drink milk?

SANDHYA: It's because of the special way his body works. Right after Jimmy was born, his doctor looked at some of his blood and found out that certain kinds of foods—some of them are things like meat and milk that most of you have every day—are bad for Jimmy.

CARLO: But Mrs. Lee told us that meat and milk are growing foods.

SANDHYA: For most children they are. But sometimes the same foods that make most people healthy, make other people sick. That's the way it is with Jimmy.

CHRISTOPHER: How will Jimmy grow up to be big and strong if he can't eat his growing foods?

SANDHYA: Well, there are lots of healthful foods Jimmy *can* eat, like salads, vegetables, and fruits. There are even some foods made especially for people like Jimmy.

KIM: Is that why Jimmy always brings his lunch and snacks with him from his home?

SANDHYA: That's why. His mother makes him sandwiches with a special kind of bread that is a little different from the bread we use here. Since he can't have milk, he brings his own drink too.

CHRISTOPHER: And sometimes he even has cookies. He gave me one. They taste good!

SANDHYA: Jimmy's cookies are special cookies, but that doesn't mean that they don't taste good.

KIM: Will Jimmy ever be able to eat regular food?

SANDHYA: Probably. In a few years, the doctor will look at Jimmy's blood again. If his body is able to handle the foods that bother him now, then Jimmy will be able to eat the same foods as everyone else.

CHRISTOPHER: When that happens, I think Jimmy will be sad.

SANDHYA: Why do you say that, Chris?

CHRISTOPHER: Because if he gets to eat the same food as all the other kids, he won't be able to bring his cartoon lunch box!

How would you explain things like PKU, blood tests, and special diets to four-year-olds? Could it be done in a different way? Did Sandhya do a good job of explaining that although Jimmy has PKU, he is not sick like someone who has a cold or a stomach virus?

lactose in those products has been broken down into units they can metabolize. Some children can drink special lactose-altered milks available at certain supermarkets.

Caregivers should be sensitive to the fact that milk may truly cause discomfort in some children. Lactose intolerance is common in several ethnic groups, including African Americans, Asians, Middle Eastern Jews, and Native Americans.

Phenylketonuria.   Children with *phenylketonuria* (PKU) are unable to metabolize properly the essential amino acid phenylalanine. Excess amounts of this amino acid build up in the blood. This disease affects mainly white children. If these children are not put on a phenylalanine-restricted diet, they may become severely retarded.

Since phenylalanine is an essential amino acid, it cannot be totally eliminated from a child's diet. Management of PKU involves maintaining a level of phenylalanine sufficient for growth and development, but not high enough to cause damage. Special infant formulas are available for children with PKU. Older children with PKU generally bring special food from home. If a processed food is being used for the class, caregivers should check the label for phenylalanine and get the approval of the child's parent before serving it to a child with PKU. Babies born in hospitals in the United States are routinely screened for PKU.

Children with Developmental Delays

Children with developmental delays or physical disabilities need the same nutrients to grow and develop as do other children. Physical or mental delays or disabilities, however, may sometimes interfere with a child's ability to eat. And since children with developmental delays often have other health problems, evaluating their nutritional needs may be difficult. Children who are confined to a wheelchair, for example, will probably need fewer calories than children who walk. Caregivers need to work with health care professionals to ensure that the diets of these children will meet their nutritional needs.

Children with Feeding Problems

Babies who are developmentally delayed may have difficulty sucking, chewing, or swallowing. As toddlers and preschoolers, these children may still be unable to feed themselves. Because of these problems, children who are developmentally delayed often eat inadequate diets.

In such a situation, parents and caregivers must modify a child's diet to take into consideration his particular abilities. Caregivers also need to recognize when the child is developmentally ready to move on to new food textures. The age at which developmentally delayed children are ready to accept new foods will probably differ from the average age for other children. The developmental sequence of food acceptance that progresses from

Children with physical disabilities need the same nutrients to grow and develop as do other children. Caregivers may need to modify children's diets if they have difficulty feeding themselves.

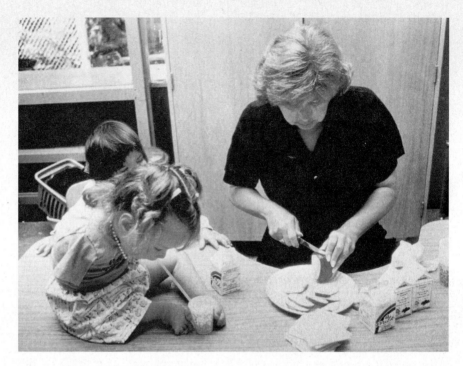

sucking liquids to eating strained foods and then coarser foods, however, is the same. Caregivers should be alert to signs that disabled children are ready to begin to self-feed and support their efforts.

Some disabled children may be overfed as an expression of parental love and concern. Others may be undernourished because caregivers or parents stop feeding before the child has eaten enough. In the day-to-day care of a developmentally delayed child, it may be difficult for a caregiver to plan for enough time, several times a day, to feed adequately a child who eats more slowly and laboriously than other children. Special planning regarding daily eating routines is, therefore, important.

Caregivers and Developmentally Delayed Children

With implementation of the Americans with Disabilities Act, caregivers may see more children with developmental delays mainstreamed into regular child care settings. Caregivers who work with developmentally delayed children need to develop sensitive communication skills to work effectively with parents and health care professionals.

Working with disabled children requires extra patience, a slower approach, and appreciation that what is a small step forward for the average child may be great progress for a child with a disability. Developmentally delayed children require extra attention and time, so it may be necessary for child care centers to hire additional staff and/or provide special training for caregivers who work with these children.

Low Birth Weight Babies

Low birth weight babies are babies born weighing less than 5 pounds. Most of these babies are premature (less than 38 weeks gestation, or development in the uterus), but some may be full-term infants who are small for their gestational ages. Low birth weight babies have higher nutrient requirements than heavier, full-term babies. These infants need more nutrients because they are growing rapidly and because they have smaller amounts of nutrients stored in their bodies.

Feeding Low Birth Weight Babies

Making sure that low birth weight babies obtain adequate nourishment is a challenge for health care professionals. Babies who are too weak to suck are fed intravenously. This means that nutrients are taken directly into the bloodstream and that they bypass the digestive system.

Once babies are strong enough, they can be fed so that the food passes through the intestines where nutrients are absorbed. Food can be placed directly in the stomach through a feeding tube. Babies strong enough to suck may be bottle-fed or breast-fed. All premature and low birth weight babies need frequent, small feedings.

Special formulas exist for premature infants. When possible, mothers are encouraged to breast-feed. Breast-feeding has value not only for nutritional reasons but also because of the close physical contact between mother and child and the immune protection supplied by breast milk. Some premature infants receive expressed breast milk.

Continued Growth of Low Birth Weight Babies

Most premature babies catch up with full-term babies in growth and development by age two. Once this period of catch-up growth concludes, the growth rates and nutritional needs of the child who was born prematurely are the same as other children's. A similar pattern is generally seen with low birth weight babies who were full term.

While they are growing extra quickly, premature and other low birth weight babies have special nutritional needs. These needs will vary with the age and health of the child. Calcium and protein requirements will be higher, for example, during the catch-up period. The additional needs will gradually lessen as the growth rate normalizes. Caregivers need to know if children enrolled in the child care facility were premature or low birth weight babies.

Caregivers may find that parents of children who were low birth weight babies or who were seriously ill as infants tend to worry excessively and overfeed these children. Because of their initial concerns about the health and survival of their babies, parents of these children may continue to feed them very frequently and encourage them to eat more than they need at each meal long after this extra concern is appropriate.

SUMMARY

- Nutritional deficiencies can result from inadequate diet, behavioral problems, homelessness, underlying illness, certain medications, or physical disabilities that make eating challenging.

- A common nutritional deficiency in children in the United States is iron-deficiency anemia. This condition usually comes about because the amount of iron in the diet is insufficient to meet the body's need for new red blood cells.

- Infants who are formula-fed should receive iron-fortified formula or, after four months of age, iron-fortified cereal to prevent iron-deficiency anemia. Toddlers and preschoolers need a variety of iron-rich foods. Children who have iron-deficiency anemia may need iron supplements to correct severe deficiencies.

- Children who are rarely exposed to sunlight are susceptible to vitamin D-deficiency rickets, especially if they drink unprocessed, unsupplemented milk. In recent years, there has been an increasing incidence of this disease among urban children.

- Obesity is a common problem in both children and adults. The causes of obesity are complex and include genetic, cultural, life-style, and psychological factors.

- Obesity is controlled in children by slowing the rate of weight gain rather than by weight reduction. Teachers can help children establish lifelong good health habits by encouraging them to eat nutritious foods and to exercise regularly.

- Obesity is associated with a number of medical conditions, including hypertension, hyperlipidemia, and diabetes. The attainment and/or maintenance of normal weight is essential to effective control of these conditions.

- Food sensitivities are common among preschool children. Food sensitivities include food allergies and food intolerances.

- In the case of a food allergy, the body's immune system reacts to a food substance as if it were an attacking organism.

- Common allergens include cow's milk, eggs, wheat, corn, soy, peanuts, chocolate, citrus fruits, strawberries, fish, and shellfish. The best way to control a food allergy is to eliminate the food from the child's diet.

- Food intolerances do not involve an immune response; they occur when the body lacks the enzyme(s) needed to properly metabolize or break down, a specific food for use by the body. Lactose intolerance and phenylketonuria are examples of food intolerances.

- Children with developmental delays need to have their diets evaluated by a health care professional to ensure that the diets will promote optimum growth and development.

- Extra time and patience are needed to feed adequately children with developmental delays and some other physical handicaps. Caregivers must be sensitive to a developmentally delayed child's readiness to move on to new food textures.
- Low birth weight babies have special nutritional needs during the period of catch-up growth until about age two. Once their growth rates have normalized, their nutritional needs are generally the same as those of other children of the same age.

ACQUIRING KNOWLEDGE

1. List two behavioral conditions and one social condition that can contribute to the development of a nutritional deficiency.
2. What is anemia? How is it diagnosed?
3. Identify the four causes of anemia.
4. What is the most common cause of iron-deficiency anemia? Why are children from lower socioeconomic groups more likely than others to suffer from this deficiency?
5. What are the symptoms of vitamin D-deficiency rickets? Why are children who are kept indoors much of the time more likely to suffer from this condition?
6. What is cystic fibrosis?
7. Explain how obesity occurs.
8. Identify three of the physical causes of obesity.
9. Identify two life-style factors that can cause obesity.
10. Identify two psychological causes of obesity.
11. In children, how is obesity controlled?
12. Explain why food should never be used as a reward for any child.
13. What is hypertension and how is it related to obesity?
14. What is hyperlipidemia and what other disease is it linked to?
15. What is diabetes and how is it controlled?
16. What is the difference between a food allergy and a food intolerance?
17. What are three symptoms of food allergies?
18. Why are food allergies sometimes difficult to diagnose? How are they generally diagnosed?
19. What is lactose intolerance and what are its symptoms?
20. How can children with lactose intolerance receive the nutrients found in milk and milk products?
21. What is phenylketonuria (PKU)?
22. List the feeding problems of developmentally delayed children that may lead to nutritional deficiencies.
23. Compare the nutritional needs of low birth weight babies with those of babies who are average weight.

24. Describe two special feeding methods for low birth weight infants.
25. By what age do most premature and low birth weight babies catch up to other children developmentally?

THINKING CRITICALLY

1. How might caregivers help to make sure that children on vegetarian diets receive a sufficient supply of iron?
2. Suppose that you believe that a child in your care has an emotional or social problem that is leading to a nutritional deficiency. How could you best handle the situation?
3. How can you distinguish between normal differences in weight and true obesity? Is there potential harm in paying excessive attention to a child's weight? If so, how can this be avoided?
4. It is recommended that obesity in children be controlled by reducing the rate of weight gain rather than by weight reduction. Why? How might this be accomplished?
5. It is common for young children to be allergic to many foods. Why is it important for caregivers to be aware of the food sensitivities of the children in their care?

OBSERVATIONS AND APPLICATIONS

1. Observe people eating in a restaurant or in a mall's food court. Observe the food choices made by three children eating a meal (not a snack). Write a general description of each person (for example preschool-age boy, extremely thin). Note what each child is eating. Does there appear to be any relationship between the weight of the child and the amount and type of food the child is eating? How much food does each child throw away at the end of the meal? Note the food choices made by the adults who are with each child. Do children who order large meals tend to be accompanied by adults who order large meals? Do thin children tend to be with thin adults and heavy children with heavy adults?
2. Observe three other children eating with their families. Note how much the children finish and how much they leave on their plates. Do you observe any adults encouraging children to finish everything they ordered (even if it is food of low-nutritive value)? What foods are left over? Do you observe any children who leave their main meals but finish all their desserts? Is leftover food packed up to take home, thrown away, or eaten by someone else in the group?
3. Suppose that at the child care center where you work parents are responsible for sending in snacks for the whole class. At a parents' meeting before school begins, you pass out a list of suggested snacks to the parents. One parent raises his hand and says that his daughter is allergic to many of the items included on the list. She is allergic to dairy products, wheat products, and citrus fruits. What should the policy of the center be

regarding sending in snacks that children in the class are allergic to? Should food choices be changed because of the allergies of this child? Should the center provide a separate snack? In such a case, should the parent be responsible for providing snacks for his child?

4. Mrs. Perry asks your advice. She gave birth to her daughter six weeks before her due date. Her daughter is fine, but she weighed only 4 pounds at birth and had to stay in the hospital for some time until being sent home. Now, at three months of age, she still needs to be fed more frequently than other babies. Mrs. Perry was granted a three-month leave and now needs to return to work. She is concerned about leaving her daughter in a child care setting. What advice and assurances can you give to Mrs. Perry about her daughter's care?

FOR FURTHER INFORMATION

Coffin, L. A. (1984). *Children's nutrition: A consumer's guide.* Santa Barbara, CA: Capra Press.

Cooper, K. H. (1991). *Kid fitness: A complete shape up program from birth through high school.* New York: Bantam Books.

Kendrick, A. S., Kaufmann, R., & Messenger, K. P. (Eds.). (1991). *Healthy young children.* Washington, DC: National Association for the Education of Young Children.

LeBow, M. D. (1991). *Overweight children: Helping your child achieve lifetime weight control.* New York: Plenum Press.

Martens, R. A., & Martens, S. (1987). *Milk sugar dilemma: Living with lactose intolerance* (2nd rev. ed.). Bloomington, IL: Medi-Ed Press.

Orenstein, N. S., & Bingham, S. L. (1988). *Food allergies.* New York: Putnam Publishing Group.

Taylor, J. F., & Latta, R. S. (1993). *Why can't I eat that? Helping kids obey medical diets.* Saratoga, CA: R & E Publishers.

PART 3

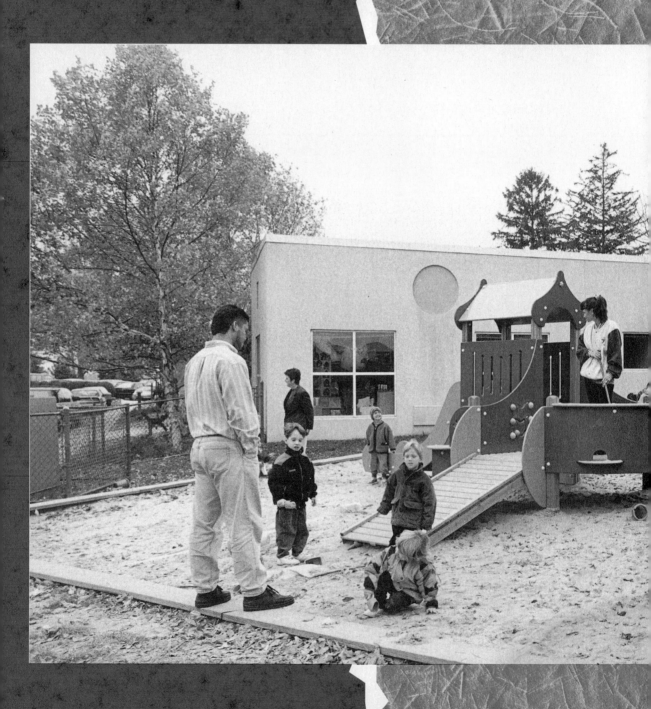

Health and Safety Concerns

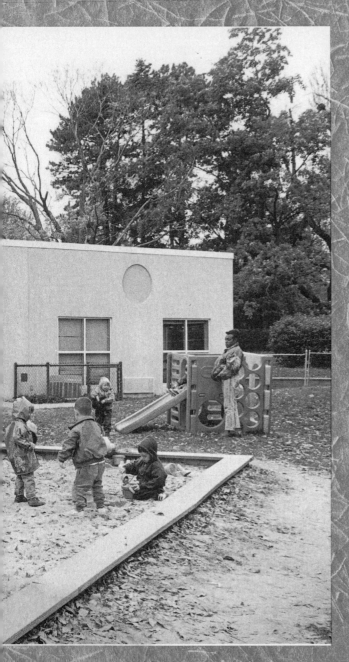

223

10

Health Awareness and Special Needs

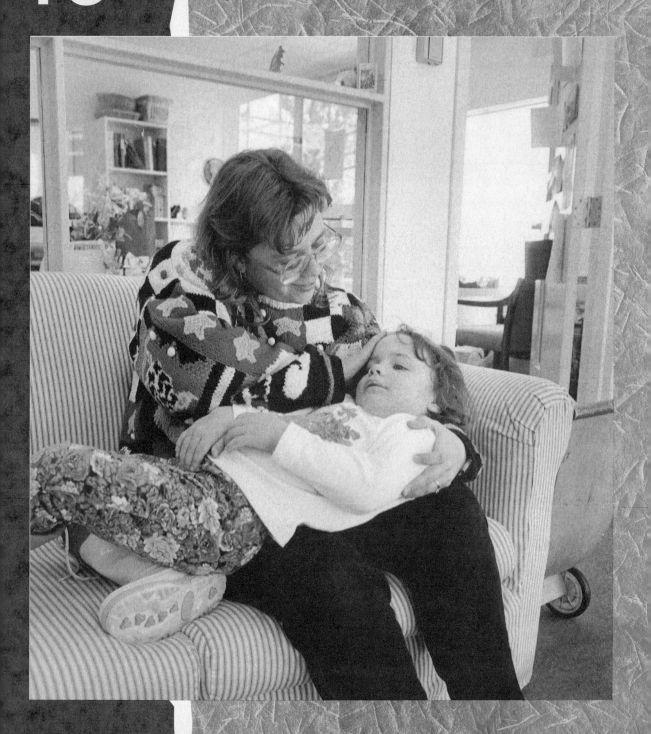

OBJECTIVES

Studying this chapter
will enable you to

- Describe ways that caregivers can
  promote children's health and
  prevent disease
- Explain the importance of health
  records and of following the
  health policies of the child care
  center
- Describe ways to recognize
  common disorders
- List strategies for protecting the
  health of children who have
  chronic disorders
- Describe ways to work effectively
  with children who have special
  needs
- Explain why caregivers should
  take care of their own health on
  and off the job

CHAPTER TERMS

asthma
chronic
fetal alcohol syndrome
hemophilia
immunization
otitis media
screenings
seizure disorder
sickle cell disease
sudden infant death syndrome

IT was early morning circle time for Margaret's prekindergarten group at the Creative Play Child Care Center. As Margaret read a story to the group, she noticed that Tiffany, usually the first to shoot up her hand with a question or comment, stared blankly at the floor. The child looked uncomfortable and pale, and Margaret decided to speak with her after the story.

While Karen, the other teacher, helped children put on their smocks for a painting activity, Margaret sat down with Tiffany and asked her if she felt okay.

"My throat hurts. My head hurts too. Right here," Tiffany said as she rubbed a spot in the middle of her forehead.

Margaret touched Tiffany's head gently and could tell immediately that the child had a fever. Just yesterday Tiffany's older brother, Shawn, had been diagnosed with strep throat. Tiffany's symptoms pointed in that direction too.

Margaret knew that a strep infection could easily be passed from child to child in the center. She also knew that Tiffany needed her attention. The Creative Play Center policy called for the teacher to stay with a sick child while the center director took over the teacher's duties. Margaret called the director on the intercom. When the director arrived, Margaret took Tiffany to the director's office, where there was a couch. After making sure that Tiffany was comfortable, Margaret called Tiffany's mother.

"I had a feeling this would happen!" Tiffany's mother said with a sigh. "I'll call our pediatrician and take Tiffany over for a throat culture right away."

Twenty minutes later, Tiffany's mother was bundling her into their station wagon. Margaret walked back inside to fill out an illness report. She was glad to have spotted Tiffany's illness early so that the child could be well soon and back with the class. Margaret hoped that her action had helped to protect the health of the rest of the class—and of the teachers as well.

Promoting Health and Preventing Disease

So far, the chapters in this book have focused on the role of nutrition in promoting the overall health of young children. But there is more to health than sound nutrition. Promoting health means recognizing illness and helping to prevent the spread of disease, as Margaret did at the Creative Play Child Care Center. It means protecting children from environmental hazards. And promoting health calls for a concern with all the aspects of health—the mental, emotional, and social well-being of children. This chapter considers the caregiver's role in promoting children's health and provides information on some common health problems and how to recognize and deal with them.

Awareness and Education

Caregivers are in a unique position to promote the health of the children in their care. Caregivers can provide a healthful environment for children, helping to prevent disease from spreading. They can provide an "early warning system" for certain kinds of problems—such as vision or hearing disorders—and can share their observations with parents or guardians. They can also help children to form healthful habits and attitudes by their examples and through the activities and routines of the child care center.

While the children are in the child care center, the caregiver is said to be *in loco parentis*, meaning that she takes the place of the parent. This role requires constant health awareness. Caregivers need to be aware of the health status of each child. And they need to consider how each child's health affects the others, since illnesses and infections can spread easily among a group of young children.

Caregivers spend a great deal of time with children, from a couple of hours several times a week to eight or ten hours each day. Caregivers may be the first to observe a problem with speech development or the frequent breathlessness that may indicate an asthmatic condition. By communicating these observations and insights to parents, caregivers can help to safeguard the health of the children in their care.

Caregivers can also help young children to learn about their bodies and about staying well. This kind of learning can give children a feeling of greater control over their lives and so contribute to their self-esteem.

Simple facts about health are the most appropriate for young children. Instruction for children should cover basic health practices, such as washing their hands, brushing their teeth, and getting enough sleep and exercise. Children can also be taught concepts that encourage social health, such as sharing with others and accepting children who have short-term or long-term health problems. They can carry a drink for a child with a broken arm or help a child with a mental disability learn a new song.

Promoting Health

Health promotion refers to the many behaviors and attitudes that strengthen a child's own resources for well-being. For example, a child who eats a healthful diet generally has greater resistance to disease and will recover from illness or injury more quickly than a child who does not. As the earlier chapters of this book have established, nutrition plays an essential role in a child's well-being. Many other behaviors and attitudes also strengthen a child's resources for overall health.

Exercise is very important for proper physical development. If the muscles are not adequately exercised, the heart and blood vessels—even the skeletal structure—can be affected. Exercise also helps the body use food energy properly. This lessens the likelihood of excessive weight gain.

Rest is crucial as well. Much of the actual development of the body occurs during rest and sleep, when the muscles recover from use and grow. Even for older children, who rarely sleep during the day, periods of rest are an important part of the center routine. Both rest and exercise are good ways to deal with the negative effects of stress. Stress is a person's response to any stimulus, physical or mental, that is seen as a threat (Jewell, 1988). Young children may experience stress in their homes, such as when a parent goes away on a business trip, when a new sibling is born, or during a long illness. In the classroom, stress can be caused by something as simple as an argument over a toy. Rest periods allow children to slow down and recover from the day's frustrations. Exercise is also an excellent remedy for stress, partly because it uses up some of the chemicals that stress causes the body to produce (Brown & Siegel, 1988).

The feelings that children have about themselves, often called their self-esteem or self-worth, are essential to their overall health and development. Children who feel appreciated by those around them and able to have an effect on their surroundings will be happier and more resilient than those who feel unloved or powerless. Caregivers can contribute to positive self-esteem by helping children to gain independence and by praising them for their accomplishments.

Throughout early childhood, children are developing social skills. Even skills that may seem simple to adults contribute in important ways to a child's social health. For example, during their early years, children spend a

Adequate exercise is important for physical development. Exercise affects the heart and blood vessels and helps the body use food properly.

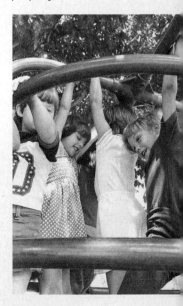

great deal of time and effort learning to share and take turns. Achieving this allows them to play together successfully, feel good about themselves, and view the world as a friendly place. Caregivers enable such skills to develop.

Preventing Disease

Health promotion includes many positive actions that contribute to overall health. However, caregivers must do more than just promote health. They must also work to prevent disease from occurring and spreading in the child care environment.

There are many basic techniques—handwashing is a simple example—that caregivers use every day to prevent the spread of disease. Chapter 11 discusses these techniques in detail. To prevent disease effectively, however, caregivers must also work with parents to make sure that children have regular attention from health care professionals. In addition, caregivers must be aware of environmental hazards to health and prevent exposure to such hazards whenever possible.

Medical and Dental Checkups.   Regular checkups are an important way for health care professionals to monitor normal development and identify health problems for diagnosis and treatment. Caregivers can be an important element in this process. First, they can encourage parents to schedule checkups regularly. Caregivers can help children recognize the importance of these visits with field trips to doctors' offices. These trips familiarize children with routines and make their checkup experiences less threatening.

Even children who have regular health examinations benefit from the observations of the caregiver. A health care professional sees the child only briefly whereas the caregiver often sees the child all day, every day. The observations of a caregiver, related to a parent, may be a key element in helping a health care professional diagnose a problem when a child becomes ill.

Regular dental checkups, too, are an important element of a child's health care. Caregivers can also help children learn good dental hygiene. In some child care centers, children brush their teeth after meals and snacks. This is an excellent time for caregivers to reinforce the importance of regular brushing. Caregivers should always monitor this activity, however. Excessive fluoride produces mottling, or discoloration, of the teeth. Swallowing excessive amounts of fluoridated toothpaste can lead to mottling. Caregivers should, therefore, discourage children from swallowing toothpaste.

Immunizations.   Immunization has been a major element in the successful advance of medical science against infectious diseases in the twentieth century. *Immunization* is a process that stimulates the immune system to make substances that protect the body from specific infectious diseases. Thanks to immunization, illnesses such as polio and diphtheria that used to cause many cases of death and disability have become rare occurrences. In recent years, however, there have been outbreaks of some diseases thought to be under control, such as measles and whooping cough. In some cases, these outbreaks have occurred because people have failed to have their children immunized.

Disease presents a great risk to young children. That is why every state requires that children be immunized before they attend public school. More than 95 percent of children receive their immunizations by that time. Many states demand proof of immunizations for preschool programs as well. Still, less than 60 percent of children under the age of two have received the immunizations that public health officials recommend (Brody, 1993). Some parents assume that because certain diseases are now rare, protection against them is no longer necessary. However, the protection by immunization against these diseases remains essential. Without adequate protection of the population, those rare diseases will become common once more. Caregivers can contribute to public health by sharing important immunization information with parents.

Environmental Risks. Because young children are growing and developing rapidly, they are especially sensitive to environmental risks. Indoor and outdoor air pollution, water pollution, spoiled food, and other dangerous substances all pose serious health risks for young children.

Regulations at federal, state, and local levels address these public health issues. Federal and state laws govern the release of industrial wastes into the air and water and the treatment of municipal sewage, garbage, and trash. State laws and local ordinances set construction and plumbing standards and rules about food handling procedures. Child care centers must meet all applicable regulations.

Caregivers must follow proper procedures for handling food (see Chapter 4) and keep all dangerous substances away from children. If hazardous substances, such as asbestos, lead, or radon, are identified in a child care center, professional removal or containment services may be necessary. It is important that caregivers also teach children the importance of avoiding dangerous substances.

Keeping Records and Following Policies

Child care centers keep many kinds of records and have standard policies to protect the health of children. Records are a source of information for caregivers on a day-to-day basis as well as when emergencies occur. Standard policies help child care centers react consistently to protect the health of all children.

Caregivers are responsible for recording information as needed, knowing where records are kept, and following the standard policies of the facility. Whenever caregivers are handling personal information about a child or a family, confidentiality is important. Information should be shared only with the center director or with another caregiver or health care professional who is involved in caring for that particular child.

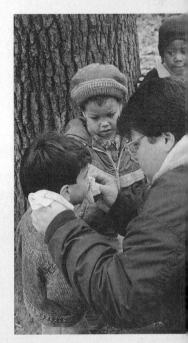

A child's health record should note even minor incidents such as a nosebleed.

Health Files

Most child care facilities ask parents for certain information about each child admitted into the program. Some of this information may be required by state or local laws. Typical information required by child care facilities includes:

- A health history
- An immunization record
- Results of a medical examination
- A list of emergency contacts

Some of this information—for example, notice of allergies to penicillin or bee stings—may be vital in an emergency. Other information may be needed for routine control or special care of conditions such as asthma, hemophilia, or diabetes. Many facilities keep records of children's height and weight. This enables staff members to track children's physical development. All of this health information must be updated regularly.

Many other pieces of information can help complete the health profile of a child. Child care centers generally include any such records that are available to them. Some examples are:

- Other measures of physical growth such as head size (for infants) or skin-fold measurements
- Specialized medical information released to the school by the parents, such as blood cholesterol levels, lead levels in the blood, or results of various screenings, particularly vision and hearing screenings

In addition, facilities generally record the daily observations of caregivers.

Emergency Information

As anyone who has been a babysitter knows, emergency contact information is extremely important. Where can the parents of a child be reached in case of an emergency or illness? Who should be called if the parents are unavailable? Who is the child's health care provider?

Child care facilities need to have up-to-date emergency information at their fingertips. The wrong telephone number or the name of a health care professional who no longer serves the child's family will be a hindrance in an emergency. Caregivers must be sure to take the files containing this information whenever children leave the facility, for example, when the class takes a field trip.

Most centers also ask parents or guardians to sign a medical release form. This is used when a child must be taken to a hospital because of an injury or illness and parents cannot get to the hospital in time. The medical release form permits authorized staff members to make decisions about the child's

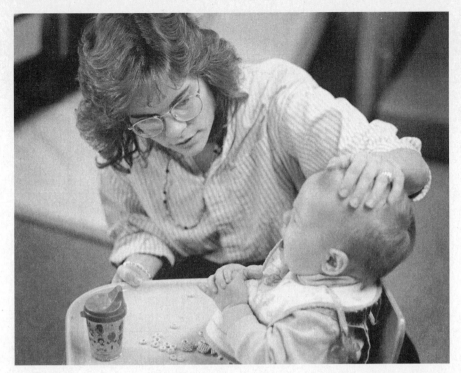

Some child care centers include health checks as part of their daily routine. Such observations help to ensure the health of the children and assure parents that their children are receiving careful attention.

medical treatment. Although most centers ask parents to sign such forms, they are used only when absolutely necessary for the health of the child. Every effort should be made to gain direct consent of the parents or guardians for *any* procedures. The religious beliefs of some groups, such as Christian Scientists and Jehovah's Witnesses, may prohibit some or all medical procedures. Caregivers must be aware of and respectful of these restrictions as well.

Daily Health Checks

Some child care facilities begin each day with a brief health check performed by the caregivers. This helps to ensure the health of each individual child and of the group. It also makes the children more aware of the importance of their own health. When such checks are part of standard policy, it is best if the people who brought the children can remain until it is completed. The health check can also assure parents that their children are receiving careful and caring attention from the staff.

Facilities that conduct standardized health checks may include the following points:

▪ Observe the child's general appearance and manner. Does the child look healthy or are there immediate signs of a problem—listlessness, paleness, or obvious discomfort. Does the child seem happy, sad, or angry?

When to Get Immediate Medical Help

Tell the parent to come right away and get medical help immediately when any of the following things happen:

- An infant under 4 months of age has an axillary temperature of 100°F or higher or a rectal temperature of 101°F or higher.
- A child over 4 months of age has a temperature of 105°F or higher.
- An infant under 4 months of age has forceful vomiting (more than once) after eating.
- Any child looks or acts very ill or seems to be getting worse quickly.
- Any child has neck pain when the head is moved or touched.
- Any child has a stiff neck or severe headache.
- Any child has a seizure for the first time.
- Any child acts unusually confused.
- Any child has uneven pupils (black centers of the eyes).
- Any child has a blood-red or purple rash made up of pinhead-sized spots or bruises that are not associated with injury.
- Any child has a rash of hives or welts that appears quickly.
- Any child breathes so fast or hard that the child cannot play, talk, cry, or drink.
- Any child has a severe stomachache that causes the child to double up and scream.
- Any child has a stomachache without vomiting or diarrhea after a recent injury, blow to the abdomen, or hard fall.
- Any child has stools that are black or have blood mixed through them.
- Any child has not urinated in more than 8 hours; the mouth and tongue look dry.
- Any child has continuous clear drainage from the nose after a hard blow to the head.

Note for programs that provide care for sick children: If any of the conditions listed above appear after the child's care has been planned, medical advice must be obtained before continuing child care can be provided.

FIGURE 10.1   When to Get Immediate Medical Help. Courtesy of the American Red Cross. All Rights Reserved in all Countries.

- Check the child for any physical signs of illness: a runny or stuffy nose, a persistent cough, a fever, a rash, inflamed cuts or sores, and so on. Some facility routines include a flashlight inspection of the mouth and throat for redness, swelling, white patches, or other unusual marks.
- Note any bruises or abrasions on a child's skin and explanations from the child or parent. Health checks aside, any observations about persistent unexplained bruising should be recorded and discussed with the director. If a child is being abused, these records will be an important factor in stopping the abuse. Recording this information also helps protect the center from charges of abuse. Chapter 13 discusses the caregiver's role in dealing with child abuse and neglect.

Caregivers must remember that they are not health care professionals and cannot diagnose illnesses or disorders in children. Their observations, however, may be very useful to health care providers when an illness is present.

Health observations are not finished when the morning health check is complete, however. Caregivers must be alert to each child's health throughout the day. A child may become irritable or may develop a cough. Diarrhea may be found during a diaper change. A child may complain about pains, a stiff neck, or a headache. Certain symptoms are a cause for special concern. Figure 10.1 lists such symptoms. These need to be taken seriously. They should be discussed with other caregivers who work with the child and the director, and noted on the child's record after any necessary action has been taken. Other symptoms are less serious but still important.

Following Center Policies

When a child seems sick, it is important to isolate him from the other children so that their health is not also endangered. Child care centers have standard procedures for dealing with illness. Parents should always be informed of a suspected illness. Sometimes the director looks after the sick child and contacts the parents. At other times, the caregiver accompanies the child to a special room while other staff members take over that person's usual responsibilities.

Caregivers should know and follow their own facility's policies on illness. Parents should also have a copy of the center's policies and procedures. This will provide clear information about the responsibilities and expectations of both caregivers and parents. In any case, caregivers should make the sick child as comfortable as possible, reassuring him that everything is being taken care of. Taking the child's temperature provides one indication of how serious the problem is (see Figure 10.2). The caregiver

How to Take a Child's Temperature

1. Wash the thermometer with soap and water, taking care not to overheat it. If the thermometer is stored in an antiseptic solution, rinse it off before using it.
2. Check the thermometer for broken edges, especially around the bulb.
3. Shake the mercury down to near the bottom of the thermometer.
4. Place a new disposable thermometer cover on the thermometer.
5a. (oral method) Place the bulb end of the thermometer in the child's mouth so the bulb rests beneath the back of the tongue. Instruct the child to close her lips around the thermometer but not to bite it. Hold the thermometer while it is in the child's mouth, and leave it there for seven minutes.

or

5b. (axillary method) Place the bulb end of the thermometer against the child's skin under the armpit. Bring the child's arm down against the side of the body. Leave the thermometer in place for five minutes.
6. Remove the thermometer and discard the cover. Read the thermometer by holding it level and rotating it until the mercury appears.
7. Normal oral temperature is 98.6°F (37°C). Normal axillary temperature may be as much as 1 degree F lower.

Notes:
- The oral method is preferred. Use the axillary method only on younger children, who may have difficulty keeping a thermometer under their tongues with their mouths closed for long periods of time without biting.
- Rectal temperature taking is not recommended because of the risk of rectal perforation.
- In addition to traditional mercury thermometers, other devices, such as digital, electronic, and plastic strip thermometers, and the tympanic membrane sensor (via the ear), may be used according to the instructions provided with them. These devices avoid problems of breakage and mercury exposure. However, plastic strip thermometers have been known to produce inaccurately high readings.

FIGURE 10.2   How to Take a Child's Temperature.

HEALTH TIPS

Common Rashes

Poison Ivy or Oak
Red, itchy, oozing
blisters

Ringworm Red, scaly,
ring-shaped rash on the
chest, abdomen, or back

Impetigo Oozy red
sores, especially on the
face, that become
covered with yellow
crusts; sometimes
accompanied by fever

Eczema Oozing red
rash, often on elbows,
wrists, and knees, and
around eyes

Prickly Heat Tiny,
uniform red blisters in
raised clusters; appear
during hot weather or
when children are
"bundled up" in winter

Chicken Pox Flat
blotches that turn into
raised, itchy blisters
that form crusts when
broken; may start on
scalp and spread to the
rest of the body, and be
accompanied by fever

Measles Pink, blotchy
rash that starts on face;
may be itchy and scaly
with possible fever or
cough

should then follow facility policies in calling the child's parents or another emergency contact person, giving as much information as possible. Some centers require that a sick child be picked up. Others are set up to care for children with minor illnesses. In any case, the caregiver should continue to comfort the child while he is at the center. He can color or draw a picture, "write" a letter to his mother or father, cuddle a blanket, or talk to his parents if he wishes. If emergency contacts cannot be reached, caregivers should work closely with the center director, following center policies in caring for the sick child and obtaining medical assistance if necessary.

All caregivers in a facility should be trained in basic first aid and CPR (cardiopulmonary resuscitation—a procedure used if a person stops breathing or has no pulse). This will allow them to deal with sudden illness or injury most effectively.

Recognizing Common Disorders

Some children may have conditions, such as poor vision, poor hearing, or internal disorders, that have not been diagnosed. Undiscovered, these conditions may have cumulative effects. Certain chemical disorders, for example, can lead to mental retardation if they are not treated.

Some conditions can be detected through screenings. *Screenings* are tests performed on apparently healthy people. Screenings are designed to detect disorders at an early stage so they can be treated effectively. A child's first screenings usually occur at birth, when health care professionals use a screening test for general alertness and health. State laws may require a number of other tests to check for conditions such as PKU (phenylketonuria) or thyroid disorders. Babies who are born at home may not have these screenings. If access to medical care is a problem for financial, religious, or cultural reasons, older children may also miss out on screening tests.

During the preschool years, common screenings include those for vision and hearing. Caregivers can supplement screening information by reporting their observations about children. By being alert for signs of vision, hearing, or speech problems, caregivers can contribute to their early detection. Once the disorders are diagnosed, caregivers can offer special support and care to the child. Some states offer assistance with testing and diagnosing some common disorders, particularly vision and hearing problems.

Vision Disorders

Common vision problems are of two types—problems with the shape of the eye and problems with muscular control of the eyes. When the shape of the eye is abnormal, the image that a child sees is out of focus. Such problems can be easily remedied by wearing glasses, but the problem must first be identified. Caregivers can watch for signs of vision problems by noting if a child makes great efforts during visual tasks—leaning forward, squinting, rubbing the eyes, holding an object very close or very far away in order to see it, or complaining of headaches. These signs indicate that a child may have a vision problem and should be checked. There are special vision tests that display pictures rather than letters for children who are too young to read.

Strabismus is the name for several eye disorders caused by improper muscle control of the eyes. The eyes fail to work together properly, leading to double vision or eyes that cross or drift. If the child compensates by using one eye over the other, vision in the less-used eye will deteriorate and blindness in that eye may result. Caregivers should report any crossing or drifting of the eyes to parents, as well as complaints of headaches. Strabismus can be treated with appropriate intervention, which may involve wearing eyeglasses or an eye patch, or doing eye exercises.

Hearing Disorders

Hearing problems may be more difficult to detect than vision problems. Sometimes a child is slow to react when spoken to or keeps saying "what?" or "huh?" She may always turn an ear toward the speaker or may carefully watch the speaker's face. A child might lose interest in stories very quickly and rarely join in conversations.

At other times, the clue to poor hearing comes from language—a child speaks unclearly and is difficult to understand. He may also speak rarely or have a voice that sounds hoarse or unusually loud. These behaviors can indicate hearing problems, though there may be other causes as well.

Hearing problems are often associated with frequent ear infections. *Otitis media*, or middle ear infection, is a common complication of colds and throat infections in young children. Ear infections can cause severe pain and temporary hearing loss. Repeated and prolonged infections can damage middle ear structures and cause permanent hearing loss.

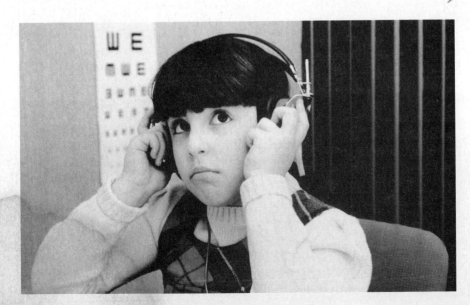

Hearing problems can sometimes be difficult to detect. Tests performed by hearing specialists can help.

Tests performed by hearing specialists can determine whether there is a hearing problem. If there is, the child can be referred to a health care professional for treatment. If a hearing problem remains undetected, it can cause delays in the development of language and affect the child's ability to learn during the early years.

Speech Disorders

Delayed speech may be the result of hearing problems or other conditions. Caregivers may be in an especially good position to notice that a child is lagging in speech development because they spend so much time observing the child along with other children of the same age.

Caregivers should remember, however, that there is great natural variation in speech development between individual children. Caregivers can, however, communicate to parents their observations about possible speech delays or difficulties. Parents can then examine the problem further with an appropriate health care professional.

Learning Disabilities

Children with learning disabilities may have difficulty with any of a number of tasks, including concentrating, memorizing, speaking, reading, writing, or performing mathematical calculations. These disabilities are often difficult to diagnose, even in older children. In children under five, they are rarely identified.

Caregivers may report to parents any unusual problems with concentration or memory, keeping in mind the developmental level of the child. Parents can then decide whether or not to have further testing done.

Working with Children with Chronic Disorders

Certain disorders are called *chronic*, meaning that they persist for a long time. Chronic disorders are not usually passed from person to person. Children and families learn to live with a chronic condition rather than expect it to be cured or go away on its own. It is important that caregivers understand and know how to care for children with the most common of these disorders. They should also request specific direction about the child's care from the child's parents or health care provider and the center director.

Asthma

Asthma is a condition in which swelling of lung tissues interferes with breathing. Most children who have problems with asthma suffer their first attacks before the age of five. An attack can be brought on by an allergy to dust, particular types of animals, or other substances. It can also be triggered by other factors, including stress, sudden temperature changes, breathing cigarette smoke, or overexertion (Mott, 1990).

FOCUS ON *Cultural Diversity*

Ethnic Home Remedies

Long before corner drugstores sold medicines for every illness, families relied on their own cures. Recipes for cough syrups, headache cures, and "spring tonics" were passed down from parents to children. Many are still used today.

People from many different ethnic backgrounds think of chicken soup when they get colds. In fact, steam from the hot broth helps unclog a stuffy nose, and the liquid goes down easily, providing needed nourishment without irritating a sore throat. Depending on the culture, noodles, vegetables, or matzo balls may be added to chicken soup.

Asians have long believed that herbal remedies can enhance health. Ginseng root, for example, is sometimes given to women after childbirth. Europeans brew tea from the flowers of the chamomile plant to relieve upset stomachs.

In some Hispanic households, tea made from an herb called manzanilla is traditionally used to treat stomach ailments. American children and adults have been given castor oil as a laxative since colonial times.

Traditional remedies are not always ingested. Sometimes they are worn on the body. Commercial eucalyptus-scented chest rubs are related to homemade rubs that use ingredients such as turpentine to relieve cold symptoms. In Mediterranean cultures, garlic, whether worn or eaten, is used to ward off illness and infection. Africans and African Americans traditionally use a strong-smelling plant called asafetida for the same purpose.

Certain traditional cures include ingredients that are used in modern medicines. Long before European settlers arrived, some Native Americans chewed willow bark (or drank willow bark tea) to relieve headaches. Salicin, a chemical found in willow bark, is related to the salicylic acid that is used to make aspirin.

During an attack of asthma, the child suddenly finds it difficult to breathe. Breathing out takes a great effort and may be accompanied by wheezing. Breathing in also becomes difficult because the lungs have not been emptied and considerable pain may be present.

A child who is asthmatic may use a vaporizer or inhaler that contains medication to help control the symptoms. Other medications may also be used to help prevent attacks. Parents need to make sure that the proper medications are kept at the child care facility. People with asthma often feel advance warnings of an attack. Caregivers should learn how the vaporizer or inhaler is used and should be familiar with the child's advance symptoms. Caregivers should also find ways to reduce exposure to substances or situations that bring on attacks.

Seizure Disorder

Seizure disorder, commonly known as epilepsy, is caused by unusually strong discharges of electricity in the brain. Isolated seizures may occur in many people, particularly young children who are suffering from a high fever.

These are unrelated to chronic seizure disorder. Seizure disorder is characterized by recurring seizures and may be caused by birth defects, genetic disorders, or injuries to the brain. Seizures may be characterized by a period of staring or blankness, or by convulsive movements of the body.

Most seizures can be controlled with medication. Caregivers need to be aware of medication schedules and follow them carefully. Caregivers should know the first-aid procedures for seizures in case they occur. The most important general instructions are to protect the child from injuring himself or others.

Circulatory and Blood Disorders

Some children may have heart conditions in which the ability of the heart to pump blood throughout the body is reduced. These heart defects may be caused by disease, as when rheumatic fever has damaged the heart valves, or may have been present at birth.

The circulatory system is also affected by hemophilia. In children with *hemophilia*, blood does not clot properly. Severe or even fatal blood loss can result. Children with hemophilia need special injections to help their blood to clot effectively. They also need to be protected from injury as much as possible, but they can participate in a number of physical activities. Caregivers should seek instruction on how to deal with bleeding episodes if they occur. Hemophilia is caused by a genetic defect.

Another genetic defect causes *sickle cell disease*. In affected children, the red blood cells do not form normally and are unable to carry the needed supply of oxygen to the body's tissues. The misshapen cells clog small blood vessels producing pain, damage to internal organs, and potentially fatal infections. Children with sickle cell disease may have joint pain, breathing difficulties, and may move slowly and sluggishly. Severe episodes, called crises, may require hospitalization.

Other Disorders

Some chronic disorders, such as diabetes, cystic fibrosis, and PKU have already been discussed in Chapter 9. Caregivers may also care for children with other disorders, such as those caused by toxic substances. These may affect the child either before or after birth and can produce serious health consequences.

Children may have been harmed during the fetal period of development if their mothers used certain drugs or drank alcoholic beverages. *Fetal alcohol syndrome* is characterized by abnormal development of the fetus, stunted growth, mental retardation, and recognizable facial irregularities that include a thin upper lip and a short, upturned nose in the child later on. There is evidence that rates of fetal alcohol syndrome are increasing (Fetal alcohol syndrome, 1993).

Lead in the environment can also cause severe health problems. Children who inhale or consume toxic amounts of lead suffer damage to the blood,

FOCUS ON   Communicating with Parents

Home Sources of Lead

Janine, the caregiver, always looks forward to seeing Mrs. Astin when she comes to pick up her two-year-old, Teddy. This evening Teddy nearly tackles his mother in greeting her. He holds the remains of the afternoon snack in his hand.

MRS. ASTIN: What in the world did you have for snack?

JANINE: It's a kumquat. We're trying to get the kids to try some new foods. I think Teddy will be a gourmet when he grows up. He'll try anything and likes almost all the foods we give him.

MRS. ASTIN: You're telling me. At home he even eats paint off the walls!

JANINE: He does? (with a troubled look) Do you live in an older building?

MRS. ASTIN: Yes, it's one of those wonderful old structures with huge rooms and windows. My apartment has so much room. Why do you ask?

JANINE: Sometimes older apartments have old paint on the walls. The paint may have lead in it. You probably know, Mrs. Astin, that lead can be very bad for children. I'm worried that Teddy may be getting lead in the peeling paint he eats.

MRS. ASTIN: I know paint isn't good for him, but I never thought of lead poisoning. What can I do?

JANINE: If your apartment hasn't been painted in a long time, you may be entitled by law to a new paint job. Find out from your landlord or the housing authority. If they do paint, make sure they scrape all the old paint off the walls, clean it up completely from your apartment, and dispose of it as toxic waste. Any paint they use nowadays is lead-free.

MRS. ASTIN: You know, my apartment hasn't been painted since I've been there, and that's over five years. I'll get in touch with my landlord immediately. I'm certainly glad you told me about this. I want Teddy to be healthy.

JANINE: There are other things you should look out for too. Sometimes old buildings have water pipes that have been put together using lead solder. If that's the case, there may also be lead in your drinking water.

MRS. ASTIN: But what can I do about that? We have to drink the water.

JANINE: The local water department is required by law to test any water that might contain lead. Give them a call and they'll tell you how to have your water tested. They can also tell you what to do if there *is* a problem.

MRS. ASTIN: Thanks so much, Janine. I'll make those calls right away.

How would you have handled this situation? Do you think Janine alarmed Mrs. Astin unnecessarily? What would you have done differently?

the kidneys, and the brain and nervous system. The main source of lead to-day is old lead paint used in homes (Whaley & Wong, 1991). One chip of lead paint may contain 500 to 1,000 times more lead than is safe for a child to ingest in a day. Lead-based paint is no longer sold in stores.

Other sources of lead are old plumbing and industrial and transportation fumes. Lead is most damaging to children whose diets contain inadequate iron, calcium, or zinc. Children who habitually eat nonfood substances, a condition known as pica, are at particular risk.

Anyone who cares for infants has probably heard about the frightening phenomenon known as sudden infant death syndrome. *Sudden infant death syndrome* (SIDS) refers to cases in which a child suddenly and unexpectedly dies in his crib. Medical professionals have been unable to explain why this happens. It is likely that there are many different causes for such a death—none of which are the result of any error on the part of the parents or care-givers. However, recent studies suggest that fewer of these deaths occur when children are laid in their cribs on their sides or backs rather than on their stomachs (Altman, 1993).

Working with Children with Special Needs

More child care programs today are including children with special needs, sometimes called children with disabilities, in their regular classes. Children with special needs include those who have chronic illnesses, family difficul-ties, and physical and mental impairments. By focusing on the abilities of children with special needs rather than on their disabilities, caregivers can contribute to the children's success and acceptance as part of the group.

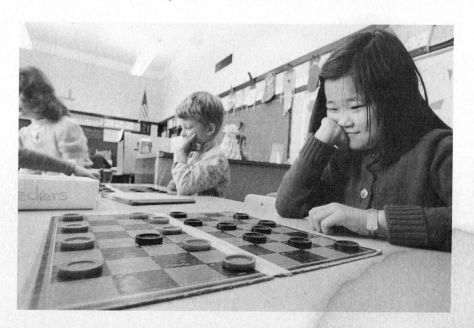

Children who have chronic illnesses may wear a Medic-Alert bracelet. Many such children require special care only during crisis periods.

FOCUS ON Promoting Healthful Habits

Including Children with Disabilities

Andy, a four-year-old in Petra's preschool class, often dominates the children's games and activities. During the two weeks since the preschool year began, Andy has been picking on Roger, an amiable child who has a physical disability that confines him to a wheelchair. Andy began by trying to exclude Roger from games. If Andy saw that Roger was the center of attention in another group, Andy would go over and belittle Roger.

Petra has spoken to Andy nearly every day about his behavior, but she realizes now that she will have to have a serious talk with the class about inclusion. This morning Andy is more abusive than usual to Roger. As Roger tries to join Andy's group, he pushes himself between Roger's wheelchair and the table. "You can't play with us. Go away!" Andy says.

Suddenly, an angry voice rings through the classroom. Marlene, one of the other children, strides over to the table. "Stop it, Andy," she cries. "Stop being mean to Roger!"

"He can't do anything right," Andy replies. "He's dumb."

Marlene places herself in front of Andy and he steps backward. "My . . . my brother," she stammers, "he's in a wheelchair too. He was born with a sickness. But he can do almost anything. My brother has a million friends. Everybody likes him. Not like you. You're mean. Nobody likes you."

Marlene stops and begins to sob. The other children seem stunned. Petra takes this moment to gather the children around her, realizing that Marlene's passionate outburst has had a greater effect on the children than anything Petra could have said. Marlene's words have affected Andy, too, who looks confused and on the verge of tears. In a soft voice, Petra begins talking about how all of us sometimes misunderstand people who are different from us. Petra knows that both children and adults sometimes act thoughtlessly, but she hopes that in time all the children, even Andy, will be much more open to including children with disabilities in their games.

Did Petra handle the situation well? Do you think she waited too long to deal with Andy? What would you have done?

Early Childhood Programs and Special Needs

The Americans with Disabilities Act (often called the ADA) was passed in 1990. It requires all facilities open to the public to provide accommodations for people who have disabilities. Sections of the law require that public services be made available to individuals who have disabilities. The law applies to child care centers as well as other public places. It requires them to take readily achievable actions to prevent discrimination against children with special needs. They are not, however, required to take actions that would put on the program what the act calls an "undue burden."

As a result, caregivers may find that the children in their care include a broader range of abilities and that more of them have special needs than in the past. Child care programs have, however, been accommodating children

Although children with physical disabilities should be given the opportunity to take care of themselves as much as possible, some situations may require that they receive special attention and care.

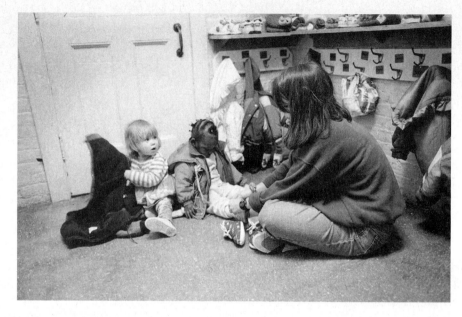

with special needs for years. The lives of all children—those designated as having special needs and others as well—can benefit from group experiences of this type.

Types of Disabilities

Most early childhood education programs share similar goals: to provide children with the opportunity to develop their skills to the fullest, to have them experience feelings of competence and high self-esteem, and to allow them to enjoy acceptance from their peers. These goals apply to all children, regardless of their individual needs.

Children with disabilities do require special care, however. Different equipment or supplies may be needed, for example wheelchairs, special bathroom facilities, or a set of crayons with pads attached that are easy to grasp. Some children may need to be steered toward the tasks and projects at which they can be successful—a child may excel at pasting but not at cutting. By understanding some of the differences in abilities among individuals with special needs, caregivers can care for them most effectively.

Physical Disabilities. Helping children who suffer from physical disabilities can be fairly straightforward. The physical space of a room can be altered to allow a child in a wheelchair to move about easily. Many adaptive tools and materials are available, from special spoons to adaptive scissors and crayons.

It is important to avoid doing too much for physically disabled children. They need to practice and experience the satisfaction of taking care of themselves as much as possible (Farrell, 1985). Caregivers should, however, be sure that these children are given adequate time to succeed as well as to rest. Some activities will be more difficult and require more effort. Displaying patience and encouraging patience and acceptance from other children are two ways of contributing to the success of children with physical disabilities.

Mental Disabilities.   Acceptance and success are also vital for the optimum development of children who have mental disabilities. Mental disabilities include mental retardation and emotional and social problems. Caregivers of children with mental disabilities should allow for extra explanation time as well as additional practice. It may be necessary to break ideas into small steps and repeat them several times. Caregivers can encourage the other children to display greater patience through their own examples.

Children with emotional and social problems benefit from a carefully structured environment. Rules must be realistic but consistently enforced. Caregivers need to be especially sensitive to these children in order to read the cues that indicate their feelings. Many difficulties can be avoided by recognizing a problem as it develops.

Multiple Disabilities.   Multiple disabilities can occur for various reasons. Children who are affected by one disability may begin to develop others if the first is not identified. For example, apparent learning disabilities may appear in a deaf child if the hearing impairment is not diagnosed. Some prenatal influences affect more than one aspect of fetal development so that slight physical irregularities may be accompanied by emotional or mental disabilities. This is the case with fetal alcohol syndrome.

Caregivers of children with multiple disabilities must take their various needs into account. However, the need these children have to develop their abilities, to experience success and competence, and to be recognized and accepted as a valuable member of the group remains the same.

The Caregiver's Health

Caregivers can get so caught up with the health of the children in their care that they lose sight of their own health needs (Kendrick, Kaufmann, & Messenger, 1991). This can have serious consequences. For example, caregivers of young children are exposed to a wide variety of diseases. Certain childhood diseases such as rubella (German measles) can cause severe defects in a developing fetus. Pregnant caregivers who have not had rubella must take preventive measures against contracting the disease.

Caregivers who do not take care of their health may suffer frequent illnesses and loss of time at work. This affects the children they work with as well as the caregivers themselves. The children in their care lose the security of knowing that the same people will be there each day. Caregivers who come to work sick may spread illnesses among the children. And caregivers cannot devote their full attention to the children when they themselves are not feeling well.

To prevent back injury, caregivers should learn the proper way to lift a child—by bending the knees, holding the child close, and lifting with the leg muscles.

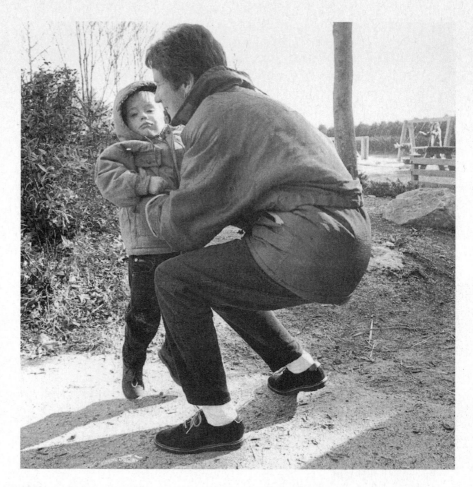

Caregivers who take wise health precautions act in everyone's best interest. They are also setting good examples for the children enrolled in their programs.

Applying for Work

Because the health of caregivers is so important, most child care centers pay particular attention to health issues in hiring new staff members. Most facilities inquire about the applicant's immunization status and history of childhood diseases. Facilities may require a medical examination before the person is hired. Centers may also ask about back injuries and other physical problems that can make it difficult for prospective caregivers to provide sound care to young children.

Because of caregivers' responsibilities to their jobs, they should be especially careful to seek and follow the advice of health care professionals. The center will usually require that staff members have periodic health examinations and see a health care professional if they have been ill or other health concerns have surfaced. The health requirements for employment in a child care center should be available in writing for review. Caregivers should understand that health requirements exist for their protection as well as to protect the children in the center.

Illness and the Caregiver

It is particularly important that caregivers stay away from work if they become sick, even if they think that they caught the illness at the center. When they consult a health care provider, caregivers should indicate that they work with young children. This information can be an aid to diagnosis and an important factor in the determination of medical advice on when to return to work. With diseases such as strep throat and impetigo, caregivers may be allowed to return to work once they are on medication. However, other conditions may require caregivers to stay away for longer periods of time. For this reason, caregivers should review the health policies at a particular center *before* accepting a job there. What are their sick leave policies? Do they have adequate backup policies if a staff member is sick so that workers will not feel pressured to come to work when they have health problems? Does the center require up-to-date immunizations for the children? All these are important questions for caregivers to find out the answers to.

Promoting Health at Work

Finally, caregivers need to be aware of how their own behaviors affect health during the working day. Adopting certain practices and precautions helps protect everyone's health. It also sets a tone for healthful living that can influence the children's behavior.

Some behaviors that affect health and safety are covered in the following chapters. Chapter 11, for example, discusses various precautions to take when handling substances that may be infectious. Chapter 12 discusses storage of dangerous substances. When handling any potentially harmful substances such as paint or cleaning fluids, caregivers should wear rubber gloves. They protect the skin and prevent caregivers from spreading any harmful materials after they finish the work. Caregivers should never work with such materials when children are present. Aerosol sprays are especially hazardous because the droplets get into the air and can affect children who are some distance from the user.

Caregivers can minimize the possibility of back injuries by following sensible procedures. They should lift children (and heavy objects) by holding them close to the body with the knees bent, then lifting with the leg muscles. Leaning forward and lifting with the back and shoulders can cause injury. Whenever possible, caregivers should sit on adult-sized chairs. Sitting awkwardly often contributes to back problems.

Caregivers should allow time for rest and relaxation outside work. They should also take advantage of break periods during the day. Caregivers who take care of their own health will be better able to take care of the health of children as well.

SUMMARY

- Caregivers can promote health by being observant, reporting their observations, and helping children learn simple health concepts.

- Both exercise and rest are crucial for physical and mental health. They help children deal with the effects of stress in their lives.

- Caregivers play an important role in helping children develop high self-esteem and healthy social relationships.

- Immunization of children helps prevent the spread of disease. Many states require proof of immunization for school (and sometimes preschool) admission.

- Up-to-date emergency information must always be readily available.

- Daily health checks performed by caregivers can protect everyone's health and are one way to monitor children's health status.

- Caregivers should follow center policies concerning treatment of sick children. Caregivers should make sick children comfortable and contact their parents.

- Special screening procedures can uncover hidden disorders so that they can be treated. Caregivers can supplement these screenings with their observations.

- Caregivers should be alert to the signs of vision disorders, which may be signaled by great efforts during visual tasks or complaints of headaches.

- Caregivers should watch for signs of hearing disorders, such as lack of response to sound or unclear speech. Repeated ear infections may cause hearing loss.

- Caregivers should report to parents any speech delays they note, but they should recognize the wide variety in speech development.

- Learning disabilities may appear in a number of areas, but they are rarely identified before the age of five.

- Caregivers should know how to protect the health of children with chronic disorders, such as asthma, seizure disorder, hemophilia, and sickle cell disease.

- Caregivers need to be responsive to children with special needs in their programs. The abilities of these children may vary widely.

- For caregivers' sake as well as the children's sake, caregivers must take care of their own health.

- Child care employers must take health issues into account when hiring employees and may request a medical examination or health-related information.

- Caregivers must seek professional help when ill and avoid spreading disease within the center.

ACQUIRING KNOWLEDGE

1. What are the two parts of the caregiver's role in promoting health and preventing disease?
2. Identify two reasons why exercise is important.
3. Why are rest and sleep important?
4. Describe the caregiver's role in helping children achieve high self-esteem and social health.
5. How can caregivers contribute to the work of health care professionals regarding medical and dental checkups?
6. What problem can arise when children routinely swallow large amounts of fluoridated toothpaste while brushing their teeth?
7. Define immunization. Why is it especially important that children be immunized?
8. What must be done if asbestos, lead, or radon are found in a child care center?
9. List two ways in which caregivers might use health records kept at the child care facility.
10. What types of information should be included in a child's health file?
11. What information must be available to caregivers in case of an emergency?
12. What is a daily health check? List three things caregivers might do during a daily health check.
13. Identify two elements in a typical child care center's policy on children's illnesses.
14. What are screenings? Give two examples of screenings children may have.
15. Describe three symptoms of vision problems.
16. What is otitis media? What more serious problem can otitis media lead to?
17. How should caregivers respond to apparent problems with speech development or learning?
18. What is asthma?
19. What causes seizure disorder?
20. Describe the symptoms and causes of fetal alcohol syndrome.
21. What impact has the Americans with Disabilities Act had on child care facilities?
22. What are three categories of disabilities?
23. List two reasons why caregivers should take good care of their own health.
24. Explain how health issues could become important in applying for a child care position.
25. What special precautions should caregivers take when they are ill?

THINKING CRITICALLY

1. By the time they reach school age, more than 95 percent of children have received their required immunizations. Less than 60 percent of children under the age of two have been immunized, however. Why do you think so many parents delay having their children immunized? What motivates them to finally immunize their children?

2. Why is it important that records and health information about children be kept confidential?

3. React to the following statement: "Early detection and intervention of developmental problems is important in order to prevent one problem from developing into multiple problems."

4. Children with a variety of health-related problems may be together in a preschool class. How can a caregiver be prepared to handle the problems of an asthmatic child, for example, as well as that of a child who suffers from seizure disorder?

5. As a result of the Americans with Disabilities Act, child care centers will be more likely to accept children who have disabilities into regular programs. What advantages do you see in including children who have disabilities in preschool classes?

OBSERVATIONS AND APPLICATIONS

1. Observe children at a child care center during a rest period. What are the ages of the children you observe? How many of the children actually sleep during the rest period? Do children who are not sleeping rest quietly on their mats? Do all the children lie down or do some play? What is the noise level in the room? What do caregivers do during the rest time?

2. Observe children as they are dropped off at a child care center in the morning. Note the interactions between the adults and the caregivers concerning children's health. Note health-related interactions between caregivers and children as well. What do parents and caregivers say to one another concerning children's health? (For example, a parent might say: "Scott went to bed very late last night so don't be surprised if he is grouchy this morning. He's not sick. He's just tired.") Do the caregivers perform a health check? If so, what is included?

3. Suppose that Reggie is a three-year-old child in your preschool class. You notice that he speaks very loudly and unclearly, and that he is frequently unresponsive when you speak to him. What problems might you suspect? What would you say to his parents about what you have observed?

4. Imagine that four-year-old Kieran comes to you complaining that she is not feeling well. You feel her forehead and it is hot. You send her to the office where her temperature is taken. She has a fever of 102°F. The school director calls her mother at work. She is told that Kieran's mother no longer works at that office. She then tries to call her at home. There is no answer. She is unable to reach anyone listed on the emergency form. What should be done? How can this situation be prevented in the future?

FOR FURTHER INFORMATION

American Academy of Pediatrics & American Public Health Association. (1992). *Caring for our children—national health and safety performance standards: Guidelines for out-of-home child care programs.* Elk Grove Village, IL and Washington, DC: Author.

American Lung Association. (1990). *Asthma alert for teachers.* New York: Author.

American Lung Association. (1992). *Open airways for schools.* New York: Author.

Barnes, K. E. (1982). *Preschool screening: The measurement and prediction of children-at-risk.* Springfield, IL: Charles C. Thomas Publisher.

Burnette, J. (1987). *Adapting instructional materials for mainstreamed students.* Reston, VA: The Council for Exceptional Children.

Deitch, S. R. (Ed.). (1987). *Health in day care: A manual for health professionals.* Evanston, IL: American Academy of Pediatrics.

Disabilities: An overview. (1987). Reston, VA: Clearinghouse on Handicapped and Gifted Children.

Dixon, S. D. (1990). Talking to the child's physician: Thoughts for the child care provider. *Young Children, 45* (3), 36–37.

Johnson, D. D. (1992). *I can't sit still: Educating and affirming inattentive and hyperactive children.* Santa Cruz, CA: ETR Associates.

Kendrick, A. S., Kaufmann, R., & Messenger, P. (1991). *Healthy young children: A manual for programs.* Washington, DC: National Association for the Education of Young Children.

Lammers, J. W. (1991). *I don't feel good: A guide to childhood complaints and diseases.* Santa Cruz, CA: ETR Associates.

Ottney, J. R. (1991). *Fetal alcohol syndrome facts and choices: A guide for teachers* (2nd ed.). Madison, WI: University of Wisconsin.

Pillitteri, A. P. (1992). *Maternal health and child nursing: Care of the childbearing and childrearing family.* Philadelphia: J. B. Lippincott.

Villarreal, S., McKinney, L., Quackenbush, M., & Scheer, J. K. (1992). *Handle with care: Helping children prenatally exposed to drugs and alcohol.* Santa Cruz, CA: ETR Associates.

11 Illness and Infectious Diseases

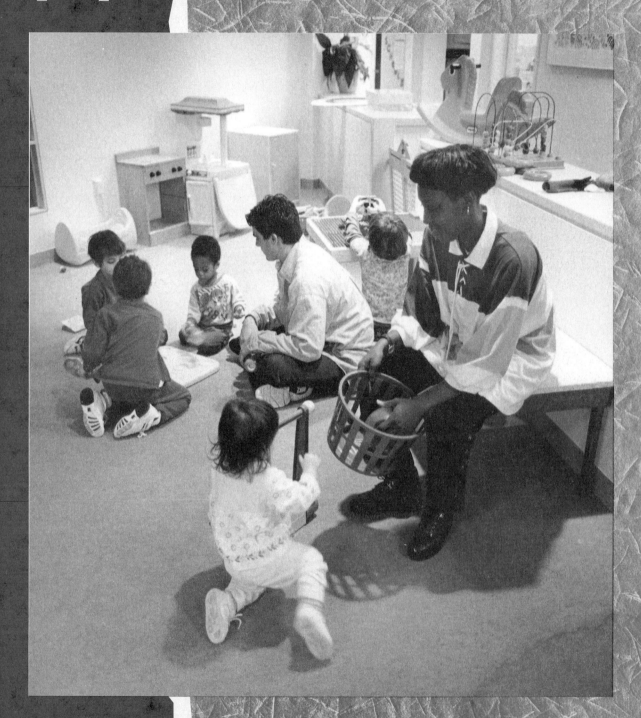

OBJECTIVES

Studying this chapter
will enable you to

- Explain why children in child care
  are at greater risk from infectious
  diseases than children at home
- Explain the difference between
  communicable and
  noncommunicable diseases
- Describe several of the
  communicable infections that
  affect children and their main
  modes of transmission
- Describe several of the
  noncommunicable infections that
  affect children and their main
  modes of transmission
- Discuss the use of vaccines to
  prevent the transmission of certain
  diseases
- Give examples of ways to minimize
  the spread of disease in a child
  care setting

CHAPTER TERMS

acute stage

carrier

communicable diseases

host

incubation period

infectious diseases

noncommunicable diseases

pathogens

prodromal stage

recovery stage

reportable disease

universal precautions

ROSE and Hector are working late at the Darby Community Center child care program. The full-day program is designed to serve children ages six months through five years. The after-school program is for children ages 6 through 12. Most of the children get picked up by 5:30, but the program remains open each day until 7 P.M. After 5:30, the few remaining children are combined into one group so that most of the caregivers can leave. Children from other rooms bring their belongings to the infant-toddler room and pile them by the door while they wait for their parents to come pick them up.

"Phew," says Rose to Hector, "I think Maurice has another dirty diaper. It's his fourth today. I wonder if there's something wrong with him. He doesn't act sick." Picking up the toddler, Rose carries him over to the changing table and begins to remove his diaper. She is still cleaning his bottom when three-year-old Joanna wanders over.

"Rose, can you please tie my shoe?" asks Joanna.

"Sure I can tie your shoe, but first I have to finish changing Maurice."

"That's okay, Rose," says Hector. "I'll help Joanna with her shoe."

Pulling up Maurice's pants, Rose lifts him off the changing table and heads for the sink. She washes Maurice's hands before bringing him back to his friends who are playing with the dump truck. Rose is still washing her own hands when Sarah's father arrives to take her home. A moment later, Darren's grandmother appears, ready to gather up Darren and his belongings.

Maurice's mother is one of the last parents to come. "Maurice has had four dirty diapers today. The last one was pretty messy," Rose tells her.

"Oh my," says Maurice's mother. "Do you think he's sick?"

"I don't know," replies Rose. "He doesn't act sick and he doesn't feel like he has a fever. But maybe he's coming down with something."

Finally all the children have gone home. Rose and Hector tidy the room. Rose gathers up Maurice's dirty diaper and the disposable table cover, which she had forgotten on the changing table when Joanna distracted her. She dumps them in the diaper pail, saying with a sigh, "I'm glad that didn't happen in the middle of the day!"

"Really!" agrees Hector. "Especially if Maurice is getting sick."

Rose wipes down the changing table with the disinfectant bleach solution and disposes of the rest of the mixture. She washes her hands, turns off the light, and follows Hector out the door.

Childhood Diseases and Health Problems

Although illness can strike at any age, certain diseases and health problems are more common in children than in adults. These range from mild colds to serious diseases such as scarlet fever. Children get some diseases because their immature immune systems provide incomplete protection. Other common childhood problems, such as ear infections, are related to children's immature physical structures. Still other health hazards, such as head lice, spread easily among children because they routinely have close physical contact when they play together.

The Changing Face of Childhood Disease

A century ago, childhood deaths from disease or illness were common. In the United States in 1900, one out of every six babies died during infancy. By 1992, the infant mortality rate had dropped to less than 1 out of every 100 live births. The two main reasons why more children are surviving today are advances in medical care and improved public health conditions.

During the early part of the twentieth century, scientists made many discoveries that resulted in the development of new medicines and vaccines. Antibiotics, such as penicillin, became widely available in the 1940s. As a result, many life-threatening infections could be controlled for the first time. Vaccines were also developed, providing immunity against infections such as polio and diphtheria. Eventually, immunization with certain vaccines became mandatory for entry into elementary school. Today, researchers continue developing new vaccines to improve the health of children and adults.

Advances in medicine were accompanied by advances in public health protection. By the middle of this century, most areas of the United States had flush toilets, public sewers, municipal water, and public garbage collection. Local and state governments established public health codes that regulated many aspects of sanitation, such as waste disposal, food preparation and storage, and water purification. Health education increased public awareness of the connection between good nutrition and health. Advances in transportation, food refrigeration, and food storage brought changes in people's diets. It became possible to have a variety of fresh fruits and vegetables year-round. The dairy industry became subject to regulations on sanitary practices and pasteurization of milk. Taken together, all these changes have drastically reduced childhood fatalities from disease.

Disease in Child Care Settings

A recent U.S. Census Bureau report shows that about 55 percent of preschool children of working mothers are cared for by nonrelatives. Most of these child care arrangements are group settings, such as child care centers, preschools, family day-care providers, and workplace care centers (Chira, 1993). Although medical and scientific advances have brought many childhood diseases under control, bringing together large numbers of preschoolers in a child care setting increases the risk that diseases will spread. Outbreaks of infectious diseases, such as Haemophilus influenzae type b (Hib), hepatitis A, and many diarrhea-causing diseases, have been reported at child care centers.

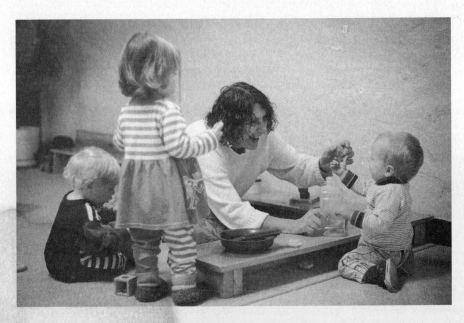

At child care centers children have more close contact with other children than they do at home. As a result, they run a higher risk of being exposed to an infectious disease.

There are several reasons why children in child care settings are more at risk from infectious diseases. Children at centers come in contact with many more people than children at home do so they are far more likely to be exposed to various diseases. And the risk of disease is high because of the child's stage of development. Very young children have immature immune systems. Infants and toddlers do not have control of their bowels or bladders, and they are not able to keep themselves clean. They drool, mouth almost everything, and sneeze and cough in each other's faces. Parents, too, sometimes contribute to the problem. To avoid missing work, parents may feel pressure to send their children to child care when the children are not entirely well. Likewise, staff members may feel pressure to come to work when they are not well. (Chapter 10 discusses health concerns for caregivers.) All of these factors contribute to the spread of infectious diseases.

In order to promote health among children and caregivers, child care centers need to have firm, reliable policies for preventing and controlling disease. For such measures to be effective, every caregiver needs to understand how diseases spread and what routine sanitary measures and illness policies can help to prevent the spread of disease.

The Nature of Infectious Diseases

Infectious diseases are diseases that are caused by organisms capable of entering the body and damaging tissue. The disease-causing organisms are called *pathogens*. Infectious diseases may be communicable or noncommunicable. *Communicable diseases* can be passed from one person to another. These include illnesses such as chicken pox, strep throat, and the common cold. *Noncommunicable diseases* are infections that do not pass from person to person. These include middle ear infections, Lyme disease, and some food-borne illnesses.

The Causes of Disease

Infectious diseases are caused by pathogens, commonly known as germs. The idea that germs cause disease is relatively new in human history. Before the mid-1800s, when scientists were able to see pathogens under microscopes, people thought infectious diseases were caused by bad air, bad blood, or an imbalance in the body. Other people thought diseases were a form of divine punishment. Since people did not know what caused diseases, they were unable to take steps to slow or stop their spread. Today, we know that we can control the spread of the pathogens that cause diseases.

There are several different categories of pathogens. Viruses are the smallest of these disease-causing organisms. Viruses invade healthy cells and use the resources in these cells to reproduce themselves. Once a person is ill with a viral infection, there are few medicines that can interrupt the course of the disease. The body must make antibodies, special substances designed to kill a particular invader. During the time it takes the body to make enough antibodies, a person shows symptoms of the infection.

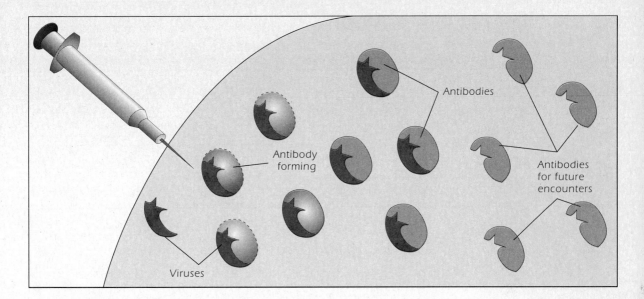

People can be immunized against some viral illnesses, such as polio, hepatitis B, and measles. Immunization exposes the person to a weakened or killed strain of the virus. This enables the body to form protective antibodies against the virus without getting the symptoms of the disease. Once a person has been immunized, his body has the antibodies to kill the virus before illness can occur.

Bacteria are another category of pathogens. Bacteria are found on and in virtually every object and living thing in the world. The great majority of bacteria are not ordinarily harmful. Many bacteria assist in the breakdown of food and perform other necessary functions in the body. Some bacteria can cause disease, however. Most disease-causing bacteria can be killed by medicines called antibiotics, but not every bacterium is killed by the same antibiotic. And some people have serious allergic reactions to some antibiotics, such as penicillin.

The body's immune system works against bacterial, as well as viral, infections. It produces antibodies against specific disease-causing bacteria once it has been exposed to them. Thus, people can be immunized against many bacterial infections, for example, diphtheria, tetanus, and whooping cough. Figure 11.1 shows how the body forms antibodies that protect it against viruses and bacteria.

Other diseases are caused by parasites. Parasites get all their nourishment from their *host*, the person or animal on which they live. Fungi are one category of parasites. Some fungi live on the skin and cause infections such as ringworm and diaper rash in children. Other fungi can be inhaled and cause respiratory diseases. Other kinds of parasites can live in the intestinal tract. Intestinal parasites, such as giardia, often cause diarrhea and are highly communicable. Parasites such as head lice and pinworms also spread easily in child care settings.

FIGURE 11.1 How Immunization Works. Injected serum contains enough of a killed or weakened disease-causing organism to stimulate the body to produce antibodies, but not enough to cause disease. The next time the virus (or bacterium) enters the body, antibodies are already present to counter the attack.

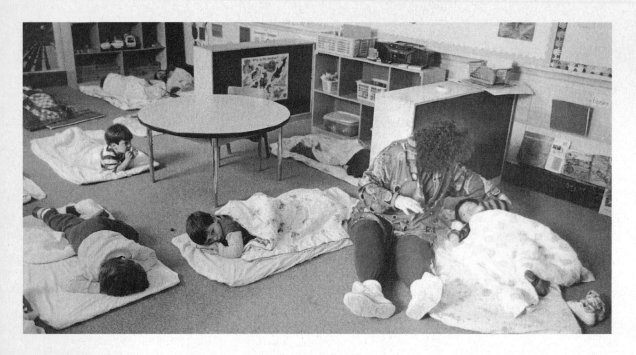

Proper nutrition and plenty of rest, including naps during the day, can help children resist infections.

Transmission of Diseases

Pathogens can be found almost anywhere—in people, on environmental surfaces, in the soil, and on and in living creatures ranging from mammals to tiny insects. When people come in contact with a pathogen, they may or may not become infected. When infection does occur, for example with the virus that causes chicken pox, the disease may produce mild symptoms in one person and severe symptoms in another.

Several factors determine whether a person exposed to an infectious disease will become ill and, if she does get sick, how seriously. Some factors involve the nature of the disease and whether the person has other medical conditions. Other factors can be directly influenced by behavior. Eating a healthful, well-balanced diet and getting plenty of rest, for example, helps children and caregivers resist infections. And understanding which diseases are communicable and how they are transmitted or passed from person to person allows child care providers to take preventive measures to control the spread of disease.

Communicable diseases are transmitted from person to person in four basic ways: respiratory droplets, fecal-oral contamination, direct contact, and body fluids. These methods of transmission and some of the diseases associated with them are described in detail later in this chapter. A person can contract a noncommunicable disease from the bite of an infected mammal, tick, insect, or other animal. Some noncommunicable diseases can be contracted by eating contaminated food or by contamination of a puncture wound. Some infections are noncommunicable because of their locations, for example, in the middle ear.

Stages of Illness

All infectious illnesses follow a similar pattern. Once a person has become infected, an *incubation period* follows during which the pathogen multiplies inside the body without giving any signs that the person is infected. Incubation periods can range from hours to weeks, depending on the disease. Many infectious diseases are communicable during the incubation period despite the absence of symptoms.

The second stage, called the *prodromal stage*, begins when a person starts showing nonspecific signs of illness. This is the stage when you may hear people say, "I think I'm coming down with something." Children may be cranky, restless, or clingy; complain of headache; or have a runny nose or a low-grade fever. People in this stage of most communicable diseases are contagious, that is, capable of passing the disease to an uninfected person.

In the *acute stage* of an illness, a person is definitely sick and shows symptoms typical of a specific infection. These symptoms may include fever, a rash, a sore throat, or a cough. This is the stage at which a health care provider can usually diagnose the disease. With most communicable illnesses, a person remains contagious until the acute stage of the disease is over.

Finally, the ill person reaches the *recovery stage*. Symptoms begin to disappear and health gradually returns. During this period for some communicable diseases, the person remains contagious even after he feels completely well.

The period of time and the stages of illness during which a person is contagious do vary with the particular disease involved. Health care professionals should be consulted for specific guidance in this matter during outbreaks of communicable diseases.

It is possible for someone to carry a disease and spread it to other people without ever showing symptoms of the disease herself. This person would be called a *carrier*. Carriers, as well as people in some stages of most communicable illnesses, are contagious despite the absence of symptoms. Because it is often impossible to tell who is contagious, routine preventive hygiene, such as handwashing, covering the mouth when sneezing or coughing, and not sharing eating utensils, is very important in controlling the spread of disease.

Infectious Diseases Affecting Children

Preschool children get sick whether they are at home or in a child care center. However, there is evidence that children who enter child care centers during infancy experience more illness during their first year of life than children who remain at home (Andersen, Bale, Blackman, & Murph, 1986). Caregivers must be able to recognize when a child is ill, evaluate the severity of the illness, and accurately report the child's symptoms to parents or health care professionals. Caregivers are not expected or qualified to diagnose specific illnesses in children.

TABLE 11.1
Common Infections of Childhood

Illness	Incubation	Period of Communicability
AIDS (acquired immune deficiency syndrome)	6 weeks to 10 years	lifetime
Chicken pox	10 to 21 days	1 to 2 days before onset of symptoms to 5 to 6 days after rash appears
Cold	12 to 72 hours	1 to 2 days before onset of symptoms and up to 2 to 3 days after symptoms begin
Conjunctivitis (pinkeye)	1 to 3 days	while symptoms are present; for bacterial form, up to 24 hours after treatment begins
Cytomegalovirus	not known	up to several years
Giardiasis	1 to 4 days	while parasite is present in stool
Haemophilus influenzae type b (Hib)	2 to 4 days	while symptoms are present, until 2 days after medication given
Hepatitis A	2 to 7 weeks (average 25 days)	2 to 3 weeks before onset of symptoms until 7 days after onset of jaundice
Hepatitis B	7 to 26 weeks (average 17 weeks)	variable—late incubation period, prodromal and acute stages, may remain a carrier for years
Impetigo	2 to 10 days	until sores heal or up to 24 hours after medication begins
Influenza	1 to 4 days	2 to 3 days before and after onset of symptoms
Lice (head)	nits hatch in 7 to 10 days, reach maturity within 2 weeks	while lice remain alive on infected person or clothing; until nits have been destroyed
Pinworms	life cycle of worm is 3 to 6 weeks; person can reinfect himself	2 to 8 weeks or as long as a source of infection remains present

(continued)

TABLE 11.1
Common Infections of Childhood (continued)

Illness	Incubation	Period of Communicability
Ringworm	1 to 4 days	while rash is present
Salmonellosis	6 to 72 hours	while symptoms persist, may remain a carrier for months
Scabies	2 to 6 weeks	until mites and eggs are destroyed
Shigellosis	1 to 7 days	while symptoms persist and stool samples show infection
Strep throat	2 to 5 days	from onset of symptoms until 24 hours after treatment begins

Communicable Infections

Communicable infections vary considerably in their frequency and severity, as well as their period of communicability (see Table 11.1). A few of these infections are discussed below to give caregivers an idea of the types of childhood illnesses they are likely to see, their severity, and how the spread of such diseases can be minimized.

Infections Transmitted by Respiratory Droplets.   Diseases such as the common cold, influenza, strep throat, chicken pox, and haemophilus influenzae type b (Hib disease) are spread through tiny droplets of respiratory secretions. These diseases are very common in child care centers. As a person talks, sings, coughs, or sneezes, millions of tiny droplets are released into the air that other people are breathing. When these droplets contain disease-causing bacteria or viruses, other people can become infected.

Saliva or nasal mucus of an infected person also spreads disease. If an infected child mouths a toy and another child picks the toy up and puts it in his mouth, the second child can become infected. Some viruses live for several days on toys, clothing, and other surfaces. Frequent handwashing and frequent washing and disinfection (see later section on sanitizing surfaces) of toys helps prevent the spread of infections by this means.

Upper respiratory infections, or colds, account for 60 to 75 percent of all infectious illnesses in children. Colds are caused by viruses. Healthy children may have six to ten colds each year. Infants enrolled in child care centers have more colds than those who remain at home (Andersen et al., 1986).

The common cold is relatively mild and virtually impossible to prevent, except by severely limiting contact with other people. One study found that cold-causing viruses could be found on 15 percent of the objects handled by an ill child, and that viruses survived up to 48 hours (Taylor & Taylor, 1989).

Other diseases spread by respiratory droplets include strep throat, chicken pox, and Hib disease. Strep throat is a bacterial infection. If left untreated, it can lead to rheumatic fever—an inflammation of the heart, joints, and other tissues—or to inflammation of the kidneys. Strep throat accompanied by a red rash and a fever is called scarlet fever.

Children with strep throat usually complain of a sore throat and have a fever. They may also have headaches, stomachaches, and swollen lymph glands. Many viruses cause these same symptoms so children suspected of having strep throat need to have a throat culture done by a health care professional. Strep throat is treated with antibiotics. Children are generally not contagious after they have taken the antibiotic for 24 hours.

Chicken pox is a common viral illness of childhood. Most children develop a mild fever and pimplelike rash that then breaks open and scabs over. Children are contagious for a day or two before the rash appears and for five or six days after the rash begins.

About 4 million children in the United States get chicken pox each year. For most children, the disease is mild. Other children develop secondary bacterial infections, pneumonia, or encephalitis (an inflammation of the brain) as a complication of the disease. Chicken pox is a serious disease for children who have weakened immune systems, such as those with leukemia or AIDS, and for some normal adults. One exposure to chicken pox creates a lifetime immunity. However, 40 to 90 chicken pox deaths occur each year (Centers for Disease Control, 1992). A vaccine to immunize against chicken pox is currently in the final stages of testing and approval.

Hib disease is a bacterial disease with flulike symptoms. It is dangerous because it can lead to serious infections or inflammations of the throat, joints, lungs, blood, and coverings of the brain. Immunizations for Hib disease are recommended starting at two months of age.

Infections Transmitted by Fecal-Oral Contamination.   Other diseases spread when pathogens from the feces of an infected person are carried to another person's mouth. This may sound unlikely, but it can happen quite easily and it is known as fecal-oral contamination. Diseases that are spread by this means include hepatitis A and giardia. Uninfected persons touch a part of the body, clothing, or a surface contaminated with feces, then later put their hands to their mouths. Pathogens are so small they cannot be seen without a microscope. A surface contaminated with feces may not look dirty; caregivers need to remember that. Children who are not toilet trained and caregivers who change diapers are at greatest risk for acquiring infections by fecal-oral contamination.

Many fecal-oral infections are caused by bacteria such as salmonella and shigella, certain viruses, or parasites. Such pathogens grow in the digestive tract and cause vomiting or diarrhea. Children and caregivers can get most of these diseases repeatedly. Outbreaks of diarrhea-causing illnesses are especially common in infant-toddler groups and in centers where infants and toddlers are mixed with older children. In the opening story, Rose and Hector had good reason to be concerned that Maurice's dirty diaper got left on the changing table. To prevent the spread of fecal-oral infections, caregivers should practice proper diaper changing and disposal (as discussed later in

FOCUS ON Cultural Diversity

Beliefs About Illness

It is helpful for caregivers to be familiar with diverse cultural attitudes toward disease. Some cultural beliefs about illness are described below.

Asian American Chinese: Disease results from an imbalance of two energy forces called the yin and the yang. Restoring balance restores health. Herbs, acupuncture, acupressure, and diet are used to treat disease.

Asian American Japanese: The ancient Japanese *Shinto* religion teaches that illness is caused by contact with polluting agents, such as blood, corpses, and skin diseases. Treatment is similar to the Chinese. Modern Japanese adhere to the modern germ theory of illness.

Vietnamese American: As with Chinese, the belief is that energy imbalance causes disease. Living in harmony with the universe and pleasing benevolent spirits ensures health. Treatment of illness is first attempted at home by the family through ritual or prayer before professional help is sought.

African American: May believe illness is due to punishment for resisting God's will. Some beliefs include evil influences as the genesis of disease. Folk medicine or spiritualists may be the first avenue for treatment. Many African Americans accept the modern germ theory of disease.

Puerto Rican American: May believe in an imbalance of hot and cold in the body as a cause for disease. Some illnesses may be caused by evil spirits. Folk healers using herbs and rituals are preferred for treatment.

Native American: Believe health is a state of harmony with the universe. All illnesses have some supernatural aspects that may include the violation of a religious taboo. Health and religion are strongly linked. Medicine people are sought for diagnosis and treatment, and may use herbs and rituals to cure disease.

this chapter), disinfect surfaces that could be contaminated with feces, and keep food preparation and serving areas separate from diaper-changing areas. It is best if caregivers who change diapers do not prepare food.

Hepatitis A is far more serious for caregivers than for children. In children, the hepatitis A virus usually causes mild, flulike symptoms. Adults affected by the hepatitis A virus often become tired, nauseated, feverish, and develop jaundice—a yellowing of the skin and the whites of the eyes. They can be sick for weeks or months.

Since children become only mildly ill and the incubation period of this virus is two to eight weeks, the first sign of an outbreak of hepatitis A in the child care setting is often illness among the caregivers. Injections of immune globulin within two weeks of exposure to the hepatitis A virus will prevent the disease, and one attack of the disease produces permanent immunity. Centers with cases of hepatitis A should notify their local boards of health (see the section on reportable diseases).

Pinworms are parasites that live in the intestines and emerge at night as threadlike worms to lay their eggs around the anus. Pinworms can cause intense itching in the anal area. It is estimated that 5 to 15 percent of all Americans are infected with pinworms (Kendrick, Kaufmann, & Messenger, 1991). Pinworms are passed from person to person when their eggs are introduced into the mouth through contact with contaminated fingers or objects. It is possible for a person to reinfect himself as well as others. Pinworms can be eliminated with medication.

Giardia is an intestinal parasite that can cause several symptoms, including diarrhea, gas, weight loss, and fatigue. However, as many as one-quarter of the children in child care centers may be infected with giardia but show no symptoms (Andersen et al., 1986). Most giardia infections originate with contaminated water sources. In child care settings, giardia spreads through the fecal-oral route. Giardia is a leading cause of diarrheal illness in child care centers. Diarrhea is also a symptom of a number of viral diseases. All diarrheal illnesses are of concern to child care providers because of the danger of dehydration, especially among infants and toddlers. Mild dehydration can be treated by giving children extra clear fluids (such as clear broths or soups, ginger ale, noncitrus juices, or commercial electrolyte solutions), as appropriate for their ages. However severe dehydration, in which the child becomes drowsy or listless, should be treated immediately by a health care professional.

Infections Transmitted by Direct Contact.   Some diseases must be spread by direct contact. An uninfected person must touch an infected person or object. Conjunctivitis (pinkeye), impetigo, head lice, scabies, and ringworm are spread this way. Because of the close physical contact among young children and between children and caregivers, the transmission of illness by direct contact is common in child care settings. These diseases are not life threatening, but they must be treated and controlled for good health.

Conjunctivitis that is communicable is caused by both viral and bacterial infections. The eye becomes red and itchy, discharging pus or watery fluid. Conjunctivitis is highly communicable. It is spread by contact with the discharge. When the infection is caused by bacteria, it can be treated with antibiotics. Children remain contagious until they have received the antibiotic for 24 hours or have no more discharge from their eyes. During this time, they should be excluded from child care. Noncontagious conjunctivitis can be caused by allergies. However, caregivers should treat all cases of pinkeye as if they were contagious until a health care professional determines otherwise.

Impetigo is a skin infection caused by bacteria. It begins in a cut or other break in the skin. Soon red, oozing sores appear that become covered with a yellowish crust. The rash often appears first on the face and may be itchy. It is easily passed from one child to another by direct contact.

Head lice are found worldwide in all socioeconomic groups. Their presence does not indicate poverty or a lack of cleanliness. These parasites infest the scalp and lay their eggs, called nits, along the hair shaft, close to its roots. Children who scratch their heads frequently should be checked for lice. If one child has lice, all other children and caregivers must also be checked.

FOCUS ON Communicating with Children

Personal Hygiene and Eating

It is the first full day of the new school year at the Atlantic Nursery School. Mrs. Ross, the head teacher in the four-year-old class, is helping a group of children get ready for lunch.

MRS. ROSS: In a few minutes it will be lunchtime. Can anyone tell me the most important thing we have to do before we eat?

CURT: Get our lunch boxes?

MRS. ROSS: Even before that.

MARISA: We have to wash our hands!

MRS. ROSS: Right, Marisa. Even if our hands don't look dirty, they may have dirt on them—dirt that we don't want to get on our food and into our bodies. (leading them toward the bathroom) I know that you all know how to wash your hands, but let's go over the way we do it here. Curt, will you be my helper?

CURT: Sure!

MRS. ROSS: First you step right up to the sink and turn on the water. Use warm water—cold water doesn't do the job. Now push down on the top of the soap dispenser. (Curt pushes enthusiastically, and a large blob of soap squirts into his hand. The other children laugh.)

MRS. ROSS: (smiling) Not quite so hard! You only need a little. Now rub it all over your hands, and keep rubbing under the running water until you've counted to ten. The next part may be a bit different from what you're used to. After you've rinsed off the soap, take a paper towel, dry your hands, and use the towel to turn off the water.

LORI: Why do we have to do that?

MRS. ROSS: When you turned on the water, your hands had dirt on them, and some of that dirt got left on the handle. Now that your hands are clean, you don't want them picking up that dirt again. (The children wash their hands.) While you are washing your hands, let's talk about a few other ways we can keep from getting sick.

LORI: My mom says you can get sick by drinking out of someone else's cup.

MRS. ROSS: Your mother is right, Lori. You should never use a cup or fork or spoon that has touched someone else's mouth, unless it has been washed first. You shouldn't finish a piece of food that someone else has taken a bite out of either. And one more thing. Does anyone know the first place we should all go after lunch? Right back to the bathroom to wash our hands again.

CURT: I'm sure glad we have a nice bathroom at this school, because we're in here a lot!

Are there other food and hygiene issues that Mrs. Ross could have discussed with the children? Would you have explained the idea of dirt and illness any differently?

Head lice are killed by special shampoos. Most schools and child care centers also require that the nits remaining in the hair be removed with a fine-tooth comb. To prevent reinfection, bedding, clothing, brushes, and anything that may have touched the child's head needs to be laundered or dry-cleaned at the same time the lice-killing shampoo is used. Things that

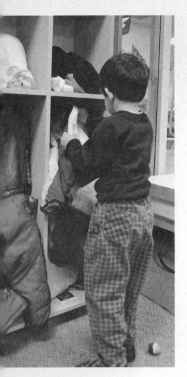

Providing individual cubbies for storing children's coats and other clothes can help to control the spread of lice.

cannot be washed can be stored in plastic bags for two weeks until the lice are dead. All members of a household where one person has head lice should be checked for lice and treated if necessary.

Caregivers can help control the spread of lice by eliminating hats from dress-up play, laundering dress-up clothes often, discouraging children from sharing hairbrushes or touching each other's heads, and providing individual cubbies for storing coats and other clothes. Parent education and cooperation is important in ridding the center of lice and preventing reinfection from home.

Scabies and ringworm are both skin diseases. Scabies is caused by a member of the spider family called a mite. The mite tunnels under the skin to lay eggs. The body reacts to the parasite with a rash and intense itching. The rash looks like red bumps and lines, which follow the mite's egg-laying burrows. Ringworm is caused by a fungus. It produces a flat, ring-shaped, itchy rash. Ringworm on the scalp can cause loss of hair. Both of these diseases are contagious until treated.

Infections Transmitted by Body Fluids.   Diseases spread through body fluids include the human immunodeficiency virus, HIV, which causes acquired immune deficiency syndrome (AIDS). HIV is spread by the entry of infected body fluids directly into the body of an uninfected person. Most commonly, HIV is transmitted during sexual activity. The virus can also be transmitted if the blood or sexual fluids of an infected person directly enter the body of an uninfected person through a break in the skin. It can also be transmitted from an infected pregnant woman to her unborn child. HIV cannot live outside the body and is *not* transmitted by hugging, shaking hands, or sharing a bathroom or clothing with an infected person.

Children infected with HIV at birth often appear normal for some period of time but develop symptoms of AIDS during the first two years of life. Because HIV attacks the immune system, these children are highly susceptible to infections of all kinds. The parents of children who are known to have HIV infection should be informed of any occurrence of communicable disease in the child care center for this reason. About half of all children with HIV infection have neurological impairments that result in developmental delays or regression of development as repeated infections affect the nervous system.

Cytomegalovirus (CMV) is less familiar than HIV but far more common. This virus is found in the saliva, urine, and tears of many children and eventually infects almost the entire adult population. About 2 percent of all babies are infected from birth. In some child care centers, as many as 70 percent of one- to three-year-olds have CMV in their body fluids (Andersen et al., 1986). Children born with CMV infections can excrete the virus in their body fluids for years and they can transmit the infection during this period. There is no effective treatment for CMV, but infection does produce permanent immunity. Most CMV infections produce a few minor symptoms (swollen lymph glands, fever, or fatigue) or none at all. However, people whose

immune systems are impaired, for example by other infections or chemo-
therapy, can develop cytomegalic inclusion disease, which can be fatal. This
disease can severely damage the nervous system and internal organs. Since
fetuses can be infected if their mothers are actively infected with CMV, pregnant women should avoid contact with children known to be infected with
CMV and should routinely follow good handwashing procedures. Pregnant
caregivers may want to be tested for CMV immunity. In fact, a caregiver who
is pregnant or who is considering pregnancy should consult her health care
provider, explaining that she works with young children and wants to know
what steps she should take to protect herself and her child.

Hepatitis B is another communicable disease passed through body fluids.
Most transmission is through sexual activity or through tainted blood. The
symptoms of hepatitis B are similar to those of hepatitis A, except that they
are more severe and long-lasting. Because the disease can cause permanent
liver damage, the American Academy of Pediatrics recommends that all
children receive the vaccine for this illness (see Table 11.2 on page 269).

Because body fluids can be infected with HIV, CMV, hepatitis B, and other
viruses, caregivers must treat all body fluids as a potential source of infection. This will be discussed later in the section on universal precautions.

Noncommunicable Infections

Not all infections are passed directly from person to person. Some are carried by animals. Others are found in contaminated food or water. Although
these infections can make children very sick, they do not spread from person
to person in child care environments. Children with noncommunicable illnesses do not have to be excluded from the child care setting. They should
be permitted to return to the center if they feel well enough to participate in
activities.

Infections Carried by Animals.   Some diseases are transmitted to people through animals, small and large. Ticks and mosquitoes can inject their
infections into people when they bite and break the skin. Lyme disease and
Rocky Mountain spotted fever are both carried by ticks.

Lyme disease is most common on the East Coast. It is spread by tiny deer
ticks. People who have Lyme disease often show a red bull's-eye rash
around the spot where the tick was attached. Later, they may develop fever,
fatigue, and flulike symptoms. Lyme disease is treated with antibiotics. Left
untreated, serious complications involving the joints, the heart, the brain,
and other tissues can develop. A vaccine against Lyme disease is in the initial stages of development.

Rocky Mountain spotted fever is carried by larger dog ticks. It causes a
rash, fever, and, occasionally, encephalitis or inflammation of the brain. Encephalitis can also be carried by mosquitoes.

Preventive measures for these diseases include wearing long-sleeved
shirts and long pants tucked into socks when walking in tick-infested areas,

FOCUS ON ✦ Promoting Healthful Habits

Sudden Fever in an Infant

When Renata put four-month-old Benjamin down for his nap at 10 in the morning, he seemed fine. At 11:05, however, he awakens fussy and crying. When Renata picks him up and holds him close to her, she notices that he feels very warm.

"Sabrina," she calls to the other caregiver. "Can you call the director, please, so she can take over for me? Benjamin just woke up from his nap and he feels hot. I want to take his temperature."

Renata puts Benjamin back in his crib for a moment as she finds the mercury thermometer. She shakes the thermometer gently until the mercury is below the 95-degree mark. Then she places the thermometer back in its holder and begins to unsnap the top buttons of Benjamin's playsuit. Renata gently removes the playsuit from Benjamin's left arm and shoulder. Then she takes the thermometer, slips a disposable cover over the bulb, and places the tip in the infant's armpit. She keeps the thermometer in place by holding Benjamin's elbow against his chest, talking to him all the time.

Five minutes later, Renata reads the thermometer. "Oh, my," she exclaims. "His temperature is 101 degrees. Sabrina!" she calls. "I have to call Benjamin's mother right away. He has quite a fever."

Over the telephone, Renata calmly tells Benjamin's mother about his fever. The caregiver explains that while a fever does not necessarily mean a serious illness, a fever in such a young child is cause for concern. Renata offers to call Benjamin's pediatrician while Benjamin's mother comes to pick him up. "I'll tell Dr. Taylor about the fever and warn her that you're on your way," Renata says. Renata collects Benjamin's belongings for his mother and comforts him until his mother arrives.

Do you think Renata did the right thing or was she overreacting to the infant's fever? What would you have said to Benjamin's mother and to the pediatrician?

and checking the body for ticks upon returning home. Mosquitoes are best kept out of living quarters and classrooms by using screens on doors and windows.

Turtles and parrots also carry diseases that can be transmitted to humans; therefore, they should not be kept as classroom pets. Rabies is transmitted through the bite of infected animals, including cats and dogs as well as raccoons and other wild animals. This disease has become epidemic in some parts of the country, making it essential to immunize pets and teach children never to approach wild animals.

Food-Borne Illnesses.   Food-borne illnesses are caused by bacteria or toxins, or poisons, that they make as they grow. Noncommunicable food-borne illnesses are generally those in which the toxin produces the symptoms of food poisoning. An example is botulism—a rare, sometimes fatal form of food poisoning. There are two food-borne types of botulism. One is caused by eating improperly processed canned foods in which the bacterium has been growing. Caregivers should never open cans that are leaking or bulging because that is a sign that botulism toxin may be present. Chapter 6 discusses the second form of this illness, infant botulism. In this case, botulism spores, an inactive form of the bacterium that would be destroyed in a more mature digestive system, grow and produce their toxins in the intestine of an infant. Honey may contain botulism spores; honey or foods made with honey should never be given to infants.

Illnesses cannot always be neatly categorized, however. Food-borne illnesses can be caused by bacteria that can be passed from person to person. Examples are salmonella and the strain of *E. coli* (a bacterial type normally found in the human digestive system) that caused widespread illness when infected beef was served in a fast-food restaurant chain (Implications for day-care, 1993). These infections are communicable by the fecal-oral route once a person has become infected by bacteria in the food.

Signs of food poisoning include nausea, vomiting, and diarrhea. Many bacteria that cause food-borne illnesses grow best at room temperature. To avoid food-borne illnesses, keep hot foods hot and cold foods cold. Wash hands and food preparation surfaces frequently. See Chapter 4 for a detailed discussion on safe food handling.

Other Noncommunicable Infections. Some infections can be associated with a child's physical stage of development or can occur because a wound becomes contaminated. Caregivers are likely to see middle ear infections because they are fairly common in infants and toddlers. These infections occur because the eustachian tube, connecting the middle ear and the throat, closes, often as a result of inflammation or swelling of surrounding tissues from a cold. Because the tube is quite small in infants and toddlers, it doesn't take much swelling to squeeze it shut. This closure prevents fluids in the ear from draining. Bacteria or viruses that have traveled up the tube from the throat while the tube was open can then grow rapidly in the trapped fluid, producing infection.

Middle ear infections can cause severe pain, discharge from the ear, and/or fever. These infections occur most frequently in children between 6 and 18 months of age (Roberts, 1993) and are treated with antibiotics. Special tubes are sometimes inserted in the ears if the infections do not respond to antibiotics or recur so frequently that hearing and language development are endangered.

Diaper rash caused by a yeast infection is another noncommunicable infection caregivers may see. Prolonged exposure to urine and feces, especially when a child has diarrhea, can irritate skin and make it vulnerable to infection by yeast—a fungus normally present in the digestive tract and the general environment. (A yeast infection that occurs in the mouth is called thrush.) Keeping a baby's bottom clean and dry helps protect against diaper rash from yeast. Once the rash is present, it may be necessary to leave the baby's bottom exposed to the air whenever possible. Occasionally, the use of a special ointment or oral medication may be prescribed by the child's health care provider. Plastic pants and diapers that trap moisture should not be used on children who have diaper rash.

Tetanus, or lockjaw, is a potentially fatal disease caused by a bacterial toxin. Although the bacterium is common in the environment, it only infects damaged tissue. Puncture wounds, burns, and crushed tissue are especially susceptible to tetanus. Immunization against tetanus is part of the recommended childhood series.

Preventable Infectious Diseases

Some infectious diseases can now be prevented through the use of vaccines. There are nine major childhood diseases for which vaccines are available. These diseases are: polio, diphtheria, pertussis (whooping cough), hepatitis B, mumps, measles, rubella (German measles), tetanus (lockjaw), and Haemophilus influenzae type b (Hib).

Vaccines stimulate the body to make antibodies that provide protection against a particular disease, but the period of immunity varies. The variation depends on the vaccine, the age of the person being immunized, and other factors. Table 11.2 shows the immunization schedule recommended by the American Academy of Pediatrics for infants and children. The DTP immunization protects against diphtheria, tetanus, and pertussis; MMR immunization protects against measles, mumps, and rubella. Immunizations are normally given as soon as the body is able to make lasting antibodies against the disease. Most immunizations require multiple exposure to the vaccine to be completely effective. For children who have not been immunized as infants, different immunization schedules are recommended.

Caregivers who have not been immunized against any of these diseases should talk to a health care practitioner about adult vaccination. Caregivers should also note the recommendation that tetanus-diphtheria (Td) boosters be repeated every ten years throughout adulthood.

It is important for child care centers to require that the children in their care receive all their immunizations at the recommended times. All nine vaccines are safe and effective in preventing debilitating, sometimes fatal, diseases. The rate of serious side effects caused by vaccination is very, very low. Nevertheless, the percentage of children receiving all their immunizations on schedule has decreased in recent years. The incidence of diseases such as whooping cough has increased as a result.

Some parents do not have their children vaccinated for religious reasons. But there are a variety of other reasons why parents fail to have their children vaccinated. Parents sometimes underestimate the damage these diseases can do or think that, since everyone else's child is vaccinated, their child is not at risk of becoming ill. Some parents may be concerned about the cost of immunizations; others may be fearful of side effects from the vaccines. Caregivers can help children by providing information to parents about the serious consequences these diseases can have, about the benefits

TABLE 11.2
Recommended Immunization Schedule

	DTP[1]	Polio[2]	MMR	Hepatitis B[3]	Haemophilus[1]	Td
Birth				✓		
1 to 2 months				✓		
2 months	✓	✓			◆	
4 months	✓	✓			◆	
6 months	✓				◆	
6 to 18 months				✓		
12 to 15 months					◆	
15 months			✓			
15 to 18 months	●	✓				
4 to 6 years	●	✓				
11 to 12 years		□		#		
14 to 16 years				#		✓

[1]The HbOC-DTP combination vaccine may be substituted for separate vaccinations for Haemophilus and DTP.
[2]Children in close contact with immunosuppressed individuals should receive inactivated polio vaccine.
[3]Infants of mothers who tested seropositive for hepatitis B surface antigen (HBsAg +) should receive hepatitis B immune globulin (HBIG) at or shortly after the first dose. These infants also will require a second hepatitis B vaccine dose at 1 month and a third hepatitis B vaccine injection at 6 months of age.
◆ Depends on which *Haemophilus influenzae* type b vaccine was given previously.
● For the fourth and fifth dose, the acellular (DTaP) pertussis vaccine may be substituted for the DTP vaccine.
□ Except where public health authorities require otherwise.
Where resources permit, the hepatitis B vaccine series of three immunizations should be given to previously unimmunized preadolescents or adolescents.
Used with permission of the American Academy of Pediatrics.

and risks of vaccination, and about free or inexpensive vaccination programs available in the community.

Reportable Diseases

A *reportable disease* is one whose occurrence must, by law, be reported to local or state public health agencies. There are three categories of reportable diseases. Serious, life-threatening diseases such as diphtheria, Haemophilus influenzae type b, and polio, are in the first category. Any occurrence of these diseases must be reported immediately by telephone. The second category generally includes diseases such as hepatitis A, whooping cough, and Lyme disease. Cases of these diseases should be reported by mail. The third category consists of diseases such as chicken pox and strep throat for which isolated cases are not considered a threat to the public health. However, local outbreaks (when more than 10 percent of a particular population of children are absent with the disease) should be reported by mail.

Accurate, timely reporting of the occurrence of serious illness helps public health officials track and minimize the spread of disease. During outbreaks, they may recommend additional precautions to stop the illness from spreading. Parents should also be informed when their children may have been exposed to an infectious disease or food-borne illness. Notifying parents is discussed later in this chapter.

Child care centers should keep on hand a list of reportable diseases, the telephone numbers of the appropriate public health departments, and the forms necessary to file the reports. Requirements and procedures for reporting vary from state to state. The center's health policy should ask that parents of an ill child inform the center about the child's illness and any specific diagnosis by a health care provider. Parents should provide this information as soon as the child becomes ill rather than wait until the child returns to the child care center. The center needs to know if others have been exposed to a communicable disease in order to take steps to prevent its spread.

Dealing with Sick Children in Child Care Settings

Children do become sick while in child care. Minimizing the spread of disease is the first line of defense against outbreaks of illness at a child care center. Policies on when to exclude sick children and how to care for mildly ill children are also necessary in order to maintain good health in both children and members of the staff.

Minimizing the Spread of Communicable Diseases

Minimizing the spread of communicable diseases involves establishing good hygiene practices that apply to all of the children and all of the staff all of the time.

Physical Considerations.   The design and arrangement of a child care setting can either hinder or encourage the spread of disease. Caregivers should set up the physical environment in ways that reduce the possibility of infection. For example, cots and cribs can be arranged so that children sleep head to foot. Alternating the children's positions in this way ensures that they will not breathe in each other's faces while they sleep.

Children need an adequate amount of space and ventilation to remain healthy. Crowded, closed environments make it easy for germs to spread. Rooms should be kept at temperatures between 65° and 75° F (18.4° and 23.9° C) in the winter and 68° and 82° F (20° and 27.8° C) in the summer. Air conditioners and vaporizers must be cleaned regularly to prevent the buildup of germs and dirt. Whenever possible, rooms where children sleep, eat, and play should be aired daily, even in cold weather.

Each child needs an individual storage cubby for personal items. Piling children's personal belongings together, as was done at the Darby Community Center in the opening story, encourages the spread of disease. Young children should always have a change of clothes from home. Soiled clothing should be sealed in plastic bags and returned to the parents to be washed.

Diapering areas must be separated from eating and food preparation areas. The diapering area should be near running water so that it is easy for caregivers to wash the children's hands and their own hands. Dirty diapers and diaper wipes should be discarded in a covered container lined with a plastic bag. Dirty diapers and trash should be removed from the room daily.

Most caregivers cannot control the design of every aspect of their work space. But if they understand how diseases spread, they may be able to see where improvements can be made to minimize the spread of illness. For example, the Darby Community Center's practice of bringing the infants, toddlers, and older children together at the end of the day was far from ideal. Mixing groups, especially when some children are in diapers, encourages the spread of communicable diseases. A better arrangement would have been for one caregiver to join the older children in their classroom while the other caregiver remained with the infants and toddlers. Maintaining a proper child-staff ratio might have required that additional caregivers remain at the Darby Community Center later.

In addition to adequate classroom space, every child care facility needs a space where children who become ill can be kept apart from other children until their parents arrive. If the center routinely cares for mildly ill children, this space should be used exclusively for that purpose.

Diapering. Caregivers must be very careful during the diapering process since it poses health risks to both caregivers and other children. The previous section explained concerns for caregivers in setting up diapering areas. All supplies should be within easy reach so that caregivers can keep one hand on the child at all times. To change a diaper properly, caregivers should follow these steps:

1. Place a disposable cover on the diapering surface.
2. Lay the child down on her back. Put on disposable gloves.
3. Remove necessary clothing and the soiled diaper. Fold disposable diapers to the inside and reseal them with the plastic tapes. Fold in the sides of cloth diapers to contain the stool.
4. Place disposable diapers in a lined, covered trash can that can be opened with the foot. Cloth diapers should be placed in one plastic bag and then within another plastic bag that is labeled to be sent home. Soiled clothing should also be double-bagged.
5. Clean the child's bottom with a disposable wipe. Always wipe from front to back. Pat the child's bottom dry with a disposable towel.
6. Dispose of the wipe in the lined, covered can. Discard disposable gloves. Wipe your hands with a disposable wipe and discard it in the can.
7. Dress the child. Pick her up and wash her hands. Take the child back to the rest of the group.
8. Remove the disposable covering from the diapering surface. Disinfect the surface. Wash your own hands thoroughly.

HEALTH TIPS

Diarrhea

A child has diarrhea when his stools are both frequent and loose. Without proper precautions, the germs that cause diarrhea can be spread to others.

Handwashing is the best way to keep diarrhea from spreading. Children and adults should always wash their hands after going to the bathroom and before and after eating. Caregivers should wear disposable gloves when changing diapers.

If a child has mild diarrhea, handwashing is the only precaution necessary. Children with severe diarrhea should remain at home until the stools are normal again.

If a caregiver suspects that a child with diarrhea has touched toys or surfaces with unwashed hands, those toys or surfaces should be disinfected as quickly as possible.

Frequent handwashing is the most effective way to minimize the spread of disease. Children should be taught proper handwashing as early as possible.

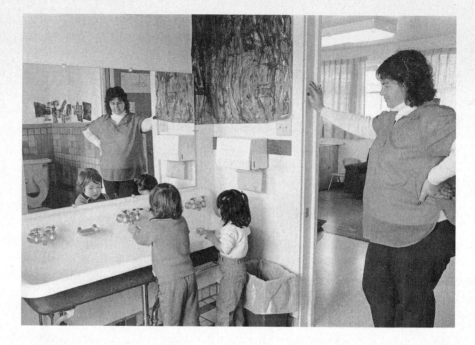

Handwashing.   Frequent handwashing is the most effective way to minimize the spread of disease. Caregivers should wash their hands upon arriving at work, before and after handling food, and after all of the following: changing diapers or helping a child use the toilet, touching a child who may be ill, handling and feeding pets, cleaning up blood or vomit, providing first aid for minor cuts and scrapes, and wiping runny noses. Children's hands should be washed before and after handling food, and after diapering or using the toilet, touching another child who may be ill, handling and feeding pets, sneezing, and wiping a runny nose.

To wash hands properly, caregivers should use warm running water—never a shared pool of water such as a dishpan. Soap is essential and liquid soap is easier for young children to handle than bar soap. The caregiver's or child's hands should be rubbed together vigorously under running water for about ten seconds. It's important to wash not only the palms but also the backs of the hands, the wrists, between the fingers, and under the fingernails. Hands should be well rinsed, then dried on a paper towel or with an automatic warm-air hand dryer. Cloth towels that are used more than once are not sanitary and should not be used. A paper towel should be used to turn off the taps, since the taps will be a source of whatever germs the unwashed hands brought with them.

Caregivers need to set an example by washing their hands at all the appropriate times and making handwashing part of the center's routine. Children need to be taught proper handwashing as soon as possible. Younger children's hands should be washed by the caregiver. The use of hand lotion can prevent drying and cracking of skin from frequent handwashing.

Sanitizing Surfaces.　Diaper-changing areas, tabletops, high chairs, crib rails, toys, sinks, and places where a child has bled, vomited, or had a leaky diaper can become contaminated. These areas and items should be disinfected routinely as well as whenever obvious contamination has occurred, as when a toddler sneezes on a toy. Bathrooms and food preparation areas should be cleaned daily.

An inexpensive but effective disinfectant that kills germs can be made using ¼ cup bleach to 1 gallon of water or 1 tablespoon per quart if less volume is needed (Kendrick et al., 1991). This solution must be made daily to maintain its strength. It can be stored in spray bottles for easy use. Ideally, the surfaces of the child care center will be durable and nonporous, making them easy to sanitize.

Universal Precautions.　The term *universal precautions* refers to preventive measures people should take in order to avoid infection. The potential for infection with viruses such as those that cause hepatitis B and AIDS has made it necessary to take universal precautions when cleaning up blood or blood-containing body fluids. Because many pathogens are shed in the stools of children with diarrhea, caregivers should use universal precautions when changing a diaper or assisting with toileting of a child with diarrhea.

When faced with a situation where universal precautions are necessary, for example stopping a bloody nose, caregivers should do the following:

1. Put on fresh disposable rubber gloves.
2. Clean up the body fluids using disposable materials, such as paper towels, tissues, or diaper wipes. Dispose of these materials in a plastic bag that is placed inside a plastic-lined, covered container. Soiled clothing should be put in a labeled plastic bag and sent home.
3. Wash the contaminated area with soap and water.
4. Sanitize the area with a disinfectant solution.
5. Remove rubber gloves and dispose of them along with the other soiled material.
6. Wash hands well.

Excluding Sick Children

Generally speaking, children who are too sick to benefit from routine activities at the child care center or who are contagious with an infectious disease should not be admitted. Often the decision about whether a child is too ill for child care on a particular day, however, is not clear-cut. Symptoms of illness develop rapidly in young children. Early morning sniffles can develop into a full-blown cold and sore throat by afternoon. Health policies need to provide guidance concerning which children to exclude from care while being flexible enough to treat each illness and child individually.

Exclusion Policies.　Each child care center should have access to a health consultant to help the center director develop illness policies, to evaluate preventive hygiene measures, and to provide guidance during outbreaks of illness. The role of the health care consultant is not to be a health care provider to children in the program, but to help establish policies that ensure the health of all children and staff. It is up to the director to see that health policies are consistently enforced.

Excluding children from child care is a sensitive issue. Many parents will miss work if their children are not admitted. Although few parents want to send a truly sick child to child care, many feel pressured to ignore mild symptoms in the hope that they will not worsen during the day. Child care centers need a written policy that outlines:

- When sick children should be kept home
- When and how the center will notify parents if their children become sick during the day
- The policy for readmission after an illness
- The circumstances in which medication will be administered
- The circumstances under which emergency care will be sought
- How parents will be notified about exposure to communicable diseases
- How parents should notify the center about reasons for absence

At the time the child is enrolled in the center, the health policy should be discussed with the parents and they should be given a written copy of it. This is also the time to obtain the health and emergency information, discussed in Chapter 10, that makes up the child's health file.

In general, children with a fever of over 100°F (37.8°C) orally or 101°F (38.3°C) rectally in the past 24 hours should remain at home. Other reasons to exclude children include undiagnosed rashes, vomiting or diarrhea, pink or inflamed eyes, discharge from the ears, open sores that cannot be covered with a bandage, and a severe cough or cold. Any child who feels too ill to participate in activities at the center should stay home. Caregivers who show these same signs of illness should not come to work.

Sudden Illness. When children become sick at the child care center, a decision must be made about how to handle the situation. Generally, parents should be contacted to pick up children who develop any of the symptoms that are specified in the exclusion policy. Some of these symptoms require only that the child be kept isolated from healthy children until a parent can come for him. Other symptoms, however, require immediate attention by a health care professional (see Figure 10.1 in Chapter 10). In addition to serious symptoms of illness, cuts where bleeding cannot be stopped by pressure, chemical burns, possible fractures, and certain other injuries (see Chapter 13) require immediate medical attention.

Informing Parents About Communicable Diseases

Letters notifying parents that their children have been exposed to a communicable disease should be sent home each time an exposure occurs. Strep

---

Sample Letter Format

Dear parent or guardian:

A case of _____ **(name of disease)** _____ has been reported at the child care center. Your child may have been exposed to this illness.

Please do the following:

1. Watch your child for the next _____ **(give incubation period information)** for symptoms of the illness, which include _____ **(list symptoms here)** _____ . Do not send your child to the program if any of these symptoms appear.

2. Call your health care provider if _____ **(list any symptoms that would require medical attention)** _____ are present.

3. You can keep this disease from spreading within your family by _____ **(list any precautions parents can take to avoid spreading the disease)** _____ .

4. _____ **(List here any special notes or precautions, as needed, such as not giving aspirin to children with chicken pox)** _____ .

_____ **(Include a paragraph here that describes the illness generally—what it is, how it is spread, how long it lasts and how serious it is, home and medical treatment methods, any complications not mentioned above and so on)** _____ .

Feel free to call the center with any questions about this illness or your child's participation in the program.

Thank you.

FIGURE 11.2 Sample Letter Format. This letter suggests a format that child care centers can use to inform parents about communicable diseases. Information about a particular disease can be inserted as needed.

---

throat, chicken pox, and head lice are all common communicable diseases that require letters to parents.

These letters should provide adequate information about the disease without frightening parents unnecessarily. Warning parents that their children may have been exposed to a specific communicable disease increases parents' awareness of early symptoms.

A sample letter format is given in Figure 11.2. These letters should use clear, simple language to explain the nature of the disease and its effects, its symptoms, preventive measures, and steps to take if symptoms appear. The center's health care consultant can be called upon to help develop such a letter. If a child's parents do not speak English, an appropriate translation of the letter will be needed.

Caring for the Mildly Ill Child

Some child care programs choose to care for mildly ill children. The decision is usually made on a case-by-case basis unless the center has separate facilities that are used exclusively for ill children. Often, family day-care providers are asked to care for a mildly ill child, such as one who is recovering from chicken pox but whose blisters have not yet scabbed over.

The issue of whether a mildly ill child should be accepted in the child care setting can be emotionally charged. Parents of sick children often have no alternate means of care except missing work and losing pay. While ill children need more rest and quiet play than healthy children, they do best in familiar settings with familiar caregivers who can give them adequate attention. This can mean that healthy children may receive inadequate attention from caregivers if ill children come to school. And parents of healthy children do not want to risk having their children become ill.

The decision to accept a mildly ill child into a program or family day care must be made on an individual basis. Questions to consider include:

- How sick does the child act?
- Can the child participate in routine activities?
- How contagious is the child to other children?
- Is the program housed and designed so that the ill child can be separated from healthy children?
- Is there a large enough staff to give needed attention to the ill child without compromising the safety or well-being of the other children?
- What alternate means of care are available to the parents?
- Is there someone on the staff who is knowledgeable about the care of ill children?

The final decision has to be made on an individual basis. It should always be based on health policy guidelines. Child care centers and family day-care providers should never feel forced to accept an ill child when it is not in the best interest of their programs. Some centers head off many problems by asking parents at the time of enrollment if they have sick child care arrangements. Center policies about illness can be clarified at that time.

Administering Medicine

State regulations vary concerning the giving of medicines to children at child care centers. Caregivers should know and obey the regulations of their states. Only when child care providers have specific written permission from the parents should they give children medicines, including any nonprescription medicines, and only if state regulations allow. All prescription medicine must be in its original container with the pharmacy label giving the name of the child, the name of the medicine, and the doctor's instructions for administration. Nonprescription medicines must be in their original containers with age-appropriate dosage information. Many centers require physicians' instructions for nonprescription medicines as well.

One person should be responsible for receiving medications, keeping them safely locked away from children, and administering them. Caregivers who give medicines to children should check the label several times to be sure they are giving the medicine to the correct child and in the correct dosage. Keep a written record of the time, the amount, and the child to whom the medicine was given.

SUMMARY

- Children in child care settings are more at risk from infectious diseases than children at home because they are exposed to more people.
- Young children are at greater risk from infectious diseases than older children because of their stage of development.
- Infectious diseases are caused by pathogens—disease-causing viruses, bacteria, parasites, and fungi.
- Communicable diseases can be passed from one person to another; noncommunicable diseases cannot.
- Communicable diseases are spread four ways: by respiratory droplets, fecal-oral contamination, direct contact, and body fluids.
- Noncommunicable diseases can be transmitted by the bite of an infected animal, through contaminated food, and by deep-wound contamination.
- Infectious illnesses follow a similar pattern: incubation period while the pathogen grows, symptoms are absent; prodromal stage while symptoms are nonspecific; acute stage while symptoms of a specific infection are present; and recovery stage while symptoms recede, health returns.
- Infections transmitted by respiratory droplets include the common cold, influenza, strep throat, chicken pox, and Hib disease.
- Infections transmitted by fecal-oral contamination include hepatitis A, pinworms, and giardia.
- Infections transmitted by direct contact include head lice, impetigo, conjunctivitis, scabies, and ringworm.
- Infections transmitted by body fluids include HIV, which causes AIDS, hepatitis B, and cytomegalovirus (CMV).
- Noncommunicable infections include Lyme disease, Rocky Mountain spotted fever, botulism, middle ear infections, and diaper rash.
- Immunization prevents people from becoming ill with certain diseases.
- Some diseases must be reported to local or state public health agencies.
- Measures to minimize the spread of disease in a child care setting include physical considerations in the center itself, proper diapering technique, thorough and frequent handwashing, sanitizing of surfaces, and the use of universal precautions.
- Illness policies are designed to ensure the health of all children and caregivers.
- Parents should be notified if their children have been exposed to a communicable illness.
- Some centers may choose to accommodate mildly ill children.
- Medicines, including nonprescription medicines, may be given to children only with specific written permission from the parent.

ACQUIRING KNOWLEDGE

1. What are the two major reasons for the drastic drop in infant mortality during this century?
2. What are infectious diseases?
3. What is the difference between a communicable disease and a noncommunicable disease? Give an example of each type.
4. Define pathogens. What is the more commonly used term for pathogen?
5. Explain what happens when a virus invades a person's body and how immunization against a viral illness prevents the disease.
6. How can disease-causing bacteria be killed?
7. What are two problems with the use of antibiotics?
8. What is a parasite? Identify three diseases caused by parasites.
9. What are the four basic ways communicable diseases are transmitted from person to person?
10. Briefly describe the four stages of an infectious illness.
11. What is a carrier?
12. Identify three diseases spread through respiratory secretions.
13. Why are colds so difficult to prevent?
14. Why is it important that strep throat be identified and properly treated?
15. How does fecal-oral contamination commonly occur?
16. What is giardia? In child care settings, how is it most frequently spread?
17. What is conjunctivitis and how is it spread?
18. Explain how HIV is transmitted from one person to another.
19. Should children with noncommunicable infections be excluded from child care? Explain your answer.
20. How can caregivers help lower the risk of diaper rash from yeast?
21. Why are the majority of vaccines given more than once?
22. Describe the three categories of reportable diseases.
23. Identify three ways child care centers can be arranged to help discourage the spread of illness.
24. What areas of a child care center should routinely be sanitized?
25. When is it necessary to inform parents about illnesses at the center?

THINKING CRITICALLY

1. Explain the importance of handwashing to preventing the spread of disease.
2. Why is it important for caregivers to practice universal precautions?
3. If a child runs a fever of 101° F (38.3° C) in the evening but is normal the next morning and exhibits no other signs of illness, should the child be sent to school? Why or why not?
4. Children in child care centers run a higher risk of becoming ill than do children cared for at home. Are there steps caregivers can take to lower this risk? If so, what are they?
5. Parents who work full time need good child care for their children. However, children in child care centers run a higher risk of becoming ill. This may cause parents to miss work. How can parents deal with such conflicts?

OBSERVATIONS AND APPLICATIONS

1. Observe children in a child care center. Note how many of the children have runny noses. During a 20-minute period, how many children and caregivers sneeze? How many cough? Do any children cover their mouths when they cough? Do you observe caregivers wiping the noses of any of the children? Do caregivers wash their hands afterwards? If the facility has a diaper-changing area, observe caregivers changing diapers. Do caregivers wash their hands after each diaper change? Are diapers disposed of in a covered, plastic-lined pail?

2. Observe the sanitary precautions taken at the center. You may have to come before or after normal school hours to observe some of these procedures. Is the diaper table sanitized? After each use? Once a day? Once a week? What about the toys? What about the dress-up clothes? What about the tables where food is served? Where children work?

3. Suppose that Sophia is a child in your class at a child care center. She has been sent to school sick on more than one occasion—twice while running a fever. When questioned, her parents say that she seemed fine in the morning. Sophia confides to you that her mother cannot afford to miss any more days of work and is aware that she is sending her child in sick. The center has a strict policy on illness. You feel the policy must be enforced in order to minimize the number of illnesses in the class. However, you do not want Sophia's mother to lose her job. What should you do?

4. Jerry has been scratching his head all day. You check his head and realize that he has head lice. What should you do?

FOR FURTHER INFORMATION

American Academy of Pediatrics. (1987). *Health in day care: A manual for health professionals.* Elk Grove Village, IL: Author.

American Academy of Pediatrics & American Public Health Association. (1992). *Caring for our children—national health and safety performance standards: Guidelines for out-of-home child care programs.* Elk Grove Village, IL, & Washington, DC: Author.

Andersen, R. D., Bale Jr., J., Blackman, J., & Murph, J. (1986). *Infections in children.* Rockville, MD: Aspen Publishers.

Kendrick, A. S., Kaufmann, R., & Messenger, K. (1991). *Healthy young children.* Washington, DC: National Association for the Education of Young Children.

National Association for the Education of Young Children. (1987). Lice aren't nice. *Young Children, 42*(3), 46.

Taylor, J. M., & Taylor, W. S. (1989). *Communicable disease and young children in group settings.* Boston: Little, Brown.

Whaley, L. F., & Wong, D. L. (1991). *Nursing care of infants and children* (4th ed.). St. Louis, MO: Mosby–Year Book.

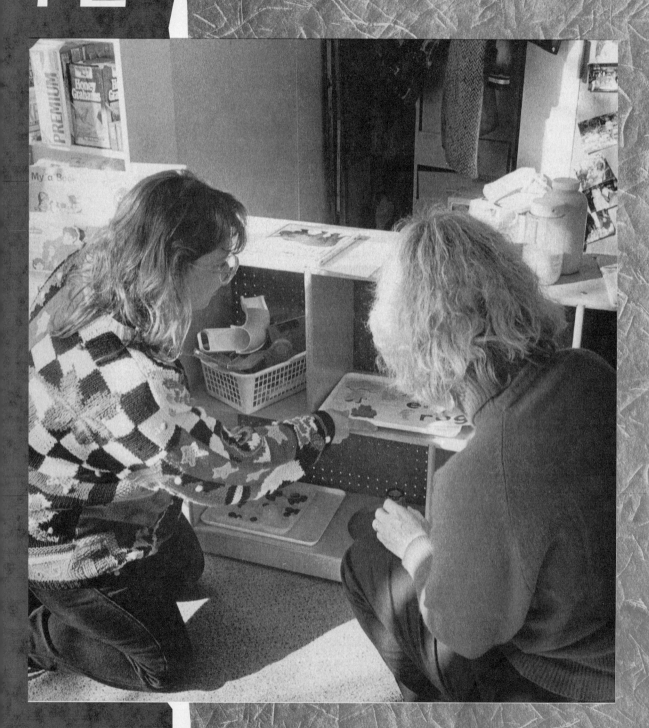

OBJECTIVES

Studying this chapter
will enable you to

- List the most common causes of
  unintentional injuries among
  infants and children
- Describe the most common types
  of unintentional injuries that affect
  infants and toddlers and list ways
  of preventing such injuries
- Describe the most common types
  of unintentional injuries that affect
  preschool and school-age children
  and list ways of preventing such
  injuries
- Describe ways to create safe
  indoor and outdoor environments
  for infants and young children

CHAPTER TERMS

attractive nuisance
drowning
entrapment
flame-retardant
mechanical suffocation
toxic
unintentional injuries
usable space

STEPHANIE and Michelle were excited about their first year as caregivers at Cornerstone Church's new child development center. Concerned about the growing need for child care in its lower middle class neighborhood, the church had converted some of its space into a child care center. The new center would be able to accommodate 40 toddlers and preschoolers.

A week before the center opened, Stephanie and Michelle were working to get the classroom in shape. It would soon be filled with 18 active four- and five-year-olds. They were unpacking supplies and working on a plan for arranging the room.

"Why don't we put this cabinet over by the bookshelf?" asked Stephanie.

"Okay," said Michelle. "No—wait a minute. If we put it there, that corner will be cut off from the rest of the room."

"That's true. If we bring the cabinet out from the wall, we won't be able to see into that space from here. But if we put it next to the bookshelf and against the wall, we could make that the quiet corner since the books and puzzles are back there already."

"Good idea!" Michelle agreed. "Then we can set up the easels and the art table over by the sink. That will make cleanup easy, and children involved in art activities won't be disturbed by children playing with blocks." Michelle frowned slightly. "We can't put the block bin near the window though. It's too easy to climb on."

The sound of the center's doorbell interrupted their conversation.

"That's probably the fire inspector," Stephanie said. "Someone is supposed to come check the facility today."

Stephanie and Michelle admitted the inspector. He examined the area, checking the smoke detectors and fire extinguishers as well as a number of other items. The inspector was impressed that the center had one of the new carbon monoxide detectors. After he finished, he handed the teachers a completed checklist.

"Please remind the director that before you open, each classroom needs a map showing the layout of the building and the route the class should take to get outside in case of fire. You'll also need to hold a fire drill during the first week you're open and regular fire drills every month. Otherwise, everything looks good."

"Great!" said Michelle. She turned to Stephanie. "I can hardly wait for the children to get here!"

Children are naturally curious. They learn about their world by exploring, by trial and error, and by imitating the behavior of others. Young children's drive to learn about their world combined with their lack of practical experience often puts them in hazardous situations. Most of the time, they are unaware that they are in danger at all. Because children cannot evaluate the risks involved in their own behavior, adult caregivers must provide a safe environment and adequate supervision. This is a primary consideration for caregivers who are acting *in loco parentis* (in place of the parent) while children are in their care.

Unintentional injuries, or accidents, are injuries that could have been foreseen and possibly prevented. Many injuries can be prevented by creating a developmentally appropriate environment. It is also important to be aware of possible hazards in the environment and work to eliminate or minimize them. Teaching children about safety makes a positive difference as well, but there is no substitute for alert adult supervision.

Causes of Death and Unintentional Injuries in Children

The death rate among children has decreased dramatically during this century. This has been due in large part to the development and widespread use of antibiotics, vaccines, and other medical advances.

Today, unintentional injuries are the leading cause of death in children over one year old. In fact, accidents cause more deaths and disabilities in children over the age of one than do all disease causes combined (Whaley &

Wong, 1991). Automobile accidents account for about half of all accidental deaths among children and are also the single largest cause of injuries during childhood. Currently, all 50 states require the use of safety restraints (car seats or seat belts) for young children in motor vehicles, although the ages for which car seats are required vary from state to state. Safety restraint laws have led to a steep decline in the number of childhood motor vehicle fatalities (Public Health Service, 1991). However, failure to use child restraints or to use restraints properly is the cause of many injuries each year.

Other common causes of fatal injuries during childhood include drowning, fires and burns, poisoning, falls, and suffocation. *Mechanical suffocation* occurs when oxygen cannot get to the lungs because an object (such as a pillow or a plastic bag) is covering the mouth and nose or there is pressure on the throat or chest. Mechanical suffocation can also occur when a child is trapped in an airtight enclosed space such as a refrigerator or other large appliance. Infants and young children can also suffocate by aspiration. This is when they inhale foreign substances into their lungs or choke on food or other objects that block their airways. *Drowning* is suffocation by submersion in water or another liquid.

The frequency with which fatal injuries from particular causes occur varies with such factors as the age and gender of the child and where the child lives. For example, more than half of all poisonings occur in children under the age of two years (Whaley & Wong, 1991). More drownings are reported in warm states, where beaches and swimming pools are common, than in colder northern areas.

It's important to realize, however, that only a small percentage of childhood injuries each year result in death. Many more children suffer nonfatal injuries that require medical attention and hospitalization. About 16 million children are seen in emergency rooms in the United States each year. Thirty thousand of these children suffer from permanent disability as a result of an injury (Division of Injury Control, 1990). Many others have their normal activities temporarily curtailed.

Safety for Infants and Toddlers

Infants and toddlers cannot assess the security of their environments. They have no sense of danger and will regard a smooth, rounded baby rattle and a sharp, pointed pair of scissors with a similar degree of interest. To infants, both are objects to explore.

Since infants and toddlers will touch, mouth, and eat almost anything, the only way to prevent unintentional injuries in children of this age is to limit their access to hazards. To do this effectively, caregivers must be aware of the children's level of development and be able to anticipate what they might do. A baby who cannot yet crawl can still reach an attractive object by squirming. Children who can walk can also climb. To prevent unintentional injuries, the caregiver must see the world from the child's point of view. Sitting on the floor often reveals hazards unnoticed when adults are standing in or walking around a room.

SAFETY TIPS

Electrical Safety

"What are these interesting holes in the wall? Let me see if this spoon handle will fit. . . ."

There's no doubt about it—small children find electrical outlets *fascinating*. Adults need to protect young children by putting plastic outlet covers on all unused outlets. Even outlets that have appliances plugged into them may have to be covered to protect plug-pulling youngsters.

It is hard for young children to understand the dangers associated with electrical outlets and appliances. Appliances and tools should not be left plugged in and unattended. Adults are advised to inspect plugs and cords regularly and to repair or replace them whenever necessary.

Abilities, Mobility, and Unintentional Injuries

"I only turned my back for a second and Emily pulled a cup of coffee off the table and got burned."

"I had no idea Ben could climb up on the counter and stick a fork in the toaster." When people talk about their children's accidents, they often mention how sudden and unexpected the injury was.

Infants and toddlers become more coordinated and mobile with each day that passes. Many unintentional injuries occur because an adult underestimates the physical skills and determination of a young child. Others happen because an adult overestimates the child's ability to understand and remember the hazards of a situation. Just because a toddler has been told to stay away from the fireplace does not mean that, absorbed in play, he will remember the rule—or even be able to associate the heat of the fire with danger and pain.

Infants.   Unintentional injuries rank sixth as a cause of death in infants. Many accidents occur because infants do the unexpected. During the first four months of life, infants cannot direct their movements, but they *can* move. They kick, wiggle, thrash, and may roll over. Their movements are often unpredictable and may take a caregiver by surprise. Falls, therefore, are a danger from birth.

Infants are especially vulnerable to suffocation because they cannot direct their movements to get away from anything that interferes with their breathing. Infants' bedclothes and anything else infants come in contact with should be evaluated as a potential suffocation hazard.

Babies are also at risk of inhaling foreign material. They cannot stop excess liquid from flowing out of a bottle, for example, and without help will choke and breathe the liquid into their lungs. This is one reason why babies should always be held when they are fed.

After four months of age, infants become increasingly mobile and rapidly gain control over their movements. They begin reaching for and grasping objects. They may, for example, lunge toward a cup of hot coffee or try to grab a pair of scissors carried by a caregiver. As babies gain control of their hands, more and more small objects go into their mouths, increasing the risk of choking. Certain foods are especially hazardous, including nuts, grapes, popcorn, hard candy, and improperly cut hot dogs.

During the second half of the first year, creeping turns to crawling, and then walking and climbing. Babies are avid explorers of their environments. It is the job of caregivers to anticipate hazards in environments and either remove them completely or keep them well out of babies' reaches. The chance of an accidental poisoning increases as babies move more freely. Falls occur frequently with children who are learning to walk.

Babies love to climb. They may climb up stairs and be unable to climb down, creating the possibility of a serious fall. Or they may attempt to climb out of their cribs. For this reason, caregivers must be alert at all times to babies' movements.

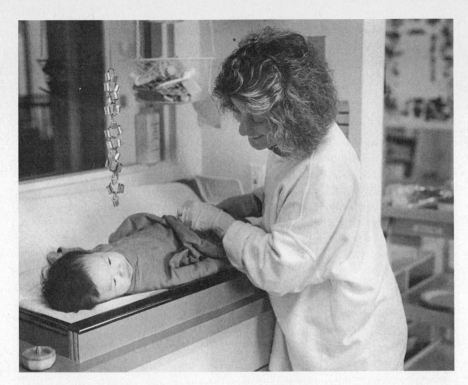

Infants' movements are often unpredictable, and falls are a constant danger. Caregivers should exercise caution when a baby is on the changing table.

Water is attractive to many children, and infants can drown in only a few inches of water. Children should never be left alone in the bath, near swimming pools, or near other bodies of water. Buckets containing only a few inches of water can be especially hazardous to babies. An infant who tips headfirst into a bucket of water will not have the strength or coordination needed to pull her head out.

Babies are also vulnerable to some types of unintentional injuries that are not directly related to developmental abilities. These include motor vehicle accidents, house fires, and sunburn.

Toddlers. More childhood deaths from unintentional injuries occur between the ages of one and four than among any other age group except adolescents (Whaley & Wong, 1991). A caregiver's goal, however, is not to create a sterile, risk-free environment, but rather to provide a safe environment where children can take moderate, well-controlled risks and find developmentally appropriate challenges. Many accidents in this age group occur because children's abilities are not adequate to deal with their environments. Others occur because toddlers can move around and quickly get into situations in which adult supervision is inadequate.

Most toddlers are extremely active, infinitely curious, and highly unpredictable. They walk, run, and climb; they open doors, windows, and drawers. When toddlers are able to unlatch gates, they may wander into potentially dangerous areas such as pool enclosures or busy streets. This puts them at risk for serious and even fatal injuries. Toddlers can be extremely persistent and resourceful when faced with a task such as removing a safety cap from a medicine bottle or sticking a bobby pin in an electrical outlet. Toddlers can also be easily distracted. They may hear and repeat a safety rule, such as "Don't touch the hot stove," one minute and, just a minute later, reach for a brightly glowing burner. Caregivers who are responsible for a group of toddlers must eliminate safety hazards, establish limits on toddler behavior, and be ever-alert for possible dangers.

Toddlers do not like to be restrained and may strongly resist being buckled into a car seat. Insisting that the child is safely buckled in for every trip, however, is essential.

Children in this age group love to explore. They are fascinated by matches, cigarettes, electrical outlets, electrical wires, and appliances. Many a curious toddler has pulled a pot containing hot liquid down on himself because he could see and reach it. Burns rank high as a cause of death among toddlers. Buckets of water remain a serious drowning hazard.

Toddlers still explore objects with their mouths. In fact, poisonings occur more frequently during the second year than at any other time (Whaley & Wong, 1991). Before age six, children have a poorly developed sense of taste and will eat and drink things adults find revolting such as houseplants or bleach.

The possibility of unintentional injuries from choking on small pieces of food or nonfood substances continues to exist, just as it did for infants. Falls remain common, especially since some toddlers are capable of unlatching gates that block off stairways. Although most falls are not fatal, toddlers do receive more head injuries from falls than older children.

Preventing Injuries in Infants and Toddlers

Unintentional injuries can occur anywhere. At home, most accidents occur indoors. In a child care center, most accidents take place outside on the playground. Most unintentional injuries are not serious. Over 95 percent of children under the age of 17 are not permanently disabled in any way as a result of the accidents they have. About 2 percent are mildly disabled. An additional 2 percent have moderate disability and 0.2 percent are severely disabled (Pless, 1987).

At a child care center, accidents are more likely to happen at certain times than at others. They are more likely to occur when the center is short staffed, when caregivers are tired or under stress, in the late morning and late afternoon when children are hungry and tired, on field trips, and when the center's routine is disrupted. When, for example, one child is injured and requires the exclusive attention of a staff member, another child is more likely to be involved in an unintentional injury (Kendrick, Kaufmann, & Messenger, 1991).

Some children are also at higher risk for unintentional injuries than others. Boys are injured more often than girls. Children who are under stress at home from causes ranging from poverty to a new sibling to a parental divorce are also more likely to by injured (Whaley & Wong, 1991). Children who have a difficult temperament or an assertive personality may often challenge rules and may be more at risk. Recognizing when, where, and to whom unintentional injuries are most likely to occur is necessary if injuries are to be prevented.

In a child care setting, safety must be a primary concern for the sake of the staff and the center as well as the children. When unintentional injuries do occur, even temporary injuries may have serious legal consequences for the child care provider and the center. Adequate liability insurance for the center and individual staff members is an important consideration.

Motor Vehicle Injuries. Motor vehicle accidents are the leading cause of death among children. Since 1970, the rate of childhood deaths from automobile accidents has declined 41 percent for children ages one through four and 31 percent for children ages 5 through 14. This decline is the result of increased use of car seats and seat belts.

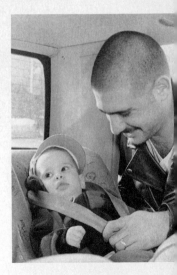

The use of infant car seats has led to a dramatic decline in childhood deaths from automobile accidents over the last two decades.

Although it has been conclusively demonstrated that car seats and seat belts save lives, some people still do not buckle up their children for every trip. And sometimes car seats are used incorrectly. An Oklahoma study of emergency room care of children under two years of age showed that 7 percent of the children had injuries related to the improper use of car seats (*Child Health Alert*, 1993).

Car seats serve three purposes. During the crash, they prevent the child from being thrown out of the car and from colliding with the interior of the car. Car seats also absorb some of the crash forces and distribute them over the strongest parts of the body. All car seats manufactured since January 1981 must meet federal motor vehicle safety standards. Car seats made before 1981 should not be used.

There are two types of approved car seats. Infant safety seats should only be used for babies weighing up to 20 pounds. Convertible car seats can be used for children who weigh as much as 40 pounds. When used with an infant under 20 pounds, the infant or convertible car seat must be installed so that the baby faces rearward. Convertible car seats for children who weigh 20 to 40 pounds are installed so that the child faces forward. Booster seats can be used to help position seat belts properly for children who weigh 40 to 65 pounds. Booster seats provide less protection, however, than infant or convertible car seats and should not be used for children who weigh less than 40 pounds.

All car seats should be secured with a seat belt according to the manufacturer's instructions. Some car seats are secured with a tethered harness that comes with the seat. In some cars, a special locking clip may be required to keep the seat belt tight and the car seat in place. The safest place for a child in a car seat is in the center of the rear seat of the vehicle.

In a child care setting, parent volunteers are sometimes asked to transport children on field trips. Before this is done, center staff should determine that the center's liability insurance remains valid in this circumstance. Every driver should show a valid driver's license, vehicle registration, and proof of

The Buckle-Up Habit

It was "Show and Tell" time for the five-year-olds at the child care center. Tommy had just wowed the class with his new pet rabbit. Lindsey showed the children a bird's nest she had found. Then Therese raised her hand and asked if she could say something. Luz, the teacher, said, "Of course."

"Well," Therese began, "yesterday my mom and I went shopping. We were driving on this big street, and there was a red light. We stopped but the car behind us didn't. It hit us in the back. We were okay but the car has a big dent."

"I'm so glad you weren't hurt," Luz exclaimed. "A car accident is very scary. Were you and your mother wearing seat belts?"

"Oh, yes," nodded Therese. "Mom won't even start the car until we're all buckled in."

"Your mother is smart," smiled Luz. "Therese, tell the class why it's important to buckle your seat belt."

"If you don't," Therese answered, "you could be hurt if you have an accident."

Therese did not seem to be frightened by her experience, so Luz asked her to describe what happened to her when the other car hit the car she was in.

"Well, there was a big bang. And the car jumped," Therese said, "But the seat belt held me still."

Luz used this incident to impress upon the children the importance of buckling up whenever they get in a car. She did not alarm them with details of what might happen to them if they did not use their seat belts. She simply told them that using seat belts is smart. "A seat belt is like a big arm holding you because it wants you to be safe," she said.

Luz asked the children, "How many of you will promise always to buckle your seat belts when you're in a car?" The response was unanimous.

Should Luz have asked Therese to describe the dent in the car? Should she have used more graphic details to impress on the children the importance of buckling up? What might you have done differently in this situation?

insurance before leaving. Centers may even want to have photocopies of these documents on file. Caregivers should review the route and explain emergency procedures to drivers. There should never be more children in a car than there are car seats and/or seat belts, as appropriate for the ages and weights of the children being transported.

Mechanical Suffocation. Mechanical suffocation can occur in various ways. As mentioned earlier, infants cannot move away from something that interferes with their breathing. For example, a thick, soft blanket could cover a baby's nose and mouth and cause suffocation. Pillows are not necessary for babies and can be hazardous. Plastic bags are also highly dangerous to infants and young children. Keep them out of the reach of children, and always knot plastic bags before throwing them away. Avoid using crib mattresses that are covered with loose plastic.

Other hazards for infants include crib slats that are too far apart and excess space between the crib mattress and the crib frame. In both cases, the child's head can be trapped and the child can suffocate. Crib slats should be no more than 2⅜ inches apart. If an adult can place two fingers between the mattress and crib frame, the mattress is too small.

Although toddlers are less at risk than infants for suffocating in cribs, they may get loose clothing entangled in furniture or play equipment and strangle. Toddlers can also strangle on curtain and drapery cords. With their increased mobility, toddlers are at risk around certain types of appliances, such as refrigerators or front-loading washing machines. *Entrapment* occurs when a child climbs into the appliance and shuts the door and then is unable to open it from inside. Once all the oxygen in the appliance is used up, the child suffocates. Appliances in storage should be positioned with their doors tight against a wall. Discarded appliances should have their doors removed.

Aspiration.   Aspiration, inhaling a foreign object into the airway, is a leading cause of fatal injury in children under one year old (Whaley & Wong, 1991). Infants and toddlers explore everything with their mouths. This is why nonfood items cause most deaths in which children suffocate by aspiration.

Marbles and other round objects smaller than 1¼ inches are particularly dangerous since they can plug the airway completely. Rigid objects are easier to expel than pliable ones, which is why uninflated or popped balloons cause more deaths in children than any other inhaled objects. These balloons should be kept away from all young children, especially those under four years old. Coins are also deadly, partly because they are so common in everyday life and partly because their size and shape tends to block the airways effectively. Other dangerous nonfood items include screws, bolts, nuts, and homemade or poorly constructed pacifiers and buttons.

Another common hazard to babies is baby powder made with talc. If inhaled, it can cause fatal aspiration pneumonia. Cornstarch-based powders are preferred over talc powders. When using any type of baby powder, caregivers should sprinkle the powder on their hands and then rub it on the baby rather than sprinkle it directly on the baby's bottom. A baby should never be allowed to play with a container of powder.

Falls.   Falls are most common after four months of age. However, from birth infants should not be left unattended on changing tables, couches, beds, or other high places. Babies make many unexpected movements, and they develop new abilities rapidly. Children who are incapable of crawling out of their cribs today may surprise you by doing it tomorrow. Caregivers should develop the habit of keeping crib rails up.

Infant walkers are considered dangerous because they are involved in so many infant falls. Walker-related falls down a flight of stairs in the home are the most common. The American Academy of Pediatrics strongly recommends against the use of infant walkers.

Falls are a common hazard in child care centers. Caregivers can help reduce the occurrence of these accidents by using nonslip pads under rugs.

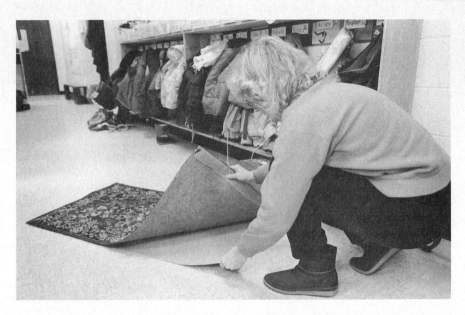

Safety gates should be placed at the tops of stairwells to prevent falls. The spacing between the slats in a gate should never be great enough to allow a child's head to become trapped or small enough to pinch fingers or toes. Gates at the bottom of stairs are also a good idea since they prevent a crawling infant from going up the stairs before she is able to climb back down.

Children who are learning to walk do their share of falling, although most injuries are mild. Padding sharp edges of furniture and securing rugs with nonslip mats helps reduce the severity of injuries and the number of falls. Remember that toddlers who can walk can also climb. Consider furniture placement, as Stephanie and Michelle did in the story at the beginning of the chapter. Arrange furniture in ways that discourage climbing. Every year, a number of children climb up on window sills and fall out of open windows. Screens alone will not keep children safe. Safety guards should be installed in all windows that can open.

Drowning.   Infants and toddlers can drown in a small amount of water. Drownings can occur both indoors and out. Never leave a young child unattended in the bath, even for a second. The bathroom is one of the most dangerous rooms in the house or child care center, and children should not be allowed to play there. As mentioned earlier, infants and toddlers can drown in just a few inches of water.

Outside, it is essential that any permanent pool in a child care facility be fenced. Gates should be childproof. Wading pools should be emptied immediately after each use. In a child care setting, sprinklers are preferred over wading pools. They not only eliminate the drowning hazard but also are less likely to spread disease. Around natural bodies of water that cannot be fenced, caregivers must either provide continuous, close supervision or remove the children from the area.

Burns. Accidental burns occur in a number of situations. Infants can be burned either by formula or other food that is too hot. They can be scalded by bath water. Even the metal attachments of car seats, after exposure to direct sun, can become hot enough to cause painful burns. Such burns can be avoided by checking the temperature of these items before allowing an infant to come into contact with them. Hot water heaters should be set so that the water temperature does not exceed 120° F (49° C). This will also prevent toddlers who can turn on the taps from accidentally scalding themselves.

Overexposure to the sun can cause serious burns as well. Infants and toddlers burn much more easily than adults. All children, even those with dark skin, need protection from the sun (see Chapter 13). Keep babies under six months of age out of direct sunlight as much as possible.

As noted earlier, many children are burned when they try to grab something hot out of a caregiver's hand. Toddlers, with their increased mobility, are most likely to be scalded by spilling containers of hot liquid on themselves. It only takes a second for a toddler to pull a cup of coffee off the table or a pot off the stove. Pot handles should always be turned in so they cannot be reached by young children.

Space heaters and fireplaces can also cause burns. Both should have protective coverings. Every house, apartment, and child care center should have working smoke detectors, and detector batteries need to be checked monthly. Centers should have two or more exits to the outdoors in case of fire. Never use an elevator in case of fire.

Poisoning. As soon as babies can grasp an object, they will bring it to their mouths. Infants and toddlers cannot distinguish poisonous from nonpoisonous substances, and they are unlikely to reject something because of its smell or taste. Most poisonings are the result of poor storage practices. No unlocked cabinet can be considered childproof. Toddlers are adept climbers and can move furniture to enable them to reach high cabinets. In a child care center, all cleaning materials should be stored in a locked closet, preferably outside of the classroom. There should also be a locked cabinet for medicines and first-aid supplies. Caregivers should create a childproof place to leave handbags and personal belongings including medicines, other poisonous substances, matches, cigarette lighters, and sharp objects.

Garage and basement areas often contain an abundance of materials that are *toxic*—that is, harmful or poisonous—to people. Paints, weed killers, turpentine, pesticides, and other common substances are all toxic. Generally, these areas are poorly childproofed because they are not places children are expected to play. In a child care center, areas like these must be physically separate from all areas to which children have access.

Many common plants found both indoors and outdoors are poisonous if eaten (see Figure 12.1). Hyacinth, daffodil, philodendron, rhododendron, and azalea are just a few examples. Many colorful berries, including mistletoe berries, are poisonous too. So are the pesticides that may be sprayed on plants. Keep poisonous plants out of the classroom and avoid using pesticides on plants that remain.

FIGURE 12.1 Poisonous Plants. Whereas some plants are only mildly poisonous, others can be fatal if ingested. This list includes some of the more common poisonous plants.

POISONOUS PLANTS
Azalea
Belladonna
Buttercup
Cherry
Daffodil
Delphinium
Dieffenbachia
Foxglove
Hyacinth
Hydrangea
Iris
Jonquil
Larkspur
Laurel
Lily of the valley
Lupine
Mistletoe
Mountain laurel
Narcissus
Nightshade
Oak
Oleander
Philodendron
Poinsettia
Privet
Rhododendron
Sweet pea
Tobacco
Wisteria
Yew

FOCUS ON Cultural Diversity

Attitudes About Toddler Independence

During the toddler years, children learn new skills every day. As soon as a child begins to walk, talk, and feed himself, he has taken the first steps down the long road to independence. Some cultures encourage a high degree of independence at an early age. Others do not.

Physical and developmental factors can influence independence. For example, early toilet training, which is encouraged in Chinese families, gives a child a feeling of control and independence. The acquisition of language skills, which enables children to make others understand their needs and wants, is also a major step toward independence. Parents in any culture who encourage a child's language skills by talking and reading to him are helping to make him more independent.

Cultural attitudes toward breast-feeding and child care also affect independence. For example, children in some African cultures are breast-fed into the toddler years. Continued breast-feeding keeps a child closer to his mother. In some African American and Hispanic cultures, young children are often cared for by members of the extended family rather than outsiders. This keeps the children closer to the family and may make them less independent than children who attend a child care center.

The sex of a child can be an important influence on independence too. In many cultures, boys are encouraged to be more independent than girls.

In any culture, parents often find that whatever they do, a child's own personality ultimately has a very large influence on how fast that child becomes independent.

Another special concern of child care centers is the safety of art supplies. Look for the notation *AP* for "Approved Product" or *CP* for "Certified Product" to indicate that these products are nontoxic. Even when nontoxic products are used, children should be discouraged from eating paste or clay or sucking on paintbrushes or markers.

In both homes and child care centers, the telephone number of the local poison control center should be posted near the telephone. Child care centers should keep an up-to-date container of syrup of ipecac on hand to use if and only if the poison control center advises making the child vomit poisonous material.

Other Causes of Injury. Sharp objects often cause toddler injuries. Discourage children from running with sharp objects or sticks in their hands. Keep knives and other sharp implements out of children's reach.

Firearms that are accidentally discharged kill children every year. In a home, guns should be kept unloaded in a locked closet. Bullets should be stored separately, also in a locked container. Guns have no place in a child care center.

Pets and toddlers do not always mix. Even the most even-tempered animal may bite or scratch if unintentionally abused by a child. At home, pets should have a place to get away from overly aggressive toddlers. In a child care setting, pet visitors must be very closely supervised. Animals can feel threatened by a pack of noisy, pushy children and react by biting.

In a child care center, safety glass should be used for all glass at children's height. Safety decals make glass more visible and prevent collisions. Install safety strips or devices that slow the closing of doors to prevent fingers from being crushed.

Safety for Preschool and School-Age Children

Preschool children face many of the same hazards as toddlers. They are still active and curious explorers. They are better coordinated, however, and are able to run faster and climb higher. Yet their ability to anticipate danger remains limited. These children frequently forget safety rules and fail to understand the consequences of their actions.

School-age children spend more time without adult supervision walking to school, playing in their neighborhoods, and playing at home. This makes them more vulnerable to approach by a stranger (see Chapter 13). Pedestrian fatalities peak in the five- to nine-year-old age group (Rivara & Barber, 1985). Many school-age children are also involved in bicycle accidents. Falls on the playground are common but rarely disabling. Unintentional poisonings decrease as does the threat of suffocation. Intentional risk-taking, however, in which school-age children knowingly engage in unsafe behavior to be accepted by their peer group, causes many serious accidents.

Abilities, Mobility, and Unintentional Injuries

Just as with infants and toddlers, the types of unintentional injuries preschoolers and school-age children are most likely to experience are directly related to their level of development. Understanding the abilities of children at different stages of development is an important part of preventing unintentional injuries.

Preschoolers. As preschoolers develop, they are rapidly refining both gross and fine motor skills. They are better coordinated than toddlers and many will be able to outwit child locks and childproof gates. This means that a swimming pool that was safely closed with a childproof gate may now need to be secured with a lock and key. Preschoolers are also able to leave the house or yard and get into unsafe situations in the street or on sidewalks.

Most preschoolers enjoy riding tricycles and want to venture out into the larger world. Children on tricycles are low to the ground and difficult for drivers to see. Preschoolers may accidentally ride out of a driveway and into traffic or lose control of their tricycles and crash when going down a hill.

Preschoolers love to climb, but they may get stuck when they're up high, panic, and fall. Windows still need safety guards because preschoolers like to climb up and look out.

Preschool is a time for teaching safety rules. Caregivers, however, can never depend on a preschooler to remember the rule or know when to apply it. The same preschooler who carefully repeats "look both ways before you cross the street" is all too likely to dart into traffic after a rolling ball. Supervision must be combined with safety education to keep preschoolers safe.

School-Age Children. It is neither possible nor desirable to limit school-age children's access to all hazards. With school-age children, safety education must gradually replace physical barriers as the chief way to prevent accidents. As they mature, school-age children become better able to recognize risks and anticipate dangerous situations. Unfortunately, some school-age children will knowingly participate in unsafe behavior as a way to be accepted by their peer groups.

Bicycle accidents are common among this age group. They account for more than half a million visits to the emergency room each year. Most bicycle accidents involve failure to follow traffic laws and failure to use proper safety equipment, particularly bicycle helmets.

School-age children are especially attracted to matches and cigarette lighters as well as firecrackers, which are legal in some states. Risk-taking behavior may also involve playing with guns. Matches and cigarette lighters should be in locked cabinets. Firecrackers and guns have no place in a child care setting.

Many falls occur on the playground where school-age children test their strength and coordination. Some children who are going through growth spurts become uncoordinated and injury prone. In addition, school-age children who have access only to preschool equipment may use the equipment in unsafe ways to make it more challenging. As children become involved in organized sports, it is important to teach them injury prevention techniques, such as warming up, as well as to see that they have proper safety equipment.

Preventing Injuries Among Preschoolers and School-Age Children

Preschool and school-age children are increasingly involved in activities away from home. This is where most unintentional injuries happen. The children are excited by speed and motion, eager to try new skills, and easily influenced by peers. These traits are at the root of many accidents. In school-age children, the injury and death rate for boys is twice that of girls (Whaley & Wong, 1991). Of course, many children pass through childhood without serious injury.

Transportation Injuries. Motor vehicle injuries remain the leading cause of death among preschool and school-age children, and car seats and seat belts continue to be the primary defense against occupant injuries. As children spend more time outdoors, they are more likely to become pedestrian casualties in motor vehicle accidents. By the time children reach the

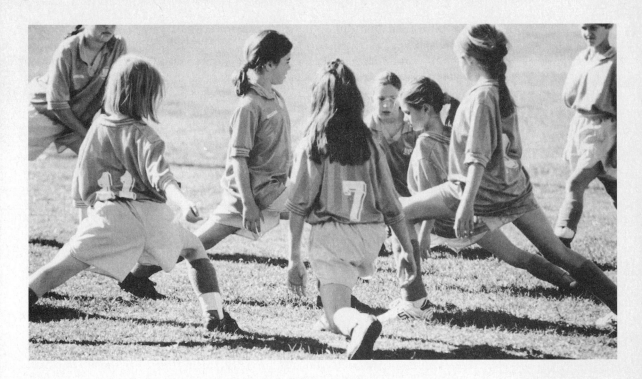

age of five, pedestrian fatalities have become two and a half times more frequent than occupant fatalities in motor vehicle accidents. Most pedestrian deaths occur among children between the ages of five and nine (Rivara & Barber, 1985). Half of these injuries occur at night and are related to the child's failure to observe traffic safety rules.

Children who play in organized sports need to learn how to prevent injuries by using the right equipment, such as the shin guards shown here.

As mentioned earlier, bicycle accidents also are frequent among school-age children. Many occur because the child loses control of the bike rather than because he is hit by a car. Most bicycle-related deaths are caused by head injuries. That is why all children should wear a properly fitting bicycle helmet that is approved by the American National Standards Institute (ANSI).

Other transportation-related accidents involve skateboards, roller skates, roller blades, all-terrain vehicles, snowmobiles, tractors, and ride-on mowers. None of these hazards should be found at a child care center or after-school program.

Drowning. Teaching preschool and school-age children to swim is a wise safety measure. Doing so gives no guarantee, however, that children will not panic when they are in the water. In natural bodies of water, unexpected currents can carry children into deep water far from shore. Many children tire more easily than they realize. Swimming instruction and flotation devices are not substitutes for careful adult supervision. Good supervision by certified water instructors coupled with teaching and enforcing water safety rules will prevent many drownings.

Although children in these age groups are not very likely to drown in a bucket of water, there are other drowning hazards that can be equally dangerous. For example, a swimming pool near a child care center, even if it is walled or fenced according to local ordinances, can be an *attractive nuisance*. An attractive nuisance is something that entices people to a restricted area or private property and may also pose a danger. Caregivers need to be aware of attractive nuisances that pose drowning or other hazards to the children in their care.

Burns.   The preschool years are a time of imitation. Many injuries occur when preschoolers attempt to imitate adult behavior. Often preschoolers are burned in attempts to "help" in the kitchen. Children of this age like to cook, but they need very direct, undistracted adult supervision and clear cooking safety rules. Older children continue to need supervision in the kitchen. They should be taught to treat the microwave with as much caution as the stove. Food cooked in the microwave can be extremely hot and may cause severe steam burns.

Other burn injuries occur when children play with matches and cigarette lighters. Preschoolers with long hair are especially at risk for setting their hair on fire. All children should be taught to stop, drop, and roll if their clothing catches fire and to crawl low to get out during a fire. Smoke and carbon monoxide detectors and fire extinguishers, such as those at Cornerstone Church's child development center, save lives. Fire drills are mandatory at child care centers and schools. Use them to familiarize children with at least two pathways out of the facility.

Other Causes of Injury.   Eye injuries caused by sharp objects are common among preschoolers and school-age children. They can be permanently disabling. Children need to be reminded many times not to run with sharp objects in their hands. Keeping the playground free of sticks and other debris will help to eliminate "sword fights."

Animals can react as aggressively toward older children as they sometimes do toward younger ones. Teach children not to approach strange animals on the street. If pet visitors are permitted at child care, supervise the pets and the children's behavior toward the pets very closely.

Safe Indoor Environments

Child care providers are responsible for creating a safe environment for the children entrusted to them (see Figure 12.2). Some aspects of safety are mandated by law. For example, Cornerstone Church needed a fire code inspection before opening its new center. Other safety considerations depend on the judgment of the program director and the caregivers. In many communities, family day-care arrangements are subject to special zoning and safety regulations and inspections. Anyone who wants to start a family day-care program needs to check with the local government about which regulations will apply.

Child Care Center Safety Checklist

INDOOR

____ The center provides at least 35 square feet of usable space (65 square feet if cribs are present) for each child.

____ Play and quiet activity areas are separated.

____ All areas of the classroom are clearly visible.

____ Office space is separated from the classroom.

____ Cleaning supplies, medicines, and caregivers' personal belongings are locked up out of the reach of children.

____ The center has working smoke and carbon monoxide alarms, fire extinguishers, and emergency lighting.

____ Window guards and safety glass are installed in the windows.

____ Stairs have handrails, safety gates, and nonslip treads.

____ Electrical outlets are covered with safety plugs.

____ The furniture and equipment are child-sized and meet Consumer Product Safety Commission (CPSC) standards or carry the Juvenile Products Manufacturers Association (JPMA) certification seal.

____ Boxes and large pieces of furniture are located away from the windows.

____ Shelves, cabinets, and other heavy pieces of furniture are anchored to the walls.

____ Space heaters and fans, if present, are well out of the reach of all children.

____ Toys are sturdy and have no small detachable parts or sharp edges.

____ Cloth toys are made of flame-retardant fabric.

____ Toy boxes, if present, do not have lids that can injure or trap children.

____ Art supplies are nontoxic. (Materials should be coded **AP** or **CP**.)

____ Houseplants are nonpoisonous.

____ There are two or more clearly marked and unobstructed exits from the classroom and building.

____ Fire drills are conducted on a regular basis.

OUTDOOR

____ Different age groups have their own play spaces with appropriate equipment.

____ Toddler and preschooler playgrounds are fenced.

____ Outdoor play areas are located away from busy streets and other hazards.

____ All areas of the play space are visible.

(continued)

FIGURE 12.2 Child Care Center Safety Checklist. If you cannot check off any of the items on this checklist, arrange to address the hazardous situation as soon as possible.

Child Care Center Safety Checklist (continued)

_____ There is adequate space around large pieces of equipment, including swings.

_____ Swings have flexible rather than rigid seats.

_____ The ground is covered to a sufficient depth with an impact-absorbing material such as sand, pea gravel, or wood chips.

_____ The play area is routinely inspected for safety hazards, such as debris, animal droppings, poisonous plants, and broken or weakened equipment.

_____ The center uses a travel rope on walking field trips.

Structures, Space, and Room Arrangement

The way in which a building is designed, the amount of space provided for different activities, and the arrangement of the equipment within that space all affect the safety of the environment. As the need for child care increases, more organizations are starting child care programs. Many of these organizations must make use of existing space, as did the Cornerstone Church in the story at the beginning of the chapter. Whether a child care facility is built for that purpose or converted from another use, various safety concerns apply. All child care facilities must comply with state and local ordinances.

Structures. Buildings that house child care programs must meet local and state building codes. These usually cover all major utilities, including plumbing, heating, and electrical systems.

Some inspections are done during building construction or renovation. Others, such as fire, safety, and sanitation inspections, occur periodically. Every child care facility should keep copies of the appropriate regulations on hand for reference. Also on hand should be any documentation that is required to satisfy these regulations.

The purpose of building and safety codes is to ensure that children are cared for in safe, appropriate environments. Minimum standards establish that the roof is watertight and the building is pest free, that there is adequate access to running water and bathroom facilities, and that the temperature and illumination are kept within a comfortable range. Regulations can be quite specific. For example, they may require that food preparation areas have multiple sinks with hot water that reaches a certain temperature for dishwashing. Because requirements vary from area to area, child care program directors should always consult local codes before making any major changes to the building.

Space. Each child in child care needs a certain amount of space to thrive. Crowding increases the chance of unintentional injuries and promotes the spread of disease. _Usable space_ is free of furniture and equipment and available for play. National standards set the minimum usable indoor space at 35

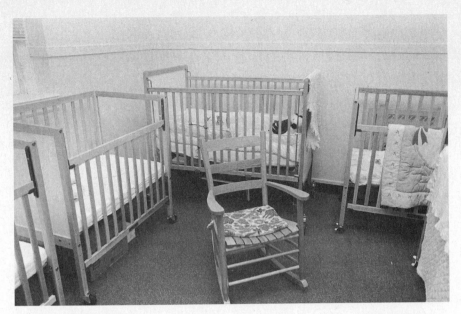

The crib space in a child care center cannot be counted toward minimum per-child space requirements.

square feet per child; 40 to 50 square feet is preferable. If cribs are used in a center in which play and sleep areas are in the same room, this space requirement increases to 65 square feet (American Public Health Association & American Academy of Pediatrics, 1992). Each child needs some individual space to store personal belongings. This gives the child a sense of privacy and security.

Each age group should have a separate classroom space. Within the classroom, there should be an area for active play and a place for quiet activities. Every center also needs a quiet space for ill or injured children. Office space should be separate from classroom space. There must be a place to lock up cleaning supplies, medicines, and caregiver's personal belongings.

Room Arrangement.   The arrangement of the furniture in a classroom affects the behavior of the children who use it. Boxes and furniture that can be used for climbing should be located well away from windows. Long, narrow aisles encourage running so they should be broken up. A partially secluded space can provide a quiet area or become a bottleneck, depending on the arrangement of the room. All areas of a classroom must be visible from other places in the room. Some arrangements in the child care setting are dictated by common sense. For example, Stephanie and Michelle at Cornerstone Church decided to put the art area near the sink for easy cleanup. Children should also be able to enter and leave the room without disrupting the entire class.

Safety Devices

Smoke and carbon monoxide alarms, fire extinguishers, and emergency lighting are safety devices that save lives. Additional safety devices can be

FOCUS ON   Communicating with Children

Playground Safety

It is the first warm day of spring at the New England Day Nursery School. Miss Simmons, one of the teachers, is getting a group of preschoolers ready to go outside.

MISS SIMMONS: Everyone remember to zip up your jackets. It's warmer than it was yesterday, but it's still chilly.

ARTHUR: You know what I'm going to do when I get outside? I'm going to go down the slide backwards!

MISS SIMMONS: Wait a minute, Arthur! Going down the slide backwards is not such a good idea. Can anyone tell me why?

ASHA: Because you can't see the end of the slide. Somebody might be there.

MISS SIMMONS: Right, Asha. It's always a good idea to be able to see where you're going. While we're talking about the slide, there are a few other rules to remember. What do we do when we're going up the steps?

JARED: We make sure not to crowd the other kids.

MISS SIMMONS: And what about when we're at the top?

ASHA: We don't fool around, and before we go down, we look to make sure the person ahead of us is off the slide.

MISS SIMMONS: Now that we all remember how to be safe on the slide, what about the swings? There's one thing that is very important to remember.

ARTHUR: My mom has told me this one about 500 times! Don't run in front or in back of the swings, 'cause if you do, you'll get hit in the head!

MISS SIMMONS: Your mother is right, Arthur. And before you start swinging, you should look around to make sure that no other children are close to your swing.

JARED: My mom says something else too.

MISS SIMMONS: What's that, Jared?

JARED: Hold on tight!

MISS SIMMONS: That's important too.

ARTHUR: Are we going to ride the bikes today? 'Cause if we are, I want the blue one.

MISS SIMMONS: I'm going to unlock the storage shed and get the bikes out. Arthur, maybe you can tell us what to remember about the bikes.

ARTHUR: One person at a time on a bike. If two kids try to get on a bike at once, they both have to take a time out.

MISS SIMMONS: And it would be terrible to have to take a time out on the first nice day of spring. What else should we remember about the bikes?

RAMONA: Don't crash them into each other! And wear a helmet!

MISS SIMMONS: That's right, Ramona. (She zips up the last child's coat.) Now I think we're ready. Oh, one more thing. That fence around the playground is there to keep us safe. It's not part of the playground equipment.

ARTHUR: That means we can't climb it, right?

MISS SIMMONS: Right!

Did Miss Simmons do a good job of explaining playground safety? Why or why not? What else would you have told the children about playground safety?

installed to prevent injuries. These include window guards on windows that open, handrails and nonslip treads on stairs, safety gates, safety plugs for electrical outlets, and safety glass. A travel rope that small children can hold onto promotes safe behavior and helps keep the group together on walking field trips. The presence of safety devices does not replace the need for supervision, but such devices make the caregiver's job easier.

As the fire inspector at Cornerstone Church noted, fire drills are an important part of the safety plan of a child care center. Children need to practice leaving the building on a regular basis so that they do not become upset or disoriented when the fire alarm rings.

Furniture and Equipment

Children are safest when furniture, bathroom fixtures, and large play equipment are child-sized. Furniture and equipment need to be sturdy and durable and should meet Consumer Product Safety Commission (CPSC) standards or carry the Juvenile Products Manufacturers Association (JPMA) certification seal. This guarantees that the products have been safety tested for use with young children.

Heavy furniture, such as a row of cubbies or a freestanding cabinet, should be anchored to the wall. This will prevent children from pulling the furniture over on themselves. Any space heaters or fans should be located well out of reach of all children. If toy boxes have lids, they should have air holes and should never be heavy enough to slam shut and injure or trap children. Shelves are preferable for the storage of toys and materials. For the comfort of caregivers, there should also be an adult-sized chair in the room.

Toys, Materials, and Other Resources

Toys and materials in child care settings need to be safe, durable, and developmentally appropriate as well as washable. If there are cloth toys for infants, they should be made of fabric that is *flame-retardant*—material that is difficult to set on fire. Dress-up clothes, puppets, and other dramatic play props that include fabric should be flame-retardant as well. (Chapter 11 discusses the importance of washing and disinfecting toys and materials.)

Most toy manufacturers provide recommendations about the age-appropriateness of their toys. This information is based primarily on safety considerations and should be taken into consideration. However, these recommendations are not always accurate and caregivers must make sure that all materials are safe for children to use. Avoid toys with small pieces that can be swallowed or lost. Look for well-made toys that will not break and cause injury. As you choose toys, keep in mind that children may not always play with them in only one way. Try to anticipate such dangers and eliminate hazards.

Caregivers must use their judgment as to the appropriateness of used or donated toys. Check these toys carefully for small pieces or sharp, broken edges. Donated toys may have been manufactured before current toy safety standards went into effect. Do not hesitate to reject donated toys that you believe are unsafe or developmentally inappropriate as well as toys that cannot be washed and disinfected.

All art materials should be nontoxic and coded *AP* or *CP*. Commercially obtained supplies should be labeled as nontoxic to children. Some art supplies to avoid are fruit-scented markers, which some children try to eat, commercial dyes that contain chemical additives, epoxy and other solvent-based glues that produce toxic fumes, and aerosol sprays.

Houseplants in the classroom can provide opportunities for learning. As noted earlier in the chapter, however, many common plants are poisonous if eaten. Before bringing plants into the classroom, check with the poison control center or your agricultural extension agent about their toxicity.

Before bringing pets into the classroom, determine exactly how much care they will need and how it will be provided. Gerbils, hamsters, mice, and rabbits need their cages cleaned frequently and cannot be left unattended during school holidays. Consider also how the animals will affect the children. All of these animals may bite. Some children may have allergies to animals such as cats or rabbits. Certain pets, including parrots and turtles, carry diseases that can be transmitted to children. These animals should not be in a child care center. Aquariums are popular and require little care, but must be placed on a strong table or counter out of the main traffic pattern to avoid accidents.

Safe Outdoor Environments

Children need to play outdoors. The playground is the place for running, jumping, and climbing. Children also develop social skills on the playground as they learn to share equipment.

Outdoor play spaces are, however, the site of many unintentional injuries. These areas need to be examined with safety in mind (see Figure 12.2). All playgrounds need routine maintenance to remain safe. The American Society for Testing and Materials (ASTM) has recently published an updated set of playground standards with many specific recommendations. It can be obtained from the ASTM (see "For Further Information" for the address and telephone number).

Play Spaces

Each age group brings different abilities and needs to the playground. Toddlers need low areas for climbing and sliding, sandboxes for digging, and open spaces for using ride-on toys. Preschoolers need more challenging equipment that can be used by several children at one time as cooperative play patterns develop. School-age children need equipment that will safely challenge their strength and coordination. Ideally, each age group at a child care center should have its own outdoor play space.

All toddler and preschool playgrounds should be fenced, as should play spaces of older children that are located near busy streets or other hazards.

The equipment should be arranged so that all areas of the play space are visible. Avoid creating hidden corners and closed-off spaces.

Large play structures need enough space around them so that children waiting to use the equipment will not interfere with children on the equipment. Swings are especially dangerous, and enough space must be left around them so that children passing by are not knocked down by swing users. All swings should have flexible, rather than rigid, plastic seats. All permanent play equipment must be anchored securely in the ground.

The surface of the playground is important in preventing injuries. The surface underneath and around all equipment should be made of material that will absorb the impact of a child falling from the highest part of the equipment. The ground, therefore, needs to be covered with approved rubber playground matting or with loose sand, pea gravel, or wood chips to a depth of about nine inches. In accordance with the Americans with Disabilities Act, playgrounds should be accessible to children with handicaps, including those in wheelchairs.

Equipment and Maintenance

Every playground needs routine maintenance and safety inspections. Persons performing these inspections should check for broken or weakened equipment, for example a splintered wood support or a rusted bolt on a climber. They should also look for foreign debris such as glass or animal droppings. Damaged equipment should be put off-limits and repaired as soon as possible.

Routine maintenance involves keeping sandboxes covered at night to keep animals out, periodically disinfecting the sand, removing sticks and foreign objects from the playground, having trees trimmed and leaves raked, and removing poisonous plants. Natural playground surfaces such as pea gravel, sand, or wood chips are much less expensive than rubber matting, but they require regular upkeep and renewal.

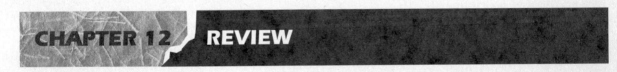

CHAPTER 12 / REVIEW

SUMMARY

- Unintentional injuries are injuries that could have been foreseen and possibly prevented.
- Many injuries can be prevented by providing a developmentally appropriate environment, being aware of possible hazards in the environment and working to eliminate or minimize them, providing alert adult supervision, and teaching children about safety.
- Unintentional injuries are the leading cause of death in children over one year old. The most common types of unintentional injuries are motor

vehicle accidents, drowning, fires and burns, poisoning, falls, and suffocation.

- Infants and toddlers cannot assess the security of their environments. Caregivers must, therefore, limit access to hazards for this age group.
- During the first four months of life, infants cannot direct their movements, but they can move. Infants are especially vulnerable to falls, suffocation, aspiration of food and other objects, poisoning, and drowning.
- Many unintentional injuries occur to toddlers because their abilities are not adequate to deal with their environments. Toddlers are susceptible to burns, drowning, poisoning, choking, and falls, in particular.
- Caregivers should be aware of the times, places, and personal characteristics of children that increase the risk of unintentional injury.
- Caregivers should know how to prevent the most common unintentional injuries among infants and toddlers in the categories of motor vehicle injuries, mechanical suffocation, aspiration, falls, drowning, burns, poisoning, and other causes.
- Preschool children are better coordinated than toddlers but still lack the ability to anticipate danger. School-age children are vulnerable to pedestrian fatalities, bicycle accidents, and injuries from intentional risk-taking.
- Caregivers should know how to prevent the most common unintentional injuries among preschool and school-age children including transportation injuries, drowning, burns, and injuries from other causes.
- Many physical aspects of a child care center are regulated by local and state building and safety codes. Structure, space, and layout considerations are important for the safety of children.
- Caregivers need to make use of safety devices and make thoughtful decisions about furniture, equipment, toys, and other resources.
- Many unintentional injuries at child care centers occur on the playground. Outdoor play spaces should be organized for maximum safety. Playgrounds need regular inspection and maintenance.

ACQUIRING KNOWLEDGE

1. Define unintentional injury. What is a term used in casual language that has approximately the same meaning?
2. What are three common causes of accidental death during childhood?
3. What is mechanical suffocation?
4. Identify two safety rules that will prevent accidental drowning.
5. Where do most unintentional injuries occur at child care centers?
6. When are unintentional injuries more likely to occur at child care centers?
7. What groups of children are at a higher risk for unintentional injuries than others?
8. Why should child care centers have liability insurance?

9. Why has the rate of childhood deaths from automobile accidents declined since 1970?
10. Describe the three purposes of car seats.
11. How does entrapment result in suffocation? Identify three other potential sources of suffocation risk for infants and young children.
12. Why is it important to keep uninflated and popped balloons away from young children?
13. Identify three nonfood items that can cause children to suffocate by aspiration.
14. Describe how to powder a baby in a way that eliminates the risk of fatal aspiration pneumonia.
15. Why should caregivers never leave infants under four months of age unattended on any high surfaces?
16. Why should wading pools be emptied immediately after each use?
17. Identify three causes of burns.
18. How can the risks of accidental poisoning be reduced?
19. What type of automobile accident involving children becomes more common as children reach school age?
20. Identify two other forms of transportation involved in accidents affecting school-age children.
21. What are two common sources of burn injuries of school-age children?
22. Identify three types of inspections conducted periodically at child care centers.
23. When choosing art supplies to use with young children, what safety precautions should be kept in mind?
24. What considerations should be kept in mind before allowing pets to be brought into class?
25. Why is special material recommended for use under and around playground equipment?

THINKING CRITICALLY

1. Explain the role of the caregiver in preventing accidents involving infants and toddlers.
2. Why is suffocation of particular concern with infants?
3. What is the difference between safety precautions needed for school-age children and those needed for younger children? What is the difference between the risks taken by school-age children and those taken by younger children?
4. Why is it important to consider the age-appropriateness recommendations manufacturers provide for toys? Why do you think these recommendations are commonly ignored by some parents when they purchase toys for their children?
5. Why should toddlers and older children have separate play areas at a child care center?

OBSERVATIONS AND APPLICATIONS

1. Visit a child care center where infants are accepted. What safe and unsafe practices do you observe? Are infants left unattended in areas where they can fall? Can they maneuver themselves to pull something over? Are caregivers watching the infants at all times? Are precrawlers, crawlers, and walkers together in one area? How many caregivers are there? How many children? What is the age range of the children?

2. Observe children at play on the playground of a child care center. Note the material used to surface the area under the equipment. Are there separate play areas for different age groups? How many caregivers watch the children? Do you observe any accidents? Do you observe any unsafe practices on the part of the children or the caregivers? What is the age range of the children you observe?

3. Suppose you are hired as a caregiver in a child care center. How would you set up your room so that the children in your care are ensured a safe, indoor environment? What special considerations and safety requirements should you be sure to remember?

4. At the child care center where you work, there is a wading pool. The children enjoy using the pool in hot weather. What safety requirements are important to keep in mind when children are using the pool and when the pool is not in use?

FOR FURTHER INFORMATION

Organizations

American Society for Testing and Materials (ASTM)
1916 Race Street
Philadelphia, PA 19103
(215) 299-5400

Art Hazards Information Center
5 Beekman Street
New York, NY 10038
(212) 227-6231

Juvenile Products Manufacturers Association (JPMA)
Two Greentree Centre, Suite 225
P. O. Box 955
Marlton, NJ 08053
(609) 985-2878

National Highway Traffic Safety Administration
NTS - 21
400 7th Street, SW
Washington, DC 20590
(202) 366-2696

National Safety Council
Family Safety and Health
444 North Michigan Avenue
Chicago, IL 60611
(708) 285-1121

U. S. Consumer Product Safety Commission (CPSC)
4330 East-West Highway
Washington, DC 20814
(800) 638-2772 or (301)504-0980

Publications

American Lung Association of Los Angeles County. (1985). *Safe at home: An early childhood safety curriculum*. Los Angeles: Author.

American Society for Testing and Materials. *Consumer safety performance specifications for playground equipment for public use*. ASTM F1487. Philadelphia: Author.

Creswell, W. H., & Newman, I. M. (1993). *School health practice* (10th ed.). St. Louis: C. V. Mosby.

National Committee for Injury Prevention and Control [American Journal of Preventive Medicine]. (1989). *Injury prevention: Meeting the challenge*. New York: U. S. Department of Health and Human Services & Oxford University Press.

National Safety Council. Various booklets and bulletins on safety issues including: *Bathroom hazards; Falls; Fire prevention; Pesticides, safe use of; Poisons, solid and liquid; Preschool pedestrian safety program; Preventing accidental poisonings*.

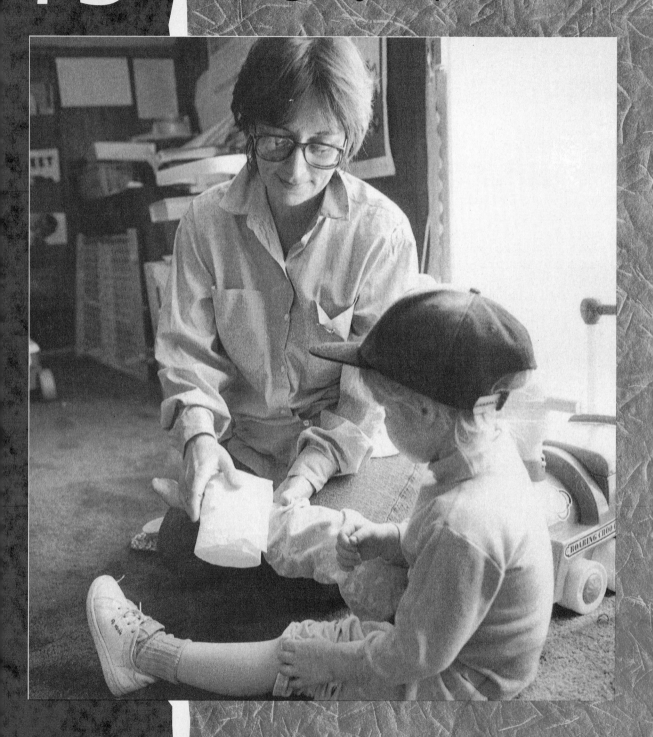

OBJECTIVES

Studying this chapter
will enable you to

- Explain how environmental and behavioral factors influence safety
- List guidelines for safe behavior in a number of child care settings
- Give examples of ways child care providers can prepare for emergencies in advance
- List the steps to take when responding to an emergency
- Describe basic first aid for a number of common emergencies
- Identify different forms of child abuse and explain measures caregivers should take when child abuse is suspected

CHAPTER TERMS

child abuse
child neglect
emotional abuse
frostbite
heat exhaustion
incest
physical abuse
sexual abuse
shock
sunburn

AT Maplewood Child Development Center, Danisha and Barbara were outdoors with the children. It was late afternoon. The children were enjoying an extra hour of outdoor play because the weather was so pleasant. Andrea was showing off her skills on the climber when a fire engine roared down the street, sirens wailing. Distracted by the fire truck, Andrea loosened her grip on the bar and fell to the resilient surface below with her leg twisted under her. As soon as Danisha heard Andrea crying, she ran toward the climber. "Where are you hurt?" she asked.

"My leg hurts," said Andrea.

"Where?"

"Here," said Andrea, pointing to her ankle. Putting her arm around Andrea, Danisha pushed Andrea's loose pants leg up and slipped off her shoe to get a better look at her ankle. It was already starting to swell.

"Barbara," called Danisha. "Could you ask Gwen to get Andrea an ice pack and then come back outside and take charge of the other children? I'm bringing Andrea inside."

309

Soon Barbara returned and Danisha carried Andrea into the classroom. Then Gwen Smith, the center's director, appeared, carrying an ice pack which she applied gently to Andrea's ankle.

"I think you should stay here and try not to walk on your leg," said Gwen. "I'll call your grandmother and see if she can come get you. I think a doctor should check your ankle."

Danisha stayed with Andrea while Gwen called Andrea's grandmother. She arrived about 15 minutes later.

After Andrea left with her grandmother, Gwen returned to Danisha's classroom. "Andrea's grandmother said she was going to take her to the urgent care center over on Rosemont Avenue. Her ankle looked pretty swollen. Here's an injury report form. Could you fill it out before you leave tonight and drop it off in my office?"

The Role of Behavior in Safety

The level of safety in a child care setting depends on two main factors: the physical environment and the behavior of the caregivers and children. Chapter 12 outlined many actions caregivers can take to create safe physical environments. This chapter will discuss safe behavior patterns. Safe behavior begins with the understanding that caregivers must be aware of safety considerations all of the time.

Safety Awareness

The main goals of safety awareness are to prevent injuries and to minimize the effects of an injury when an accident does occur. Prevention of injuries is best achieved by:

- Establishing a physically safe environment
- Consistently enforcing age-appropriate safety rules
- Providing alert supervision
- Educating children about safety issues

To minimize the effects of accidents when they occur, caregivers must:

- Have a plan to follow when an emergency occurs
- Possess the training and skills to follow the plan
- Have access to specialized resources in the community to deal with the emergency

Environmental Factors Influencing Safety.   There are two ways to create safe physical environments for children. The first is to eliminate safety hazards from the environment. This includes fencing off water hazards, locking up poisons, providing smoke detectors, and covering electrical outlets. The second way is to arrange the environment to encourage safe behavior. This means allowing enough space between equipment, breaking up long hallways that encourage running, and arranging indoor and outdoor play areas so that all parts of the space are visible to caregivers. Creating safe physical environments was discussed in Chapter 12.

Behavioral Factors Influencing Safety. The attitudes and actions of caregivers have an enormous impact on the safety of the children in their care. The way rules are enforced and conflicts are resolved, the quality of supervision, the level of risk caregivers find acceptable, and the examples caregivers set with their own behavior all influence safety. There are times, as when Andrea fell from the climber and hurt her ankle, when no amount of caregiver alertness can prevent an unintentional injury. Practicing consistently safe behavior patterns, however, reduces the frequency of injury and makes the child care setting a safer place.

Planning ahead is an important part of safe behavior. Advance planning allows caregivers to anticipate and avoid possible safety hazards. Planning ahead can be as simple as having everything within reach when changing a diaper or as complex as driving the route of a field trip in advance. Planning ahead for emergencies can mean having the telephone numbers of the fire department, ambulance, and police department posted at each telephone or practicing evacuating the building.

Every caregiver must establish rules of behavior. The goal of these rules is to keep children from harming themselves or others and to encourage desired behavior. The rules have to be put in simple terms that children can understand. In general, the younger the child, the more specific the rule must be. Young children lack the ability to generalize and apply one rule to several different situations. Language should be direct and understandable. A two-year-old will find it easier to understand "let Timmy have a turn on the swing" than "share the playground equipment with the other children."

Whenever possible, establish positive rules that tell children what to do. Say "put the scissors on the table when you are finished" rather than "don't walk around with scissors in your hand." Or say "use the ladder to go up the slide" rather than "don't walk up the front of the slide."

Rules need to be consistently enforced, both as a teaching tool and as a way of making children feel secure. And when adults behave safely, children are likely to follow their lead. For example, parents or teachers who wear bicycle helmets will have less trouble getting children to wear helmets.

In some cases, it is better to change the environment than to make a rule. For example, moving breakable objects out of a toddler's reach is more effective than making rules about not touching these things. The toddler's drive to explore is much stronger than his ability to obey the rule. In any case, rules never replace the need for supervision. Children forget or misunderstand rules. Caregivers can never count on the existence of a rule to keep a child safe.

It is always preferable to have at least two adults supervising any group of children. That way, if one child requires the exclusive attention of an adult—the way Andrea did—there is another one available to get help or continue supervision of the group. Never leave children unattended.

SAFETY TIPS

Head Injuries

When a child hits her head, be sure to watch for signs of serious injury. Always call a physician if the injured child is less than one year old. In older children, get medical help if any of the following symptoms appear:

- Pupils that are different sizes
- Confusion or a sudden, deep sleep
- Hard, repeated vomiting
- Blood or fluid from the ears or nose
- A severe headache
- Convulsions
- An inability to move part of the body

If none of these symptoms appear, apply ice to the "bumped" area. Be sure to tell parents about the injury.

The maximum number of children of each age that one adult may supervise is usually determined by state law. This represents the minimum amount of supervision required. (See Table 1.1 for suggested ratios of caregivers to children of various ages.) Depending on the activity, more adults may be needed, especially during special activities such as cooking.

Safe Behaviors

Teachers are responsible for establishing safe behavior in child care programs. Preschoolers cannot be expected to see dangerous situations or anticipate their consequences. However, creating a risk-free environment in which every activity is controlled by a rule is highly impractical. In addition, rigid control is not beneficial for a child's social, emotional, or physical development. But safety must always be a major consideration. It is possible to find safe, healthy, stimulating activities both indoors and out.

Indoor Safety.   Many aspects of indoor safety that have to do with the physical environment were discussed in Chapter 12. Caregivers should establish general rules that promote indoor safety. An example of a general safety rule is "walk when you are inside the classroom." Remember that such general rules are more understandable to older children than to younger ones.

Indoor safety is a special concern when children are cooking or using appliances, tools, or other equipment not designed for child care classrooms. For example, children can benefit greatly from classroom cooking and woodworking projects. However, close supervision during these projects is essential. Teachers should precede the activity with a discussion of how to use the equipment safely. It is also advisable to have extra adults, such as parent volunteers, present and to limit the number of children using the equipment at any one time. Teachers should always take time to explain the activity and appropriate safety rules to parent volunteers.

Indoor safety can also be affected by the conflicts between children that typically erupt in child care classrooms. The ways children resolve conflicts are strongly influenced by what they experience in their environments and in the surrounding culture. Many children, especially the 20 percent who live below the poverty line, experience violence firsthand in their daily lives (Children's Defense Fund, 1992). In addition, virtually every child in America is exposed to secondhand violence through television programming, movies, and toys such as swords and guns. Most cartoon heroes use violence to resolve conflicts. Between the ages of 5 and 15, a child will see more than 13,000 killings on television (Tuchascherer, 1988). Parents and teachers can see the effects of this exposure in their homes and classrooms.

Teachers need to develop strategies to resolve conflicts and to teach children the skills they need to handle future conflicts on their own. Giving "time-outs" to both children involved in a conflict or removing a toy that children are fighting over puts an immediate end to the conflict. Often this is the best short-term solution, especially if tempers are high. However, this approach does not teach children any skills for resolving future conflicts without adult assistance. A more successful strategy is to involve children in a discussion of the problem and let them suggest solutions while the teacher acts as moderator (Carlsson-Paige & Levin, 1992). There are many excellent professional workshops on conflict resolution available to child care professionals.

Occasionally a child's aggressive behavior will go beyond the normal level of preschool confrontation. This behavior may take the form of repeated biting, punching, hair pulling, or destruction of property. Teachers are responsible for protecting the other children in the class from both physically and emotionally abusive behavior. It may be necessary to isolate the aggressive child in order to keep other children safe.

Teachers should keep in mind that excessively aggressive behavior may be a sign of other problems in the child's life or a plea for adult help. If this appears to be the case, teachers should consult their director about referring the child and family to professional help from social service agencies.

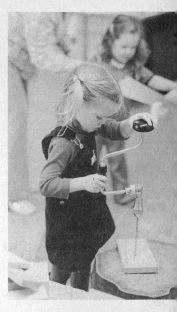

Close supervision during classroom projects, such as this woodworking activity, is essential for children's safety.

Playground Safety.   Many injuries, especially falls and scrapes, occur on the playground. Chapter 12 discussed some of the physical requirements for a safe playground. The most important of these are choosing age-appropriate equipment, arranging the equipment so that children have enough space to play safely, and covering the playground surface with a shock-absorbent material. It is important to have enough equipment of sufficient variety to meet the needs of the children. Boredom can lead to misbehavior or misuse of equipment.

The behavior of the children influences the rate of injuries on the playground. By consistently enforcing expectations of safe play, teachers can reduce the number of injuries. Rules for safe play include taking turns on equipment; limiting the number of children on a piece of equipment at one time, especially on slides and other raised equipment; and forbidding shoving and "pretend fighting."

Caregivers must be especially careful about the safety of physically or mentally handicapped children that are in the group. Their handicaps may require alternate activities or equipment. A handicapped child should be allowed to participate in playground activities as fully as possible. This may require special equipment, more individual attention, or different types of games, especially those that are cooperative rather than competitive.

Children's play periods are not a break time for teachers. Supervision of play is an active task. During playground time, teachers can observe potential behavioral trouble spots, asking questions like the following:

- Does a fight always break out around one piece of equipment?
- Are smaller children overrun by larger ones?
- Do children become lost from view in obscure areas of the playground?
- Do children seem afraid to try a particular piece of equipment?
- Do injuries seem to occur more frequently on one piece of equipment or in one specific section of the playground?

Sunburn Precautions

Denise's class of three-year-olds are ready for their afternoon at the beach. The class has been studying seashells, and they will spend a couple of hours in the late afternoon swimming and collecting shells.

Denise leads the children toward several blankets that she has smoothed out over the sand. It takes several minutes to calm the excited youngsters so they can sit quietly on the blankets.

"Before we go hunting for seashells," Denise begins, "there is something we have to do to protect ourselves so our skin doesn't get burned by the sun. Who knows what we have to do?"

"Put on sunblock!" several children call out at the same time.

"Why do we need to protect our skin from the sun?" asks Denise.

"Because sunburn hurts," says Todd.

"Because then you get red instead of brown," suggests the blond and freckled Georgina.

"Because if you don't, your skin comes off. Yuck!" contributes Jonathan with a grimace.

"You're all right," Denise replies. "We need to use sunblock because otherwise the sun will hurt our skin. Getting a sunburn not only hurts, it is bad for you too. Sunblock keeps the sun from hurting your skin."

Denise pulls bottles of sunblock out of her beach bag. Each child's parents have provided one labeled with the child's name. All the brands have an SPF (Sun Protection Factor) of 15—the minimum amount of protection doctors recommend. Denise distributes the bottles to the parent volunteers. Then the adults carefully cover the exposed parts of the children's skin with the sunblock. Some of the children try to help.

Soon the children are splashing and wading in the shallow water. Afterwards, sunblock is applied again. Then the children play, eat a snack, and compare the treasures they have found on the shore.

Do you think Denise did a good job of explaining to the children why they should use sunblock? Should she have given them more information? What might you have done differently?

If the answer to any of these questions is yes, it may be necessary to restructure the playground, remove equipment, or make other adjustments.

Safe behavior on the playground must also include consideration of the weather. During hot weather, children need to be protected against sunburn, dehydration, and heat exhaustion.

Sunburn results from prolonged exposure of skin to the sun and causes damage ranging from mild reddening to extensive blistering. Serious sunburn can cause intense pain, nausea, abdominal cramps, headache, chills, and fever. Exposure to the sun also ages skin and can cause changes that can produce skin cancer later on. Although children with light skin and eyes are most susceptible to sunburn, all children need protection from overexposure to the sun.

The sun is most likely to cause damage during midday between the hours of 11 A.M. and 2 P.M. During these hours, all outdoor play should take place primarily in the shade, especially in hot weather. Very young children should routinely wear hats that shade their faces when they are outdoors. Commercial sunblocks provide some protection against sun damage but should be supplied by parents or guardians. Written permission for use of sunblocks should be obtained. Ingredients in some sunblocks can cause skin irritation or allergic reactions in some children. Never apply sunblock to broken, irritated, or reddened skin.

Dehydration, the extreme loss of water from the body, is also a serious concern during hot weather. Sweating is a natural way for people to remove excess heat from the body, but water is lost in the process. People working or playing strenuously in hot weather may lose up to 3 percent of their total body weight through sweating (Parcel, 1989). Children are more susceptible to dehydration than adults. That is because children have a greater skin surface area relative to their body weight, and water is lost through the skin. Children should be encouraged to drink plenty of water in hot weather to avoid dehydration.

Heat exhaustion is caused by dehydration and/or the loss of salts from the body due to exposure to high temperatures for long periods of time. Heat exhaustion is a medical emergency. A person suffering from heat exhaustion usually has pale, moist skin. He may feel weak, nauseous, or faint. He may sweat heavily or complain of headache or muscle cramps. A child who is suffering from heat exhaustion should be allowed to rest in a cool place and drink plenty of cool liquids. Caregivers should seek medical advice. To prevent heat exhaustion, children should be encouraged to drink water and cool down frequently during hot weather.

If water play occurs in a child care setting, at least one supervising adult should have lifesaving and cardiopulmonary resuscitation (CPR) training. Flotation devices such as swimming rings do not replace the need for active supervision, and they may even lull children into feeling safe in deep water. Special rules apply to swimming pools in child care settings. For example, written records must be maintained showing that the water is regularly disinfected and tested. In a child care environment, sprinklers are safer and easier to maintain than wading pools.

Cold weather brings the hazard of frostbite. *Frostbite* occurs when body tissues freeze from exposure to cold temperatures. Most often, frostbite occurs in body parts farthest from the center of the body: the fingers, toes, nose, ears, or cheeks. Frostbitten skin appears white and waxy. Children may or may not feel pain. Treatment for frostbite includes immersing the frostbitten parts of the body in lukewarm—not hot—water without rubbing or massaging them. Then professional medical help should be sought.

Young children can be oblivious to cold while they are playing. For this reason, teachers should insist that parents send adequate outdoor clothing and that children keep hats, mittens, and boots on while playing outdoors. Teachers should realize, however, that long trailing scarves may become entangled in equipment and choke a child. Teachers should, therefore, discourage parents from dressing their children in long scarves or make sure that the scarves are tucked inside coats or jackets.

A travel rope with knots for children to hold is one of the best safety devices for walking trips.

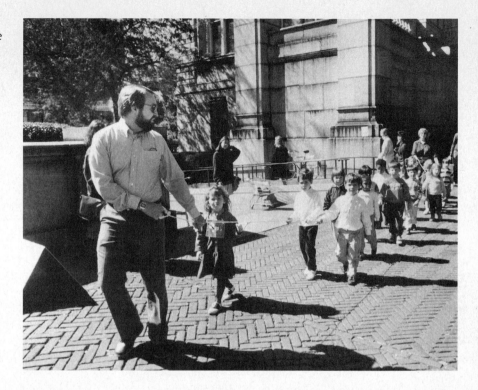

Street Safety.   Many pedestrian accidents occur because children misunderstand traffic signs or disobey common traffic rules such as crossing the street only on the green light (Whaley & Wong, 1991). Bicycle injuries are also common. Traffic safety education should begin early and should be repeated often, continuing through the elementary school years. Teachers can begin with "red means stop and green means go," and move through more sophisticated concepts such as "yellow means caution" or "watch for cars turning right on red." Street safety lessons should make children aware that they have a responsibility to behave safely as pedestrians and later as bicyclists.

Often preschools take walking trips in their neighborhoods. One of the best devices for safe walking is a travel rope. The rope, with knots every few feet, is held in front and in back by an adult. Children are instructed to keep their hands on their own knots at all times. In the absence of a travel rope, a way to control preschool pedestrians is to have them hold hands with a partner. This helps prevent dawdling or darting into traffic. During walking trips, teachers should practice safe behavior such as crossing streets only at corners. These trips can also provide opportunities to point out traffic signs and talk about their meanings.

Field Trip Safety.   Field trips can enrich children's preschool experiences. Successful field trips, however, require advance planning and adequate supervision. More supervision is needed in unfamiliar environments than in familiar ones. Parent volunteers can be of great help on field trips. You cannot, however, depend on them to supervise as closely as teachers.

Signed parental permission slips are needed whenever children leave the center, including on walking field trips. Teachers, of course, should have cleared the field trip site and plans with the center director before sending out any permission slips for signature. Permission slips should give the name of the child, the trip destination, and the approximate times of departure and return. Permission slips must be distributed and returned signed before children leave the center. Advance planning also extends to planning for field trip emergencies. Teachers should take with them a list of the children and their emergency contact cards. Taking a small first-aid kit is also a good idea.

Another part of field trip planning requires making arrangements for the care of children who cannot participate in the field trip either because of parent refusal or because their permission slips were not returned promptly. Extra staff should be available to remain at the center with nonparticipating children. Teachers should never take a child along on a trip without the written consent of her parents.

All teachers and adult volunteers should be briefed before the field trip on the route, the program, and what to do in case of an emergency. The center may provide a list of field trip guidelines that covers the major points. Adult volunteers who drive children in their own cars should show proof of a valid driver's license and insurance. Teachers should be aware that transportation of children by parent volunteers may have liability implications for both the parent and the child care center. Transportation safety and seat belt use were discussed in Chapter 12.

Teachers should also talk to children about how to behave on a field trip and what to do if they become separated from the group. Identification tags with the center's name and phone number are a good idea. They can be attached to the children's clothing. These tags should not, however, have the child's name on them because that allows a potential abductor to call the child by name.

Stranger Safety.   Of all the safety issues that worry parents, the threat of child abduction and molestation probably brings on the most vivid fears. Children need to be protected from potential dangers through a combination of vigilance and education.

Vigilance in a child care setting starts with arranging the building so that anyone entering must pass a receptionist or other responsible adult. Although parents should be encouraged to visit often, they should sign in and receive a visitor's badge or other indication that they belong on the premises. It may be necessary to lock all outside doors except one in order to control access to the center. Locked doors should always be of the type that can be opened from the inside with a pressure bar in case of an emergency.

Caregivers should require that every parent sign a form indicating who may remove their children from child care. People on this list might include the other parent, another relative or adult friend, and people who are listed as the child's emergency contacts. If there is any doubt about whether the child should be released into someone's care, caregivers should take the child along and go to the director. Caregivers should also be alert to anyone loitering outside the center at play time or dismissal. In these situations, it is better to be too cautious than not to be cautious enough.

Every year, many children are abducted by noncustodial parents or other family members. These people are not strangers, but they can be a threat to the child's well-being. In the event of a separation or divorce, caregivers should get written instructions about when each parent is permitted to remove the child from child care. These situations can be very sensitive and confusing, so caregivers should seek assistance from the center's director if there is any question about whether the noncustodial parent should remove the child. Always take the child with you while you resolve the situation.

Educating children about stranger safety begins in preschool and continues through elementary school. The education must be age-appropriate. For example, preschoolers can be taught not to talk to strangers, not to go with strangers, and to scream for help if a stranger attempts to pick them up. Part of stranger education is helping the child develop the concept of who a stranger is. Children may feel they "know" a mail carrier, delivery person, or salesclerk whom they see several times a week. Even so, they should be told not to go anywhere with such a person and to tell a trusted adult if anyone tries to force his attentions on them. Other points to make are:

- It is good to run away from a stranger.
- You do not have to obey an adult who is a stranger.
- You do not have to answer an adult's questions or requests for help.
- Appearance has nothing to do with whether a person is good or bad, safe or dangerous.
- Law officers are there for your protection and can be treated as safe strangers.
- It is very important to tell a trusted adult immediately if you have been approached by a stranger.

Caregivers in family day-care situations need to be wary of admitting strangers into their homes. Repair and maintenance people should always be asked to present identification—and they should be able to produce it readily. Door-to-door salespersons should not be admitted into the home. Children should be supervised when playing outside, and any suspicious strangers or motor vehicles should be reported to the police. Caregivers should recognize that street safety, field trip safety, and stranger safety are all ways to prevent child abuse, which is discussed later in this chapter.

Staff Qualifications and Hiring Guidelines

Licensing standards for child care programs and staff qualifications for caregivers are under state control and vary greatly from state to state. These standards reflect the minimum requirements needed to assure safe, healthful

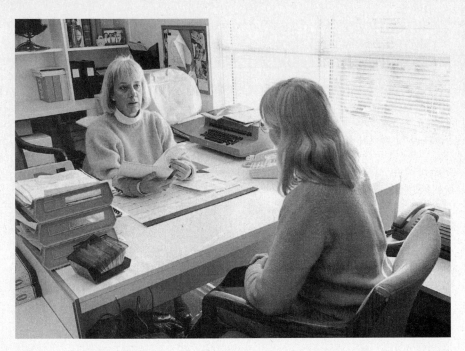

One way that a center can help to ensure the children's safety is to interview and conduct background and reference checks on potential employees.

environments for children. To achieve quality care, it may be necessary to exceed these standards, especially if the center cares for children with physical or emotional disabilities.

Some of the inspections required of child care centers were discussed in Chapter 12. In some states, family day-care providers also have the option of becoming registered or licensed. Requirements differ from state to state. National health and safety performance standards have been jointly developed by the American Public Health Association and the American Academy of Pediatrics (APHA & AAP, 1992). However, these standards are only recommendations, not requirements. Also, since 1985, national voluntary accreditation has been available through the National Academy of Early Childhood Programs established by the National Association for the Education of Young Children (NAEYC).

Many states require only that caregivers be adult high school graduates. All head teachers and center directors should take formal early childhood education and child development courses. At least one person at the center should be certified in CPR and have first-aid training.

Some states require that caregivers submit to background checks as an assurance that they do not have criminal records. Some centers may require preemployment drug testing. Personal interviews, background checks, and verification of references of prospective staff members are ways in which child care centers can protect children. On-the-job supervision of staff members is also an important safeguard. Family day-care providers should be able to provide references to new families interested in their programs.

The high level of responsibility, moderate pay, and long hours required of child care professionals often make it difficult to attract and keep qualified caregivers. Centers can improve their staff qualifications by allowing paid time to attend professional seminars, encouraging caregivers to join professional organizations such as the NAEYC, and encouraging caregivers to participate in first-aid training.

As mentioned in Chapter 11, caregivers who are sick should not come to work because they may spread their illnesses to others. Centers need to have sick leave policies that support responsible behavior from caregivers in this matter. Centers should also maintain a list of qualified substitutes so that adequate child/staff ratios can be maintained when caregivers are ill. When regular caregivers are absent, it may be wise to postpone activities, such as cooking or a field trip (even a neighborhood walk), that require intense supervision.

Lapses in Safe Behavior

As mentioned in Chapter 12, unintentional injuries and emergencies are more likely to happen at certain times of the day and in certain places. In general, the less familiar the place or activity, the greater the likelihood of an unintentional injury. Children who are tired and hungry or under stress are also more at risk. Under these circumstances, children are less apt to remember safety rules.

Caregivers themselves are not immune to stress. Lapses in safe behavior are more likely to occur when regular staff members are absent; when caregivers are tired, ill, or distracted by personal problems; when there are visitors at the center; or when caregivers must give their full attention to an injured or seriously ill child. Under circumstances such as these, caregivers are less likely to notice safety hazards, to follow safety rules, and to enforce safety rules among the children in their care.

Preventing lapses in safe behavior requires both knowledge and action. Caregivers need first to be aware of the times and situations that encourage lapses. With that knowledge, they can take action to achieve safe behavior. Taking well-prepared parent volunteers along on a field trip is a good example of recognizing a potentially dangerous situation and taking action to promote safety. Planning quiet, well-supervised activities for times when children are tired or hungry is another. Although lapses in safe behavior are always possible, awareness and advance planning can minimize their occurrences and their effects.

Emergency Preparedness

Emergencies can happen in any caregiving situation. A child care emergency is an event that requires immediate action to protect the well-being of a child. Emergencies can be environmental, such as a fire or tornado, or medical. They can affect one child or dozens of children. Not all emergencies are life-threatening, but all require calm, intelligent decision-making based on a previously developed plan. Special training can help child care professionals face and meet medical and other emergencies successfully.

FOCUS ON / **Communicating with Parents**

Home Safety Checklist

It is the third parent-teacher meeting at Penrose Nursery School. The meetings that are held every two months allow Jennifer and the other teachers to share information and concerns with parents. Tonight the topic is home safety. After opening the evening with words of welcome, Jennifer distributes home safety checklists.

JENNIFER: Tonight we're talking about home safety. Take a look at the home safety checklist I just distributed. The purpose of the checklist is to help you inspect your home to make sure it is safe for your child. Place a check next to each safety item your home has. If your home does not have a safety item, use the space next to the item to write down what you need to do to make it safe. Are there any questions?

MRS. WALLACE: What do you mean when you say wheeled furniture is dangerous?

JENNIFER: Sometimes children climb up on stools and other small wheeled furniture and then try to jump off. The furniture slides away, often causing a fall.

MRS. WASHINGTON: Everything about electrical safety and sharp objects makes sense, but I have a question about poisons. How do we know which household products are poisons?

JENNIFER: Any product that contains poison has to indicate that on its label. Sometimes the label says *CAUTION*. Sometimes it says *WARNING* or *DANGER*. You have to read the labels of every product in your house: paints, cleansers, and so on. Look for those words. If the label says any of those things, keep the product in a high, securely locked cabinet where children can't get to it. Oh, yes, I almost forgot. Some labels will also have a picture of a skull and crossbones—the picture that indicates deadly poison. Make sure your children never get near those substances.

MRS. MACHEDA: What about products that are not poison but probably aren't good for children to eat? Like dishwashing liquid, for example. I keep mine on the kitchen counter. It doesn't say it's poison, but it can't be good for Jesse to eat. Do I have to keep that locked away too?

JENNIFER: As long as Jesse can't get to it, it's okay. Although it's not poison, he'll get sick to his stomach if he drinks it. Since you don't want that, it should be out of his reach. But it doesn't need to be locked away.

MR. BOWDEN: I'm looking at the section on fire safety. Our stove doesn't have a pilot light, and I have to keep matches next to it to light it.

JENNIFER: You should keep the matches in a locked drawer or on a high shelf where Patricia can't get to them. It's worth the trouble to prevent a fire or explosion. (She pauses, waiting for further questions.) I really appreciate all your questions. I hope the checklist is useful. If, as you use it, you find you have additional questions, feel free to ask me. Are there any other issues you want to discuss?

Do you think Jennifer prepared well for the meeting? What do you think of the way she organized and ran the meeting? What might you have done differently?

Written Records

Written records must be kept for each child in child care. These records are the base on which an emergency response is built. Caregivers need at least the following information to respond effectively to an emergency:

- Permission from parents to seek medical care for the child if the parents cannot be reached in an emergency. Ideally, this should be accompanied by a signed release for treatment on file at the local hospital along with other appropriate documentation such as insurance coverage. Caregivers should always carry a release for each child along on field trips.
- Health records that indicate any health conditions or allergies.
- The name and telephone number of the child's health care professional and hospital of preference if there is more than one in the local area.
- Up-to-date emergency contact telephone numbers for parents.
- Alternate emergency contacts if the parents are not available.

In some states, permission forms authorizing caregivers to get emergency medical care in the absence of parents must be notarized to be valid. The local hospital emergency room can provide information on what is necessary and suggest wording for the forms. Caregivers in family day-care situations need to have these written records as well.

Emergency Arrangements

Child care centers and family day-care providers must have emergency telephone numbers for the police, ambulance, poison control center, and fire department posted at every telephone. Child care centers need to have a physician and a dentist on whom they can call if a child's own health care provider cannot be reached. This professional arrangement can be developed under the guidance of a health care consultant. As you learned in Chapter 10, identifying families that have religious or other beliefs that prohibit some or all medical treatment must be handled as part of the enrollment process. It is also helpful to have the telephone numbers of the gas, oil, or electric company and emergency heating and plumbing services on hand.

Teachers should know how to request emergency services calmly. They will need to state the location where help is needed, the nature of the emergency, and the number and ages of the children involved. Never hang up until you are told to do so by the emergency service dispatcher. In the classroom, teachers can instruct older children in how to call for help in an emergency.

As mentioned earlier, teachers should have emergency telephone numbers for parents and alternate contacts if parents are not available. Teachers must periodically ask parents to update their emergency information cards. Parents should be informed that the people designated as emergency contacts will probably not be able to get medical attention for the child unless they have written permission from the parents.

Evacuations and Drills

Every child care center is required to post evacuation and fire drill instructions in the classrooms. Fire drills should be held often enough that children do not become panicked by the fire alarm and can respond quickly and quietly. In occasional practice drills, an exit should be unexpectedly blocked, forcing caregivers to use the alternate exit. Procedures should also be developed for evacuating the building in the event of a natural gas leak, bomb threat, or toxic waste spill.

Some areas of the country experience natural disasters such as tornadoes and earthquakes. Tornado drills may be appropriate, for example, in some parts of the Midwest. Plans should be made for the safety of children and staff during these emergencies.

Having a written emergency response plan is a start toward appropriate emergency response, but it is not enough. All staff members should know their specific roles. Who leads the children outdoors? Who checks that everyone is out of the room? Who shuts doors and windows? Who is responsible for bringing the emergency contact cards out of the building? If there is high staff turnover, it may be necessary to drill caregivers on their specific jobs several times a year.

Follow-Up Procedures

Every unintentional injury requires a written follow-up. This is true whether the event results in calling an ambulance, asking the parents to pick up their children, or giving first aid for minor cuts and bruises. In the case of medical emergencies or unintentional injuries, an injury or medical report is written.

Injury and medical emergency reports are very important and should be written as soon as possible after the event. A typical injury or medical emergency report will ask for:

- The name and age of the child
- When and where the injury or medical emergency occurred
- A description of the injuries or medical emergency
- A description of the circumstances under which the injuries or medical emergency occurred
- The name of the supervising adult and other witnesses
- The action taken in response to the injury or medical emergency

In addition, a log should be kept describing first aid administered for minor injuries such as bumps and small cuts or any prescribed medications used for medical emergencies such as asthma attacks.

Good record keeping is useful in several ways. For example, it can help child care centers pinpoint potential danger areas. If, for example, injuries happen repeatedly on a swing set, the design of that swing set and its placement should be reevaluated. Injury reports can also be used in court should a child care center be sued as a result of an injury.

FIGURE 13.1   **First-aid Kit Items.** These first-aid supplies can help care-givers respond appropriately to a variety of emergency situations.

First-aid Kit Items
BANDAGES Adhesive bandages, various sizes Adhesive tape in several widths Elastic bandages Gauze rolls in several widths Sterile gauze pads in many different sizes
MEDICATIONS Acetaminophen Antiseptic cream, ointment, or spray Calamine lotion Isopropyl alcohol or hydrogen peroxide Syrup of ipecac
OTHER SUPPLIES American Red Cross first-aid manual Blanket Blunt-tipped scissors Disposable gloves Fever thermometer Flashlight Hot water bottle Instant ice pack or plastic bags for holding ice cubes Large triangular bandages to use as slings Safety pins Sewing needle Sterile cotton balls Tweezers

First Aid

First aid is exactly what it sounds like—the first help given to an injured or suddenly ill person. Caregivers will be the first adults on hand should sudden illness or injury occur at the center. They should be prepared to evaluate the extent of illness or injury, summon professional help, and offer basic first aid. First aid is not, however, medical treatment given by lay people. Medications should only be given as prescribed by or under the guidance of medical personnel.

The child care center or family day-care provider should have a well-stocked first-aid kit (see Figure 13.1). Some centers also maintain standing orders from physicians for medications that treat life-threatening conditions such as severe allergic reactions to bee stings or asthma attacks. There are excellent first-aid and CPR courses available at no cost or for a nominal fee through the American Red Cross or other organizations. Every caregiver should take such courses. They provide both theoretical and hands-on training. The descriptions in this book of first aid in various situations are intended only as general guidelines and do not replace first-aid training. Many centers require Red Cross certification for all caregivers.

Responding to Emergency Situations

Recognizing when to call for emergency medical services, when to call a child's parents, and when to administer minor first aid without additional care is an important part of a caregiver's job. When a sudden illness or injury occurs, there are steps every caregiver can take to bring the situation under control. These steps are:

- Remain calm. You will not be able to help anyone if you are not in control.
- Evaluate the situation. Who needs help first? Who else needs help?
- Send for assistance. Do not leave the injured child alone.
- Do nothing to make the injury worse. Do not move the injured child unless she is in immediate danger of further injury by remaining in place. This is especially important with possible neck and back injuries.
- When assistance arrives, divide responsibilities as Danisha, Barbara, and Gwen did. Let the person with the most first-aid experience take over assisting the injured child. Designate someone to make the appropriate telephone calls for help. Designate another person to supervise the other children in the group.
- The types of calls that need to be made depend on the severity of the illness or injury. Sometimes only the child's parent or emergency contact person needs to be called. At other times, the child's health care provider or emergency medical services must be contacted. If there is doubt about the severity of the situation, call for professional help.

Effective planning should prevent a caregiver from ever being the only adult present when an injury occurs. Should this happen, however, the caregiver should use her best judgment to deal with the situation. An older child may, for example, be able to call for help with instructions from the caregiver, who must remain with the injured child.

Assessing Injuries

Injury assessment can be done while help is being summoned. Follow these steps in assessing injuries.

- If the child is able to speak, find out what happened. Ask the child where he is injured and what hurts.
- If the child is unconscious, perform the ABCs of assessment. *A* stands for airway. Is it open? If not, remove any visible foreign material from the mouth. *B* stands for breathing. Is the child breathing? If not, begin artificial (mouth-to-mouth) breathing. *C* stands for circulation. Does the child have a pulse? If there is no pulse, begin CPR (cardiopulmonary resuscitation) if you have been trained in this procedure.

- Check for shock. When *shock* occurs, not enough blood is reaching important parts of the body. Is the child pale, cold, and clammy? Is breathing shallow and rapid? Put a blanket over the child to keep him warm.
- Check for injuries. Deal with severe bleeding first by putting pressure on the wound. If the injury is not obvious, begin searching at the head and work down. Never force a child to move any body part he does not want to move. Moving an injured body part could do additional damage.

General First-Aid Procedures for Common Childhood Injuries

Some injuries, such as severe bleeding and poisoning, happen rarely. Because they are life-threatening, caregivers must know how to respond to them. Other less serious injuries such as scrapes and bruises happen fairly frequently. Caregivers quickly learn how to deal with them effectively.

Any caregiver who is in doubt about what to do when an injury occurs needs to remember these important rules:

- Stay calm.
- Do nothing to cause additional harm.
- Get help.

Choking.   Choking emergencies in infants must be handled differently from those in older children. Helping an infant who is choking involves using a combination of back blows and chest thrusts that must be given carefully and correctly. Helping an older child who is choking involves giving abdominal thrusts. Other steps are necessary if the person is unconscious. See Figure 13.2 for this information. Caregivers should receive first-aid training in the use of these techniques. Child care centers are advised to have wall posters describing these techniques as a reminder for trained caregivers.

Poisoning.   Call the local poison control center. Be prepared to give the name of the poison, the amount consumed, and the age of the child. Follow the poison center's advice. Do not induce vomiting unless told to do so. With certain poisons, this could cause additional damage to internal organs.

Burns.   Immerse the part of the body that has been burned in cold water. If the skin is broken, cover the area with a clean cloth and seek medical help. Never put butter or grease on burns, because a serious infection may result. Fatty substances also retain the heat of the burn and may cause additional tissue damage to occur. Wash chemically burned skin well with cool running water and seek medical help.

Falls, Sprains, and Fractures.   Do not try to move the child. This is especially important if the head, neck, or back are injured. If the child is unconscious, apply the ABCs of first aid. If the child is conscious, look for signs of concussion. These include dizziness, confusion, and pupils—the black

If infant (birth to one year old) is conscious but choking:

1. give four back blows   2. give four chest thrusts

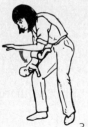 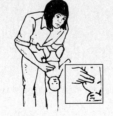

3. repeat blows and thrusts

If infant becomes unconscious:

1. look for object
2. clear mouth
3. give two slow breaths

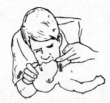

If air won't go in:

1. give four back blows
2. give four chest thrusts
3. look for object and clear mouth
4. give two slow breaths
5. repeat steps 1–4 until breaths go in or help arrives

If child is conscious but choking:

1. give abdominal thrusts

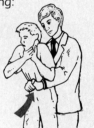

If child becomes unconscious:

1. clear mouth
2. give two slow breaths

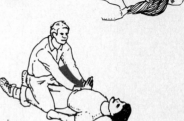

If air won't go in:

1. give up to ten abdominal thrusts
2. clear mouth
3. give two slow breaths
4. repeat steps 1–3 until breaths go in or help arrives

center of the colored iris of the eye—that are of different sizes. Keep the child warm and call for medical help.

For sprains and possible fractures, apply ice to reduce the swelling. Do not let the child use the injured body part. Seek medical help. Minor bruises can be treated with an ice pack.

Bleeding, Cuts, and Scrapes. Use universal precautions (Chapter 11) in handling injuries where there is blood. Try to stop the bleeding by applying continuous pressure using a clean cloth on the wound. Keep the child warm and watch for signs of shock. If bleeding does not stop or if the wound is severe, call for medical help.

Nosebleeds are common in child care centers. Remember to use universal precautions. Have the child sit with her head tilted forward (not back). Pinch the fleshy part of the nose and have the child breathe through her mouth. If possible, apply ice to the nose.

FIGURE 13.2   First-aid for Choking. Caregivers need first-aid training in the use of techniques for helping infants and children who are choking.

Minor cuts should be covered with an adhesive bandage once an antiseptic has been applied.

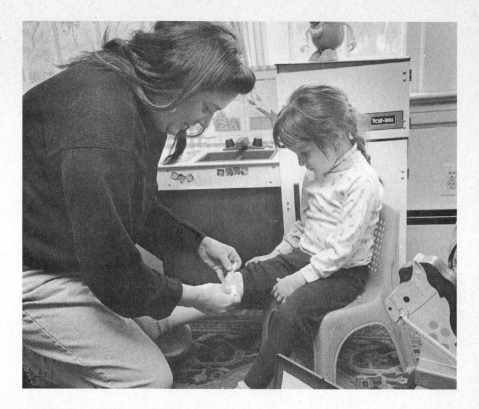

Minor cuts and scrapes should be washed gently with soap and water. Apply an antiseptic and cover with an adhesive bandage.

Insect Stings.   Remove the stinger by scraping it away from the skin with your fingernail. Do not use tweezers because that will inject more venom into the wound. Apply an ice pack to relieve pain. Watch carefully for signs of an allergic reaction. These include dizziness, faintness, nausea, problems breathing, or swelling away from the site of the sting. If a child has a history of allergic reactions to stings, seek medical help immediately and follow instructions on the use of prescribed emergency medications. In some children, insect stings can cause death.

Child Abuse and Neglect

Child abuse happens in every ethnic, racial, and socioeconomic group. It is difficult to know exactly how many children experience child abuse each year. Reporting practices vary from state to state, and many cases of suspected child abuse remain unreported. In 1990, however, more than 2.5 million cases of child abuse and neglect were reported in the United States according to the Department of Health and Human Services (Lowry & Samuelson, 1993). Most children who are victims of abuse are abused by someone they know, not by a stranger.

Since 1974, legislation has required every state to develop policies and procedures for handling suspected child abuse and neglect. Many experts feel that public awareness of the problem of child abuse has increased the percentage of cases that are reported.

Identifying Abused and Neglected Children

There is no single profile of an abused or neglected child. Even the definition of what constitutes abuse changes from state to state, making it difficult to pinpoint when an adult has crossed the line separating discipline or poor parenting skills from actual abuse. Many adults feel that they have the right to do as they please with their children in their own homes. It is only within the past 30 years that harsh treatment of children has become a public policy issue.

Types of Abuse and Neglect. *Child abuse* is defined by the National Committee for Prevention of Child Abuse (NCPCA) as a "nonaccidental injury or pattern of injuries to a child for which there is no 'reasonable' explanation" (Kendrick, Kaufmann, & Messenger, 1991). Organizations that help abused children recognize several different types of abuse. With *physical abuse*, a child is injured by shaking, hitting, beating, burning, or similar violent acts. The abuse can occur once or over a long period. With *emotional abuse*, a child experiences verbal threats and abuse. The child may be rejected, ignored, terrorized, belittled, or isolated. Often unreasonable demands are put on the child.

Sexual abuse is a form of abuse where a child is exploited for the sexual gratification of an adult. Sexual abuse includes touching and nontouching offenses. Rape, incest, any attempt at intercourse, and fondling the genitals are examples of touching offenses. Nontouching offenses include exhibitionism, voyeurism, and using a child for child pornography. It may occur once or over a long period of time. *Incest* is sexual activity among members of a family who are not married to one another. This includes sexual activities between the child and parents, stepparents, siblings, and extended family members, such as aunts, uncles, cousins, and grandparents.

Child neglect is the failure of a parent to provide for the physical care, safety, education, and emotional well-being of a child. Neglect may also involve failure to provide health care, including preventive health care. Neglect is not necessarily related to poverty. It is a symptom of family breakdown.

Signs of Abuse and Neglect

Abuse and neglect leave both physical and emotional marks on a child. Children who are physically abused often have unexplained bruises, welts, burns, cuts, or fractures. These often appear on the face, back, or buttocks and are most often seen when the child returns from a vacation, weekend, or absence. Children who are physically abused often show extremes in their behavior. They may be very aggressive or may withdraw from those around them. They often are wary and untrusting of adults and apprehensive when other children cry. They may say that they are afraid of their parents or afraid to go home. Some may even report being hurt by their parents.

Children who are emotionally abused are much more difficult to recognize. The effects of emotional abuse are cumulative and may not be noticeable until the abuse has gone on for many months or even years. Children who are abused emotionally may show habit disorders such as biting or rocking, or they may exhibit antisocial or destructive behavior. These children may develop obsessions, compulsions, or phobias.

The behavior of emotionally abused children can be extreme—either passive and compliant or aggressive and demanding. They may behave either in an overly adult or overly infantile way. They may lag behind in social and emotional growth and have low self-esteem. Some of these signs can also indicate the presence of a developmental or behavioral problem unrelated to emotional abuse.

Children who are sexually abused may have a variety of physical symptoms. These include pain in the genital area that causes difficulty in sitting or walking. Their genital or anal area may be bruised or bloody. They may have frequent vaginal or urinary infections. They may resist having their clothes changed or being helped with toileting.

Children who are sexually abused may show behavioral symptoms, including bizarre or inappropriate sexual behavior or knowledge. They may withdraw into a fantasy world or revert to infantile behavior such as bedwetting. These children usually have trouble getting along with their peers. They may even talk about their sexual activity.

Neglected children usually show more physical signs of their condition than do abused children. These children are often hungry, dirty, and tired. They may be dressed inappropriately. Often they have physical problems or medical needs that are not met. They may report that they spend long periods at home alone. Neglected children will beg for or steal food. They may try to come to school early or stay late. They also may talk about the lack of care they receive at home.

Factors Contributing to Child Abuse and Neglect

No parent starts out intending to abuse or neglect a child. Abuse and neglect represent a breakdown in parenting. Some parents begin at a disadvantage because they had poor models for parenting in their own childhoods. Others fall apart under stress and become abusive or neglectful.

Characteristics of Child Abusers.   Although child abusers can come from any socioeconomic group, they do share certain emotional and behavioral characteristics. Many child abusers were abused themselves as children. Subconsciously, they learned from their own parents that children should be handled using physical force. Others may have been taught that

Signs of Child Abuse

Caregivers should be alert to signs of child abuse or neglect, but they must also be careful about interpreting those signs. Each culture expects different things from children and has different ways of disciplining them. It is important to understand the standards of an individual child's culture before making a judgment about whether he is being harmed by his parents or other caregivers.

In some countries, all forms of physical punishment are considered unacceptable. In Sweden, for example, spanking is against the law. In other cultures, parents see nothing wrong with physical punishment. Some Taiwanese children are punished for unacceptable behavior by being made to kneel for a period of time. Spanking is used in parts of the Middle East, although very young children may be spanked less severely than older children.

Some ethnic home remedies may produce side effects that could be interpreted as signs of child abuse. "Coining," for example, is a Vietnamese practice in which the edge of a coin is rubbed on the person's back to cure a disease. The procedure may leave a mark that looks like a welt.

Good communication with both children and their parents is important. If a child shows signs of possible abuse, listen to what he tells you about the problem. Let the child know that he can trust you. Ask the parent for an explanation of the child's symptoms as well. If the child or parent comes from a cultural background that is unfamiliar to you, make an effort to ask about the methods of discipline.

Always be on guard if a parent gives vague or unconvincing explanations for a child's injury or emotional upset or tries to "cover up" the injury. If you suspect that a child's home is unsafe or that his parents abuse drugs or alcohol, tell the director of the child care center. Such situations may need to be investigated by a social worker or other trained professional.

children should be isolated or completely ignored when they are disobedient. This can result in emotional abuse of a child.

In addition, many child abusers feel that they are failures. Abusers often feel unloved and isolated from others. They have low self-esteem, have suffered frequent rejections, and have difficulty making friends and forming trusting relationships. They tend to be immature, handling stress poorly and angering easily. They express their anger directly through physical force or emotional abuse.

Circumstances that May Contribute to Child Abuse. Not every adult who has the characteristics of a child abuser becomes abusive. Sometimes a particular set of circumstances acts as a trigger for abusive behavior. Stress brought on by personal and social problems increases the chances that child abuse will occur. Such stress can be social or economic, as with unemployment, or personal, as with marital conflict. Parents under stress frequently have difficulty distinguishing between major problems and minor ones. They may react to something as minor as a child's refusal to eat breakfast with explosive anger or violence.

Drug and alcohol use or addiction also contribute to child abuse and neglect. So may an unplanned pregnancy or the presence in the family of a child who has special physical or emotional needs. Parents who are isolated and lack community support systems are more at risk of becoming abusive. For example, very young parents (preteens or adolescents) who lack the strong emotional and financial support of other family members are at risk of abusing and neglecting their children.

Helping Abused or Neglected Children

The idea that a child is being abused or neglected may be difficult to accept, but child abuse does happen. It is the responsibility of every caring adult to report suspected child abuse. In fact, the law requires that certain people in positions of trust report suspected child abuse.

Gathering Information. The suspicion that a child is being abused may build gradually. Many of the symptoms of child abuse can arise from other causes. Caregivers should keep a written record indicating anything they notice about a child that is out of the ordinary. One bad bruise may be an accident, but repeated bruising may indicate child abuse. Suspicions of child abuse should be shared with the center's director.

Before making a report, consult your state laws about what is considered abuse and neglect. No state requires that a person have *proof* of child abuse before making a report. It is not advisable to wait for such proof. Anyone who, in good faith, reports suspicion of child abuse is protected by the law from prosecution even if it turns out that child abuse is not occurring.

Reporting Abuse or Neglect. Child care professionals along with physicians, nurses, dentists, school counselors, and police officers are required by law in many states to report suspected cases of child abuse or neglect. This is a legal as well as a moral responsibility. Many states maintain hotlines for reporting child abuse. You do not need to tell the parents of the child before you make a report.

It is important to report child abuse to the proper agency. If you do not know where to report suspected abuse, the National Child Abuse Hotline handles crisis calls and offers referrals to every county in the United States (NCPCA, 1988). It can be reached at 1-800-422-4453. Police departments and hospital emergency rooms will also provide local referrals. When making the report, you will generally be asked:

- The name, address, and age of the child
- The extent of the child's injuries
- The names and addresses of the parents
- The identity of the offending adult, if known
- Often, your name and address

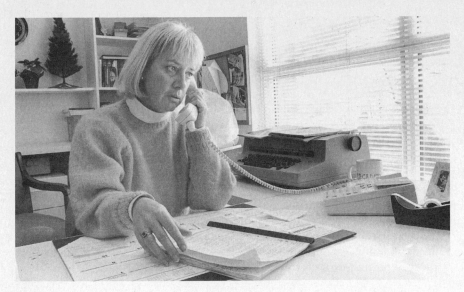

Child care professionals have a legal as well as a moral responsibility to report suspected cases of child abuse or neglect.

Providing Emotional Support.   Children who claim to have been abused or neglected need to be believed and taken seriously. The child is never responsible for the abuse and must never be made to feel that that is the case. Teachers can help abused and neglected children by establishing a secure and trusting environment where children are listened to and valued. The child care center should be a place where children are encouraged to talk about their feelings.

Teachers can also help children who have been abused or neglected in other ways. For example, they can set limits for acceptable behavior and be consistent in enforcing them. Abused and neglected children lack consistency in their lives. Providing it during the time they are in child care will benefit them greatly. Many abused children also have low self-esteem. Responding to all children in an accepting manner, praising their efforts, and helping them to develop their abilities are all ways of contributing to children's self-esteem.

Educating Children.   Teachers can help all the children in their care by educating them about child abuse. One way to educate children about abuse is to use the concepts about strangers already discussed. However, most children are abused by a person they know, not by a stranger. Important concepts for children include:

▪ Providing information about "good touching" such as hugging and "bad touching," which makes the child uncomfortable
▪ Reminding children that their bodies belong to them and they can decide who touches them and where
▪ Teaching children the difference between surprises (good secrets) and bad secrets, in which the hidden information makes the child uncomfortable or threats are made

Helping Parents

Child abuse and neglect are family problems that come about because of a breakdown in the household. Child abusers need help just as much as abused children do. Caregivers can provide informal aid by developing supportive relationships with parents and offering help with difficulties they may be experiencing in raising their children. Child care centers can provide information about child development and sponsor programs and speakers on parenting issues.

Child care centers should keep a list of community resources for troubled families. State child protective services will provide referrals to social service agencies that work with families. Crisis intervention centers and self-help groups may be useful to some parents.

Keep in mind that parents under stress may need special encouragement to seek assistance from social service agencies. Giving them a telephone number may not be enough. Caregivers may need to guide families toward sources of help more directly.

Protecting Children from Child Abuse in Child Care Centers

Several highly publicized charges of child abuse in child care settings have occurred in recent years. Child care centers must take responsibility for protecting the children in their care. One way to prevent child abuse in child care centers is to screen staff members thoroughly before they are hired. Some of the screening procedures, such as interviewing and background checks, were mentioned earlier in this chapter in the discussion on staff qualifications.

New staff members should have extra supervision for some time after they begin working. In addition, centers should be designed to reduce opportunities for a caregiver to be isolated with a child or several children.

Centers need to talk with caregivers about acceptable types of touching, such as pats on the back, hand holding, or a warm hug. Caregivers should be taught to be sensitive to a child's resistance even to acceptable touching and not to force unwanted contact. Sharing center policies on touching with parents and requesting their input will aid communication and reduce misunderstanding.

Child care centers should also have a written statement of philosophy and clear policies about discipline and its use with children. Discipline should always be aimed at helping children learn to handle interactions with other people in a constructive, nonviolent manner. Every discipline policy should clearly state that no form of physical punishment will be employed or tolerated. Physical punishment includes any measure that hinders a child's ability or opportunity to eat, sleep, relieve himself, or perform other functions important to his physical or mental health.

Every child care center should provide training on child abuse and develop a child abuse policy. Caregivers should be educated about what is considered child abuse and know that it will not be tolerated for any reason.

SUMMARY

- Safety awareness attempts to prevent injuries and to minimize their effects when they do happen.
- Caregivers keep children safe through safe physical environments, enforced rules for safe behavior, and safety education.
- Teachers can help keep children safe indoors by establishing general safety rules, providing adequate supervision, and helping children to resolve their conflicts nonviolently.
- Achieving safety on the playground requires safe equipment and careful supervision.
- Teachers need to guard against sunburn, dehydration, and heat exhaustion during hot weather and frostbite during cold weather.
- Children should be taught bicycle and pedestrian safety during the preschool years.
- Field trips must be carefully planned and supervised.
- Child care centers should implement procedures that prevent child abductions. Children should be taught how to avoid strangers and to tell an adult if they are approached by a stranger.
- Child care centers should make responsible hiring decisions and provide opportunities for staff to participate in continuing education.
- Caregivers can help prevent lapses in safe behavior by recognizing when they are most likely to occur and planning activities carefully to decrease the possibility of accidental injury.
- Written records are needed to respond effectively to an emergency. Every emergency requires a written follow-up.
- When faced with an emergency situation, caregivers should stay calm, do nothing to cause additional harm, and get help.
- The ABCs of injury assessment are A (open airways), B (start breathing), and C (establish circulation).
- Caregivers should be familiar with general first-aid procedures for dealing with common injuries.
- Children can be abused physically, emotionally, and sexually. Child neglect involves failing to provide properly for the needs of a child.
- Caregivers should be able to recognize the signs of child abuse and neglect and to understand the characteristics of child abusers and the circumstances that may lead to child abuse.
- Child care professionals should know the proper agency to contact if they suspect child abuse.
- Child care workers may be able to prevent abuse or neglect by maintaining communication with parents and offering help when necessary.

- Child care centers have a responsibility for protecting children from abuse in the child care environment. Careful hiring procedures, employee supervision, and communication with staff members and parents are important aspects of such protection.

ACQUIRING KNOWLEDGE

1. What are the two main factors that affect the level of safety in a child care setting?
2. Identify the two ways to create safe physical environments for children. Give an example of each.
3. Explain how planning ahead helps reduce the risk of accidents.
4. Identify three guidelines to follow when establishing rules of behavior for young children.
5. Why should at least two adults be present when children are being supervised?
6. What is the criticism of the use of "time-outs" as a means of ending a conflict?
7. List three rules for safe play on the playground.
8. Explain how to protect children from overexposure to the sun.
9. What is frostbite?
10. Identify three ways caregivers can prepare for a field trip.
11. How can caregivers reduce the threat of a child being taken by a noncustodial parent or by a stranger?
12. What are three ways that employers of caregivers can help ensure that the people they hire can be trusted to work with children?
13. Identify the five pieces of written information caregivers should have for each child in order to respond effectively in any emergency.
14. Identify five telephone numbers caregivers should have at hand in case of emergencies (in addition to emergency numbers for individual children).
15. Identify three types of disasters caregivers may be asked to respond to.
16. Give two reasons why injury reports are useful.
17. Describe the ABCs of injury assessment.
18. What are the signs of shock?
19. What should be done first if a child is bleeding severely from a wound?
20. What are the three most important rules to remember when an injury occurs?
21. List six categories of injuries that caregivers should know how to respond to.
22. Describe how to treat a nosebleed.
23. Why is it important to know if a child has a history of allergic reactions to insect stings?
24. Define child abuse and child neglect.
25. Identify five possible signs of physical child abuse.

THINKING CRITICALLY

1. List two indoor safety rules caregivers should establish with young children. When writing them, remember to follow the chapter guidelines for establishing rules with young children.
2. Many children are surrounded by images that clearly or subtly advocate the use of violence as a means of resolving conflicts. In what way do you think exposure to violence will affect your job of caring for children and keeping them safe?
3. Caregivers emphasize to children the importance of never talking to strangers. If, however, a child becomes lost, it may become necessary for him to talk to a stranger. What should caregivers tell young children to do if they become separated from a parent or caregiver?
4. Do you think first-aid training should be required for caregivers? Why or why not?
5. Explain the relationship between ongoing stress in parents' lives and the occurence of child abuse.

OBSERVATIONS AND APPLICATIONS

1. Observe children playing on the playground at a child care center. Note the ages of the children and how many children are on the playground. Note the behavior of the caregivers. How many caregivers are on the playground with the children? Are the caregivers watching the children, or are they engaged in conversation with one another? Do caregivers intervene when too many children are on a piece of equipment or when children play inappropriately? What safety rules do you see children following? What safety rules do caregivers point out to children while you are observing?
2. Observe children playing indoors during a free play period at a child care center. Note the ages of the children and how many children are in the class. Note also the number of caregivers watching the children. Are the caregivers primarily engaged in watching and participating with the children or are they involved in other activities—setting up for snack or an art project, for example? Do caregivers intervene in the children's play to resolve any conflicts? If so, describe what initiated the conflict and how the caregiver resolved it. Note rules you hear caregivers and children mention that involve safety. What other practices that relate to safety do you observe? Are the toys appropriate for the age of the children? Are they in good condition? Do they have small pieces that young children might swallow?
3. Mr. and Mrs. Marquez are going away for a few days. Their son Julio will stay with his friend Robert's family, the Zimmers. Julio and Robert attend the same child care center. Before leaving, what emergency and other information should Julio's parents leave with Robert's parents? What should Julio's parents tell the school?

4. Suppose you, as a caregiver, are aware that the family of Shannon, a four-year-old in your class, is experiencing great stress. The mother recently told you that the father lost his job. You notice the effects of stress on Shannon and worry that the situation is moving toward abuse. Without a suspicion of actual abuse, but feeling that the situation is almost out of control, what can you do to try to help Shannon and her parents? Should you report the situation or first try to work with the family? Explain.

FOR FURTHER INFORMATION

Organizations

Center on Children and the Law
1800 M Street, NW, Suite 200 South
Washington, DC 20036
(202) 331-2250

Children's Defense Fund
25 E Street, NW
Washington, DC 20001
(202) 628-8787

National Center on Child Abuse and Neglect
P. O. Box 1182
Washington, DC 20013
(703) 385-7565 or (800) 394-3366

National Child Abuse Hotline (a referral service)
(800) 422-4453

National Committee to Prevent Child Abuse
332 South Michigan Avenue, Suite 1600
Chicago, IL 60604
(312) 663-3520

National Safe Kids
111 Michigan Avenue, NW
Washington, DC 20010
(202) 939-4993

National Safety Council
Family Safety and Health
P. O. Box 558
Itasca, IL 60143-0558
(708) 285-1121

Trauma Foundation
Building One, Room 400
San Francisco General Hospital
San Francisco, CA 94110

Publications

Ammerman, R. T., & Hersen, M. (Eds.). (1990). *Children at risk: An evaluation of factors contributing to child abuse and neglect.* New York: Plenum.

Baxter, A. (1985). *Techniques for dealing with child abuse.* Springfield, IL: C. C. Thomas.

Baxter, A. (1986). *Techniques for dealing with child sexual abuse.* Springfield, IL: C. C. Thomas.

Besherov, D. J. (Ed.). (1990). *Recognizing child abuse: A guide for the concerned.* New York: Free Press.

Braun, L. D. (1988). *Someone heard . . . A comprehensive educator's handbook for child abuse and neglect recognition and prevention.* Winter Park, FL: Currier-Davis.

Carlsson-Paige, N., & Levin, D. E. (1992). Making peace in violent times: A constructivist approach to conflict resolution. *Young Children, 48* (1), 4–13.

Charnizon, M. (Ed.). (1990). *New York society for the prevention of cruelty to children professionals' handbook: Identifying and reporting child abuse and neglect.* New York: New York Society for the Prevention of Cruelty to Children.

Children's Defense Fund. (1992). *The state of America's children 1991.* Washington, DC: Author.

Haugaard, J. J., & Reppucci, N. D. (1988). *The sexual abuse of children: A comprehensive guide to current knowledge and intervention strategies.* San Francisco: Jossey-Bass.

Hillman, D., & Solek-Tefft, J. (1990). *Spiders and flies: Help for parents and teachers of sexually abused children.* New York: Free Press.

Mufson, S. (1993). *Straight talk about child abuse.* New York: Dell.

National Center for the Prevention of Child Abuse. (1988). *Basic facts about child sexual abuse* (3rd ed.). Chicago: Author.

National Safety Council. (1992). *Accident Facts, 1992.* Chicago: Author.

Parcel, G. S. (1989). *Basic emergency care of the sick and injured* (4th ed.). St. Louis: Mosby-Year Book.

Tuchascherer, P. (1988). *TV interactive toys: The new high tech threat to children.* Bend, OR: Pinnaroo Publishing.

PART 4

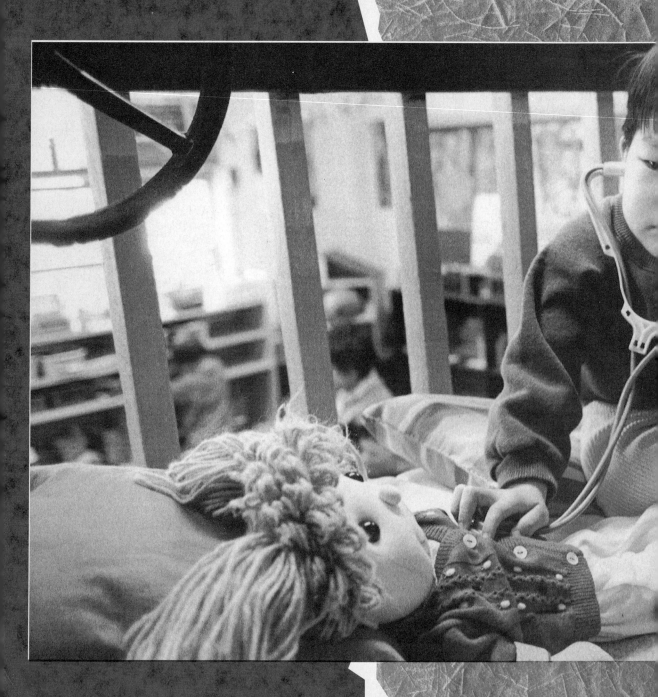

Teaching Nutrition, Health, and Safety

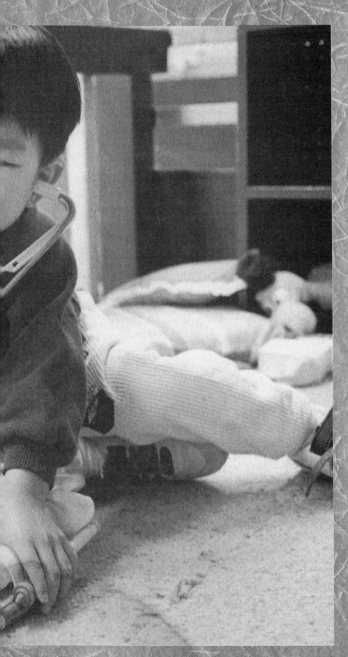

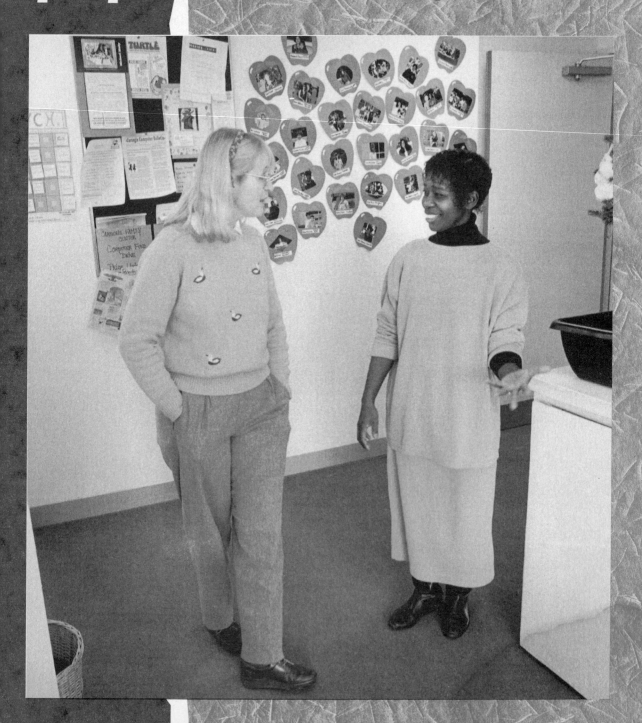

OBJECTIVES

Studying this chapter
will enable you to

- Identify the goals for a nutrition, health, and safety curriculum
- Define curriculum and describe the four elements of a curriculum
- List the five basic guidelines to be followed when teaching young children
- Explain how to prepare and evaluate lesson plans

CHAPTER TERMS

attitudes
child-initiated
curriculum
instructional objective
teacher-directed
transition times

TONYA and Elizabeth, two teachers at the Westlake Preschool, were talking as they walked together to their classrooms one Monday morning.

"My class of four-year-olds is going to make tacos for lunch today. I thought it would be a good way to reinforce the food group songs and puppet play from last week," Tonya told her coworker.

"Sounds like a good idea," said Elizabeth. "How are you going to do it?"

"I've cut out magazine pictures of taco ingredients and fruits—for dessert. They'll have pictures of meat, shredded cheese, lettuce, tomatoes, taco shells, apples, and oranges. I've made a sign for each food group to which I have pasted identical pictures of the ingredients as well as other foods in each group," Tonya said. "Each child will match a taco ingredient picture with the correct group."

"Then what?" asked Elizabeth.

"Then we all wash our hands and head into the kitchen. I chopped the vegetables this morning, but they can put them in bowls and shred the cheese with a plastic shredder. I'll warm the meat, which I cooked yesterday, in the microwave. I didn't think I could cook the raw hamburger safely with four-year-olds. We'll all build our tacos at the lunch table, family-style," Tonya explained.

"Sounds like you're all set for this event," said Elizabeth.

"Well, I will be as soon as I get the fruit sliced and refrigerated."

"Do you suppose any fruit will end up in a taco?" asked Elizabeth.

"Probably," said Tonya. "But there's nothing wrong with a little extra adventure in eating. In fact, while we're cleaning up, I plan to ask them how many foods they just ate and talk a little about why eating a variety of foods helps people stay healthy."

"Tacos really are a good way to demonstrate both the food groups and variety," said Elizabeth. "Hey—do you mind if I borrow your idea next week for my five-year-olds?" asked Elizabeth.

"Not at all," Tonya replied. "You can even use my signs. Just let me know how the activity works out with an older group."

Caring For and Teaching Young Children

Caring for young children and teaching them about nutrition, health, and safety are two closely related aspects of preschool education. When people care for children, they are keeping the children safe and healthy in the present. Caregivers perform many acts of caregiving throughout the school day. They prepare nutritious lunches and snacks for children, keep them inside a fenced area to protect them from traffic, and isolate children with colds and other communicable diseases from the rest of the group to prevent the spread of illness. Children are usually unaware of the importance of these actions for their safety and well-being. But caregivers perform them day in and day out.

Teaching, like caregiving, meets the needs of the present. But teaching also reaches into the future. It provides children with skills, knowledge, and attitudes that they can use to help keep themselves safe and healthy for the rest of their lives. For example, every time children wash their hands after toileting and before eating, they are preventing the spread of germs. But they are also forming a lifelong healthful habit that will help them to avoid many common illnesses in future years.

Goals for Nutrition, Health, and Safety Education

The goals of nutrition, health, and safety education for young children are two pronged: to promote healthful behavior during the preschool years and to motivate children to develop good nutrition, health, and safety habits for the rest of their lives. This type of education has the goal of nurturing individuals who will take care of their own bodies, relate well to others, and act responsibly in their societies.

Nutrition, health, and safety instruction can help young children learn to take care of their bodies by eating nutritious foods, exercising regularly, getting adequate rest and relaxation, and avoiding dangerous situations. Successful programs also help children to learn how to cooperate with others, communicate, and settle conflicts nonviolently. In addition, nutrition, health, and safety education strives to teach children how to make responsible decisions about matters that affect their bodies (Creswell & Newman, 1993). Learning to make responsible decisions involves the ability to assess a situation and the actions needed to protect one's health and safety. Although much of this is beyond the abilities of very young children, even toddlers can begin to develop some healthful habits, such as toothbrushing and handwashing. Children need to learn many different kinds of responsible actions in areas ranging from traffic safety to avoidance of illegal drugs and prevention of transmission of dangerous diseases.

Getting Started Early

The early childhood years are the best starting point for developing good nutrition, health, and safety habits (Cornacchia, Olsen, & Nickerson, 1991). Parents begin teaching children about food, health, and safety very early. Parents may, for example, start teaching toddlers about nutrition by talking about the colors, textures, and other qualities of foods and by offering a wide variety of nutritious foods to toddlers throughout the day. Similarly, parents and caregivers teach toddlers and preschoolers to practice good health habits such as covering the mouth when coughing and dressing warmly to go outside in cold weather. And they help them avoid many common dangers such as street traffic and electrical outlets.

Young children are quick and enthusiastic learners. They learn by observing everything around them, imitating their parents and other adults, and manipulating objects in their environments. They learn most effectively, however, when all of their emerging abilities—physical, emotional, intellectual, social, and creative—are taken into account. This chapter explores how teachers can engage those abilities to help children begin learning about nutrition, health, and safety.

The Elements of Curriculum

A preschool *curriculum* is the process of identifying goals and making plans to provide educational experiences for young children. A preschool curriculum has four basic elements. The first element is building a positive self-concept, in which the child develops positive feelings about herself and her abilities. The second element is skills acquisition; the curriculum helps children gain many kinds of skills that they can use in future situations. The third element is knowledge acquisition; the curriculum teaches children about their world. And the fourth element is attitude development. *Attitudes* are a person's feelings, beliefs, or opinions about a person, object, or event. A person's attitudes cause her to respond positively or negatively in a situation. An effective preschool curriculum helps children develop positive attitudes about themselves, others, and the world around them. Teachers should try to incorporate each of these elements into nutrition, health, and safety instruction.

WHOLESOME SNACKS

Exploring Rice

Ingredients:

3 cups uncooked rice
6 cups water

Optional Ingredients:

cooked peas (Italy)
cooked red beans (Latin America)
soy sauce (East Asia)
raisins (Southwest Asia)
cinnamon (India)

Directions:

1. Have children help to measure the rice and water and to pour it into the pan.
2. Boil uncovered, then reduce heat. Simmer covered for 15 minutes or until all water is absorbed. Cool until warm. (Note: Cook rice in kitchen, away from children.)
3. At snack time, allow children to stir their own ingredients into their rice.

Yield: 18 servings
Each serving contains:
Calories: 113
Protein: 2 g
Fat: Trace
Carbohydrates: 25 g

Source: University of Illinois at Urbana-Champaign Child Development Lab.

Opportunities to share with the group help children develop a positive self-concept.

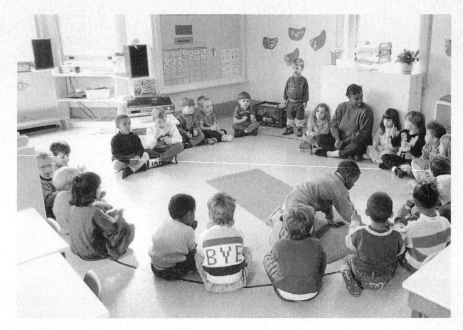

Developing a Positive Self-Concept

The preschool child is working hard to form an identity and to establish a view of herself. Many of the ways young children view themselves are based on how they believe they are perceived by others, especially by adults who are important to them such as parents and teachers. The preschool curriculum should include many opportunities, activities, and materials that encourage children to form a positive self-concept—that is, to feel successful and competent.

In order to develop a positive self-concept, children need many opportunities to master skills and to feel successful. "You're learning to use a fork very well," "I really liked the way you remembered to wash your hands before lunch," and "You're carrying the scissors pointing down just like we said" are statements that help children evaluate their own increasing skills and competence. A child's abilities to learn specific skills should not be compared to those of another child but only to his own past efforts.

Young children also need opportunities to make choices and initiate actions. Nutrition activities provide excellent opportunities to make choices. Children can, for example, choose one food over another or decide how much of a food they want to eat. Other parts of the preschool curriculum allow children to feel good about themselves by initiating actions. A child can propose a game to her classmates on the playground, for example, or suggest a direction or action in a game of "Simon Says." These kinds of experiences help preschoolers understand that they can influence their environments and that they are worthwhile individuals whose preferences and opinions are important. Over time, children are able to develop a high level of self-esteem that contributes to their emotional and social health.

Acquiring Skills

As they grow and develop, children learn increasingly complex physical, emotional, social, intellectual, and creative skills. A preschool curriculum can build on developing skills as it helps children acquire new ones.

Curriculum activities should give preschoolers opportunities to practice several different kinds of skills at one time. Tonya's taco-making activity in the story at the beginning of the chapter provided practice in a variety of skills. Physical skills were addressed as the children shredded cheese, put chopped vegetables in serving bowls, and assembled the ingredients in a taco. Such activities help develop fine motor skills, muscle control, and hand-eye coordination. The children exercised their intellectual skills as they tried to classify the taco components into the five food groups.

Tonya also considered her preschoolers' social development. The taco-making activity required the children to work together as they prepared the tacos. That gave them the opportunity to practice such social skills as communication, cooperation, and sharing. They also enjoyed the satisfaction of eating food they had prepared themselves. All these are valuable aids in developing social competence and a sense of self-worth.

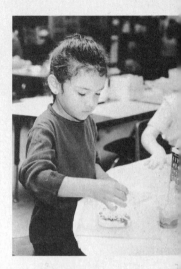

Some curriculum activities, such as the pizza making shown here, can help develop fine motor skills, muscle control, and hand-eye coordination.

Building Knowledge

Children need specific, accurate information in order to make wise choices and decisions about their nutrition, health, and safety. They can be taught such things as the names of foods and where they come from, which foods fit into which groups, and simple explanations of how different foods help children grow and develop. So, for example, they can learn what food group cheese is part of, that it is made from cow's milk, and that it helps to keep bones strong and healthy. The same level of knowledge is appropriate in the areas of health and safety. Children can learn why exercise is good for the body and what to do if the fire alarm rings.

To be useful to children, the information they are taught must be understandable and relevant to their developmental age. When Tonya indicated that she would limit her explanation about the importance of eating a variety of foods, she was making a good point. Preschoolers are not ready to learn about all of the different kinds of vitamins, minerals, and other nutrients found in foods. Yet they can begin to absorb very basic information about the food groups and why eating a variety of foods helps people get everything they need to stay strong and healthy. Matching pictures of ingredients to food groups and preparing the tacos also provided the kinds of hands-on learning that is most effective with young children.

Forming Positive Attitudes

Preschool children not only develop attitudes about themselves but also develop attitudes about other people. Many of these attitudes are strongly influenced by their parents and other caregivers. An effective curriculum

FOCUS ON Cultural Diversity

Cultural Kitchen Corner

One way to help children appreciate a variety of cultures is through something that is basic to every culture—food. It is easy to set up a cultural kitchen corner in which the foods and the eating and cooking utensils of different cultures can be displayed.

Change the exhibits in the cultural kitchen corner once a month or even more often if possible. Put up colorful posters showing scenes from a specific country or area of the world. Use shelf space to display nonperishable staple foods and unique pots, pans, and dishes.

Highlight Asian food traditions by displaying a bamboo steamer basket and wok. Encourage children to use all five senses by letting them see and smell herbs and spices used in Asian cuisine. Lemongrass, sometimes used in Vietnamese cooking, is one example. Gingerroot is another. Chopsticks made of wood, ivory, or plastic are handy learning tools. Children of Asian background might demonstrate how to use them.

Focus on the cultures of the Middle East and North Africa by displaying a couscousier, the special pot used to cook couscous (fine-grained semolina cereal). Stock the kitchen corner with foods such as canned grape leaves, chick peas, and sesame seeds. You can prepare a meal or snack using pita bread, a flat bread with a pocket in the center that is eaten throughout the Middle East.

Much "American" food is based on foods that are traditional in Western Europe. Nevertheless, children might not be familiar with the special foods of countries such as Sweden or Spain. To make the kitchen corner Swedish, try to find one of the special pans used for cooking Swedish pancakes. Stock products such as preserved lingonberries or cloudberry jam.

Children will take pride in bringing in foods or cooking utensils that are part of their families and cultural traditions. This is also a great way to involve parents in the preschool program!

encourages unbiased, inclusive attitudes toward others and an openness toward new experiences, whether in the form of trying new foods or respecting someone else's cultural or religious practices.

As toddlers, children begin to develop the intellectual abilities to classify and categorize objects and people. By the age of three, children have already begun to establish their own gender and racial identities and to notice differences in others (Katz, 1982). Between the ages of three and five, children can also begin to form negative attitudes and express stereotypical views of various racial and ethnic groups (Aboud, 1988).

Nutrition, health, and safety concepts can be important elements in curricula that help children learn about the similarities and differences between people. A good curriculum challenges the misconceptions, biases, and stereotypes that children acquire about gender roles, racial characteristics, and disabilities. Materials, activities, books, and bulletin board displays can reflect different races and cultures in a positive light. Many schools incorporate foods, traditions, and artifacts from different cultures in their curricula

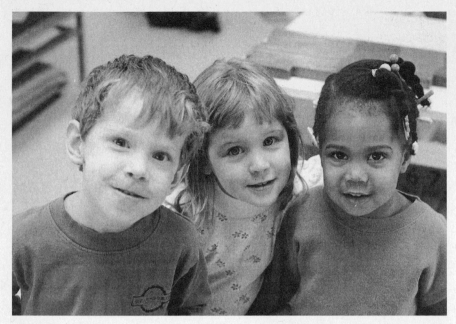

By the time they are three years old, children have begun to establish their gender and racial identities. It is important for preschool curricula to encourage unbiased, inclusive attitudes towards other people from the very beginning.

to promote multicultural diversity. A Japanese kimono, Mexican piñata, Korean meal, or a display of West African sculpture all provide information about how people in different cultures live. Teachers can use maps, pictures, books, videos, and even invited guests to show the diversity of the world's people and to promote a knowledge and understanding of other cultures. Teachers should remember that they are important role models for young children. Adults should treat all children with respect and affection regardless of their skin color, sex, religion, or ethnic background.

A good preschool curriculum should emphasize that people have many behaviors in common. People in different cultures all eat, stay healthy, and remain safe. They may, however, perform these activities in different and interesting ways. Each culture develops its own kind of grain products, for instance. In Mexico, corn is ground into flour to make tortillas; in Italy, flour is made into spaghetti and other kinds of pasta; and in China, people eat a variety of noodles. A bread-tasting or pasta-tasting activity could help children learn that each culture has many different, unique, and valuable contributions to make. Other types of activities could expose children to the many ways people stay well and remain safe throughout the world.

Guidelines for Teaching Young Children

Effective nutrition, health, and safety education does not just happen. Teachers need to devote time and energy to *making* it happen in their classrooms and with their particular group of children. The basic guidelines for teaching nutrition, health, and safety are really no different from those for other subject areas. Teaching methods, however, must be geared toward the needs, interests, culture groups, and abilities of the children involved. Five guidelines for an effective curriculum follow.

Offer Variety

No two children learn in exactly the same way, and no two children have precisely the same interests or come to school with the same prior experiences. Educators, therefore, use a variety of teaching approaches, techniques, and materials to present the information being taught. A lesson on milk and calcium, for example, could include a visit to a dairy farm; examination of a model of human teeth and a trip to a dentist's office; a dairy products tasting party with milk, yogurt, and various cheeses; a visit to a supermarket dairy case; and the use of books and posters about dairy farming and milk products. Each child will enjoy and understand at least some of those activities even if others are less appealing.

Most preschools use a combination of teacher-directed and child-initiated curriculum approaches in teaching young children. In the *teacher-directed* approach, the teacher determines and leads the lesson or activity. In the *child-initiated* approach, children are given opportunities to choose their own activities and to decide for themselves how to go about exploring new materials and pursuing new experiences.

If the children are learning about fruits, a teacher using the teacher-directed approach might lead the class in an exercise in naming different fruits in a fruit bowl or on a tour of an orchard. Later that same day, the teacher might set up materials for a child-initiated activity in which children can explore the colors, tastes, and textures of different fruits. Each child could choose from a range of activities, such as painting a picture of one kind of fruit, tasting different kinds of fruit, or categorizing fruits by color.

Plan Developmentally Appropriate Material

No one can teach children skills or knowledge that they are not yet ready to receive. Five-year-olds cannot understand the chemical changes that occur when a peach is baked, but they *can* understand that peaches are eaten raw, cooked, canned, and even dried. They cannot comprehend a nutritional analysis of a meal, but they can help plan a meal that includes food from each of the food groups.

Appropriateness also has to do with what children are interested in and what they need to know at a particular time. Nutrition, health, and safety have intrinsic appeal because they have to do with basic body processes and everyday behavior. Preschoolers, for example, generally love to run and jump and play and don't want to be sick in bed. Although they do not need to know the difference between bacteria and viruses, they will need to know about covering their mouths when coughing and washing their hands before meals.

Teachers also need to recognize and accommodate individual developmental and personality differences between children. Curriculum choices should allow children to work at their own pace as much as possible. A good mix of approaches and activities can reach children who are working at very different levels.

Keep Ideas Simple

Keeping ideas simple is important for a preschool audience. Lessons should introduce a limited number of new concepts at a time. For example, Tonya planned to introduce only two closely related ideas to her four-year-olds: foods can be classified into groups and people should eat a wide variety of foods to stay healthy.

Simple lessons should also be positive. They should emphasize the rewards of good nutrition, health, and safety practices. A lesson on the need to bathe regularly should stress that regular bathing keeps people clean and healthy and that it makes them feel good. Although recognizing dangers is necessary in some subject areas—especially the area of safety—a positive approach works best overall. Safety concepts such as "go swimming only with an adult" and "always wear a bicycle helmet when you ride" are both simple and positive.

Lessons for preschoolers should also be concrete and relevant to daily life. Avoid long lists of do's and don'ts. Instead, help children incorporate good nutrition, health, and safety practices into their everyday lives. Lessons on eating nutritious foods, brushing their teeth after meals, and wearing seat belts in the car have direct, everyday relevance for preschoolers.

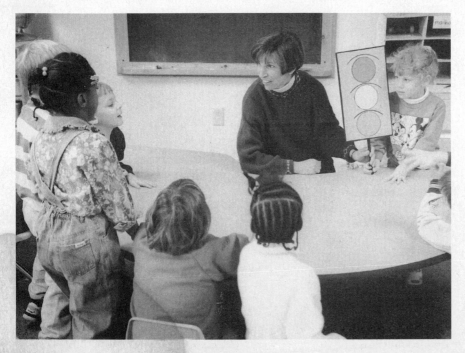

Lesson plans for young children should introduce only a limited number of new ideas at a time. Keeping the ideas simple is also important.

Use Repetition and Predictability

Young children need many opportunities to practice new skills, hear new information, and form positive attitudes about nutrition, health, and safety. One day's lesson about the importance of drinking milk or the need to cover one's mouth while coughing will not make a lasting impression. The curriculum should be structured so that children can experience information again and again in new and progressively more challenging ways (Hendrick, 1990). Each lesson plan should review and then build on concepts that have already been introduced. Eventually, children will internalize the information, and it will no longer need to be reinforced.

Predictability is another important aspect of teaching nutrition, health, and safety to young children. Predictability in daily and weekly activities is reassuring to children. They like to know what is going to happen next (Hendrick, 1992) and that their teachers will behave in predictable ways. Schedules, routines, and rules should be followed whenever possible. For example, snacks and rest periods should come at about the same time every day. Although predictability helps children feel secure in the preschool environment, it is not advisable to let routines drive a program regardless of circumstances. Teachers should also be open to adapting their plans to the needs of the children.

Repetition and predictability also involve consistency. A teacher who talks about the importance of eating a variety of foods but serves crackers for every snack is sending a confusing message to children who are trying to form their own concepts of nutrition. In other words, teachers should recognize the importance of role-modeling as a teaching method. All aspects of a curriculum should be integrated as much as possible to allow reinforcement, not contradiction, within the program.

Strive for Inclusiveness

Curriculum activities and projects should involve everyone, attracting children's interest and exciting their imaginations. Activities should challenge all children to master a new skill, solve a problem, or think creatively. Lessons should be structured so that every child experiences challenge and success as often as possible. Activities that are too easy or too difficult can produce boredom and frustration. Variety in activities as well as recognition of each child's strengths is crucial. A child who speaks Spanish can tell the Spanish names for pictured fruits and vegetables. A child who uses a wheelchair can demonstrate how to use it safely in the classroom.

Teachers should be aware of children who are holding back from participating because of boredom or shyness. Withdrawal is often a coping mechanism for children, and it should be recognized and treated sensitively (Hendrick, 1990). Teachers should make patient efforts to include a shy child in a group without forcing participation. Some young children need an opportunity to practice a skill with an understanding adult before they try it in a group of their peers.

Healthful Foods for Birthday Celebrations

It is the end of the day at the Brookdale Learning Center. Nicole's mother stops to speak to Amy, one of the teachers.

NICOLE'S MOTHER: Since Nicole's birthday is on Sunday, I thought I would bring in her birthday treat tomorrow. The problem is that this is our first year here. What kinds of treats do other people bring in?

AMY: Lots of different things. Of course, the kids love sweets of any kind, but Mrs. Rose, the director, likes the snacks to be as nutritious as possible.

NICOLE'S MOTHER: I don't know about the other kids, but if Nicole knows that something is good for her, she won't eat it—especially if I ask her to.

AMY: The other children are like that too. Even so, we manage to feed them things that taste good and have nutritious ingredients. Of course, we don't hang a sign on the food that says nutritious! We do find that all of the children seem to eat pretty well if we just don't comment about what they're eating or not eating.

NICOLE'S MOTHER: That is interesting! So what do the other parents bring for birthday treats?

AMY: Well, Eric's mother brought in some soft vanilla cookies that were made with cottage cheese. Eric helped bake them and he decorated them with colored sprinkles. Kristin's grandmother made zucchini bread—that was a real hit. Ursula's grandmother made pumpkin muffins in a special pan. They came out in different animal shapes, and the children enjoyed them very much.

NICOLE'S MOTHER: All of that sounds terrific, but I'm not much of a baker. I would hate to bring in something that Nicole and her friends didn't like. Isn't there something that I can buy that's healthful and tasty?

AMY: How about bran muffins or bagels with cream cheese? The bakery across the street makes wonderful whole wheat banana bread. What does Nicole like?

NICOLE'S MOTHER: I'm sure you've noticed that she's a very picky eater. Right now she will eat cheddar cheese, an apple slice or two, and frozen yogurt—but only vanilla or strawberry flavor.

AMY: Why not bring in some low-fat frozen yogurt? It's sweet, the children love it, and it's pretty good for them.

NICOLE'S MOTHER: That's a good idea! Tasty, nutritious, and I don't have to bake it!

AMY: If you would like to bring in some apples, I could slice them so the children could make sundaes.

NICOLE'S MOTHER: That would be great! I'll bring in those paper cups that have dinosaurs on them to serve the yogurt sundaes in.

AMY: We've had superhero napkins and ballerina plates. Dinosaur cups will really make the party!

Did Amy handle Nicole's mother's questions effectively? Would you have done anything differently? What other nutritious foods could Nicole's mother bring in?

Preparing and Evaluating Lesson Plans

The guidelines just described should be kept in mind as specific planning is carried out. Written lesson plans, including detailed procedures, are crucial organizational tools for early childhood education. Preparing a lesson plan involves five steps:

- Choosing an overall idea or concept
- Choosing a topic to illustrate the concept
- Preparing instructional objectives for the activity
- Selecting activities that achieve those objectives
- Evaluating the lesson plan

Each of these steps will be examined separately.

Step 1: Choosing a Concept

A concept is a major idea or theme that helps children to learn about themselves and their world. When children have grasped a concept, it means that they have learned to categorize or regroup information so that they think about a subject in a new way. The goal is to teach basic concepts about nutrition, health, and safety that will provide a firm foundation on which more complex concepts can later be built.

Basic nutrition, health, and safety concepts that can be taught to preschoolers include:

- Foods have different names, flavors, and textures.
- Foods come from plants and animals.
- People need a variety of foods to stay healthy.
- Exercise is fun and good for you.
- Many sicknesses are caused by germs that can be passed from one person to another.
- Children should be cautious around strangers.
- Sharp objects must be handled safely.

Step 2: Choosing a Topic

A topic is the specific subject used in a lesson plan to explain or illustrate a concept. Suppose a teacher starts with the concept that cooking changes how foods look, feel, and taste. The next step is to choose a topic that illustrates this concept. The topic, therefore, may be discovering how cooking affects popcorn or bread dough. Or it may be exploring how many ways a potato can be cooked. The teacher may decide to set up a demonstration using eggs, or he may lead a cooking activity in which the children make vegetable soup.

How does the planner choose a topic out of the many that are possible? First, the topic selected should clearly explain or demonstrate the concept for the age group involved. Topics must fit the developmental level as well as the needs and interests of the group. To teach the concept "children need to protect themselves from fire" for preschoolers, topics such as staying away from matches and lighters or planning a family fire drill would be developmentally appropriate, whereas checking clothing labels to see if flame retardant materials were used would not be appropriate for this age group. The topic should also be one for which materials or equipment are available. Another consideration in topic selection is whether the whole class can get involved in a particular topic. Food preparation projects are especially good for preschool classes because everyone can participate in making the food as well as in eating it. Finally, lesson planners should consider whether the topic has any multicultural aspects that can be developed and emphasized as part of the activity.

Tonya's taco-making fit all of these criteria. It clearly showed how a variety of foods can be included in a single meal and it did this in a way that was understandable to four-year-olds. The ingredients and equipment were readily available. With close supervision, everyone could take part in some aspect of the meal preparation. Finally, making tacos opened the way to a discussion of how Mexican Americans and others satisfy their nutritional needs.

USEFUL VERBS
arrange (in order)
classify
compare
construct
contrast
demonstrate
describe
draw
explain
identify
list
match
name
select
state

FIGURE 14.1 Useful Verbs. Using verbs like these can help make instructional objectives specific and measurable.

Step 3: Preparing Instructional Objectives

When teachers develop a lesson plan, they should have a clear idea of the instructional objectives they want to achieve. An *instructional objective* expresses the intended outcome of the lesson. It states the specific skill, behavior, knowledge, or attitude that the teacher wants the children to acquire, accomplish, or understand. Objectives tend to be most useful when they are very specific. They should, however, always reflect the long-term objective of nutrition, health, and safety education—to prepare children to make sound decisions and act responsibly to protect their own health and safety and that of others.

Each lesson plan should include a set of clearly written objectives, stated in simple language. Each objective should describe the specific content to be covered and the specific behavior that is expected. Objectives should always be measurable or observable. "Appreciates highly nutritious food" would be a poor objective because it is a skill that cannot be observed or measured. "Will name two ways to prepare apples" would be a better objective because the content is specific and the behavior is measurable. It tells exactly what the behavioral outcome is and how it can be demonstrated. See Figure 14.1 for a list of verbs that are useful for teachers who are developing instructional objectives.

What objectives might Tonya have stated for her taco-making project? They could have included these: "The children will name two ingredients of tacos," "The children will match pictures of taco ingredients with pictures on food group signs," and "The children will demonstrate how to put together a taco from the ingredients they have helped to prepare."

Step 4: Translating Objectives into Activities

The chain of concept to topic to objective should always flow logically. Note the logical flow of the following lesson plan elements:

Concept:	Foods come from many different sources.
Topic:	Plant foods
Objectives:	The children will name a food that grows on trees.
	The children will name a food that grows on the ground.

Activities to achieve these objectives may include visiting a farm, an orchard, or a produce market; collecting and tasting a variety of fruits and vegetables; identifying pictures of fruits and vegetables on a poster; planting a vegetable garden; sculpting fruits or vegetables in clay; cooking corn on the cob, making vegetable soup, or preparing a fruit salad.

Each concept should be reinforced by several activities presented over the course of a day or week, or periodically throughout the school year. Teachers should keep in mind that children are individuals who learn in different ways and come to school with different sets of experiences. A particular activity may not make much of an impression on an individual child, but another activity or a combination of activities may.

A broad mix of activities also gives children more opportunities to practice the new skills and use the knowledge they are acquiring. A child might not remember one explanation of the "stop, drop, and roll" rule to extinguish a fire on his clothing. However, a visit to a firehouse, practicing dropping and rolling himself, and listening to a story in which a child uses the skill will fix it securely in his mind.

Step 5: Evaluating the Lesson Plan

The main purpose of this evaluation is to determine whether the instructional objectives have been met. If the objectives were clear and well constructed, it will be easy to determine if the lesson was successful. Evaluation will answer questions such as: "Can the children place foods in the food groups?" and "Can the children describe two ways to leave the classroom in the event of a fire?" If one or more objectives were not met, the evaluation process allows the teacher to examine what went wrong. The evaluation process also determines:

- Whether the lesson met the needs and interests of the learners
- Whether the planned activities were appropriate and helpful
- Whether the teacher was effective in helping children to reach the intended outcomes

Evaluation is a valuable tool for improving future lesson planning and implementation. Once a lesson plan has been evaluated, the teacher can determine how to revise it to make it more effective in meeting its objectives in the future. Suppose that a teacher has taken a class of preschool children to a farm as part of the lesson on where foods come from, as described above. The farm produces corn, tomatoes, and peas. Although they have talked about foods such as apples and pears that grow on trees, the children cannot name any "tree foods" after the visit. In her evaluation, the teacher might note that the farm chosen for the visit should produce at least one of each type of food mentioned in the objectives or that the objectives should be focused more narrowly. As she plans further activities on different topics, she will keep in mind the need to show concrete connections, especially between objectives and activities.

Daily Reviews.   One of the simplest and most efficient ways to evaluate a lesson plan is to spend a few minutes reviewing it at the end of each day. At that point, the day's events are still fresh in the teacher's mind. In a daily review, children's reactions and responses to each activity should be recorded. (Refer to Figures 14.3 and 14.4 later in this chapter.) The daily review should answer such questions as:

- Did the children's attention wander?
- Did any unforeseen situations arise? If so, how were activities modified to accommodate them?
- Was everyone able to participate in the activities as planned? As modified?
- Were there enough materials?
- Did the children ask any questions that suggest additional activities?
- Should any activities be eliminated or changed?
- What activities did the children seem to enjoy the most? Least?

Answers to these questions provide valuable information for future planning.

Monthly or Quarterly Reviews.   In addition to a daily review, lesson plans should also be reviewed monthly or quarterly. The object of this review is to see how the curriculum as a whole may be revised over time to accommodate new situations. Children grow and develop, gain new skills, and become more familiar with the center's routines and the teachers—as well as with one another. Other changes may occur as well. New children may come and some may leave. The seasons may have changed since the lesson plan was last used. Different weather may call for new activities.

During the monthly or quarterly review, the teacher should take a close look at activities and objectives. Do the activities planned still meet the objectives? Are the activities still developmentally appropriate or are they now too easy? Are there other, more important objectives that should be included or substituted? Activities can be adapted to different seasons or to upcoming holidays while still illustrating the same topic and concept. If the topic is "foods that grow on vines," for example, the children could toast pumpkin

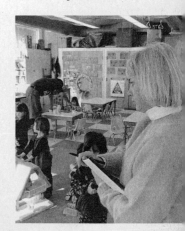

A child care center's curriculum should be subjected to a monthly or quarterly review to ensure that activities are current and developmentally appropriate and meet the center's objectives.

FOCUS ON   Promoting Healthful Habits

Holding a Fire Drill

The Buttonwood Road Preschool is holding its second fire drill of the year. Lisa's and Ashley's class of five-year-olds has just finished several lessons on fire safety. They have practiced following two possible exit routes from the building, but the drill will be a surprise. At about 10:30, the fire alarm bell rings.

All of the children are startled, and one, Danny, begins to cry. Ashley comforts Danny while Lisa helps the rest of the children to form a line. Danny quiets down almost immediately, and the children and teachers begin to file out of the room. Lisa leads the group, and Ashley follows the last child.

"We're going to go to the door that leads to the playground, just like we did last time," Lisa says. On her way past the office, Ashley slips inside to get the file of emergency information cards.

When the group reaches the door, however, they see a large sign.

"The sign says that this exit is blocked," Lisa says. "What should we do?"

Brianna, one of the children, speaks up, "I know what we do! We go to the other door." Excited at remembering the plan, Brianna turns and begins to run back down the hallway. The other children, eager to be first, turn and begin to run as well.

Ashley emerges from the office, holds up one hand, and says, "Hold on a minute, children. Remember what we said about walking during a fire drill? It's important to get out, but it's also important not to get hurt." Ashley takes Brianna's hand. "Let's go to the other exit, but let's go safely." She leads the children outside to a warm fall day.

"Good work, everyone," Lisa says as the children gather around her. "Now let's make sure everyone is out. Danny, Brianna, ..." she calls out as the children answer.

How did Lisa and Ashley handle this fire drill evacuation? Can you think of anything you would have done differently?

---

seeds in October, make pumpkin pie in November, or plant pumpkin vines in the school garden plot in June.

In the weeks and months after presenting the lesson, teachers should determine whether children remember what they have learned by conducting one or more follow-up activities. In the case of the taco-making lesson, a follow-up activity might involve additional matching and categorizing exercises in which the children are required to place foods into the five food groups.

Overall Lesson Planning Considerations

In planning a curriculum and the activities that will be included in it, teachers must keep several additional factors in mind. They include making connections to other subject areas, maintaining balance in the program, considering timing factors, and staying flexible.

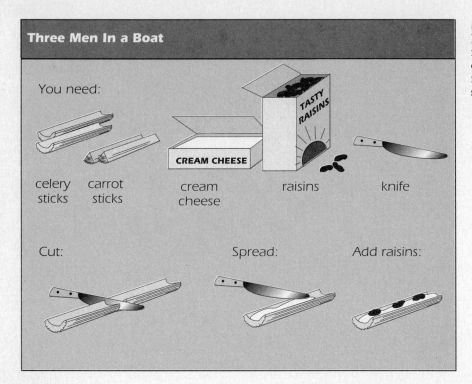

Three Men In a Boat

You need:

celery
sticks   carrot
           sticks   cream
                      cheese   raisins   knife

Cut: Spread: Add raisins:

FIGURE 14.2   Three Men in a Boat. Picture recipes such as this one can help children who do not read yet learn to follow simple directions.

Making Connections.   Teachers can make connections with other subject areas in the curriculum. Mathematics and language concepts are especially easy to introduce. Matching pictures of foods to their shapes on a flannel board, counting slices of fruit for snacks, and performing simple measurements when cooking all help promote the learning of mathematical skills. Since few preschoolers can read, a common practice is to make up recipes by drawing pictures of each step on a large sheet (see Figure 14.2). Sometimes each step is pictured on a separate card, and children arrange the cards in the order in which the steps should be followed. Whenever preschoolers listen to directions or react verbally to an activity, they are practicing language skills.

Connections can also be made through preparation and follow-up activities. Before watching a video on toothbrushing, the children might visit a dentist's office. Afterward, they could use fine motor skills to practice proper brushing techniques with their own toothbrushes.

Maintaining Balance.   Health, nutrition, and safety concepts lend themselves to a broad range of activities. Maintaining a balanced program that includes different types of activities is important. Games, art projects, block play, field trips, and visits from community representatives, such as physicians, dentists, police officers, and fire fighters, are possible teaching methods. Videos, films, television programs, story reading, and story telling are also possibilities. Dramatic play is effective with children of this age. With a

---

Lesson Plan One

Concept:	Traffic safety is important.
Topic:	Obeying traffic signals
Objectives:	1. The children will identify the meanings of the red, yellow, and green lights on a traffic signal.
	2. The children will cross the street on the green signal.
	3. The children will look both ways before crossing the street and proceed only when the street is clear of moving traffic.
Materials:	Two or three tricycles, masking tape, chalk or other material to create an intersection, homemade four-sided traffic signal with cardboard shutters that can be opened and closed so that only one color (red, yellow, or green) is displayed on each side at a time
Preparation:	Mark out a large intersection on the playground or in a large cleared space indoors. Place the traffic signal at the intersection.
Activity:	Allow children to choose to be either "drivers" or "walkers." Tell children that they will have the opportunity to change roles during the activity.
	Go over the meaning of the three colors: red means "stop," yellow means "slow down and be ready to stop," and green means "go when it is safe."
	Have the drivers, riding tricycles, approach the intersection and either stop or continue through it depending upon the traffic signal being displayed. The teacher plays "traffic cop," controlling the signal lights and providing instructions. Another teacher can instruct the walkers to look both ways and make sure traffic has come to a halt before crossing the street.
Evaluation:	The teacher found that the children enjoyed being drivers much more than they enjoyed being pedestrians. The intersection should have been constructed in a much larger space to allow the drivers enough room to turn around and approach the intersection again. The children could easily identify the meanings of the colors, but some had trouble using the signal to cross the street (Objectives 1, 2). The children consistently looked both ways before crossing (Objective 3). The teachers provided children with many opportunities to practice and gave hints whenever necessary.
Follow-up Activity:	Over the course of several days, the teachers will take two children at a time to the intersection closest to the school. Together they will cross the street safely several times to allow the children to experience a real intersection and to determine if they understand the concept.

FIGURE 14.3   Lesson Plan One.

few props, children can play hospital or go shopping in a grocery store. Empty food boxes from home and a variety of canned goods will stock the "store." The children can build roads, a firehouse, and a police station in the block area and use toy vehicles to pretend to be fire fighters and police officers responding to an emergency. Puppet activities can also be useful, especially in working through new experiences such as a first trip to the dentist. (The lesson plans in Figures 14.3 and 14.4 use a variety of activities.)

Whatever mix of activities is chosen, teachers should try to alternate between active and quiet activities and between activities that promote large muscle development and those that promote small muscle skills (Hendrick,

Lesson Plan Two	
Concept:	Different foods look, feel, taste, and smell different.
Topic:	Distinguishing between fruits
Objective:	The children will distinguish between five fruits by touch, taste, and smell.
Materials:	Several of each kind of these fruits—apples, oranges, bananas, pineapples, and pears; plates; a paring knife; a large paper bag
Preparation:	Wash all fruit. Set aside one of each type of fruit. Peel and cut the other fruit into pieces of identical size and shape. Store them in the refrigerator until they are needed.
Activity 1:	Place one of each kind of whole fruit on a table as children watch. Allow each child to feel and handle each fruit. Name each fruit several times. Place all the fruit in the paper bag. Hold the bag so the children cannot see into it. Have each child reach into the bag, touch a fruit, and name it. Then have the child take the fruit out of the bag to see if he was correct. Repeat the activity until the bag is empty. As the children watch, wash the fruit, peel it, and cut it into pieces. Offer each child a taste of each fruit as it is identified by name.
Activity 2:	Bring out the cut-up fruit. Have each child choose a piece of fruit. See if the child can identify the fruit by smell. Have the child taste the fruit to see if she can identify it by taste. Give each child several opportunities to smell and taste different fruits.
Evaluation:	The children could distinguish each fruit by sight and most by smell and taste (objective). Some of the children did not want to eat a food that had not first been identified. Teachers should assure children that all the choices are good to eat. The apple and pear were too similar in shape and texture, and several children had trouble distinguishing between them; these two fruits should not be used together in this activity.
Follow-up Activity:	Several activities involving the matching and grouping of fruits, vegetables, and other foods are planned throughout the year including visits to a grocery store and farm. Next week the school will supply real fruits in the children's play store so the children can "purchase" the fruit of their choice for snack.

FIGURE 14.4   Lesson Plan Two.

1990). Follow a vigorous large muscle activity such as dancing or an obstacle course with a quiet, small muscle one like cutting pictures out of magazines or drawing a picture. Activities should also be balanced between those that are done outdoors and ones that can be performed inside. Children should get some vigorous outdoor play every day. In inclement weather, arrange to do large muscle activities such as creative movement inside.

Considering Timing Factors.   When teachers carry out a lesson plan, timing is an important factor. Children should not be rushed through an activity so that they are forced to leave it before they are ready (Hendrick, 1990), nor should an activity last so long that the group becomes bored with it. Although the attention span of preschoolers is limited, they often need a substantial period of time to get completely involved in an activity. It is very frustrating for children who have just become absorbed in a project to be told that the time is up and that they must put it away.

The pacing of lesson plans is an important consideration. Children should be allowed ample time to complete activities, but not so much time that they become bored.

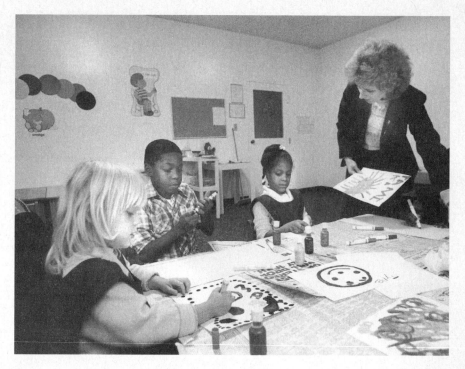

The ideal timing of any activity varies with the ages of the children, the size of the group, and the specific activity that is being carried out. Some activities, such as preparing granola for the snack, may take half an hour. Others, such as visiting a hospital or planting a flower garden, may take an entire day or even more.

Timing factors also involve being aware of the time of day and how it affects the children. When children are tired or hungry they will not want to undertake an activity requiring concentration. Teachers should learn to respect *transition times*, those periods when one activity is ending and another is beginning. Children need a certain amount of time to redirect their focus. It is therefore helpful to let children know when one activity period is about to end and another will begin. This gives them time to make the transition at their own pace. Cleanup, special music, or other signal sounds (for example, ringing a bell) can communicate a break and provide a secure framework around activities. Sometimes an activity is needed to act as a bridge. When children come in from the playground, for example, having them sit in a circle for a story helps ease their transition to a quieter activity.

Finally, timing factors include sequence considerations. Simple skills must be presented before higher level knowledge and skills are.

Remaining Flexible. Teachers need to be flexible in order to cope with unscheduled events, weather changes (rain or snow), canceled visits or field trips, and other unexpected disruptions of their lesson plans. Flexibility allows a teacher to make use of unexpected events. Such events can be teachable moments—opportunities to use the children's own interests and concerns to provide instruction.

A child whose parents are planning to move to another state provides an opportunity to teach children about packing, moving, and making new friends. It is also an opportunity to prepare the child for the move and to prepare his classmates for his absence. A group of children who discover a bird's nest laden with eggs in a tree on the playground, a new building being constructed across the street from the nursery school, or a child's recent trip to a foreign country can be rich opportunities to capture the interests and imaginations of children and teach new concepts.

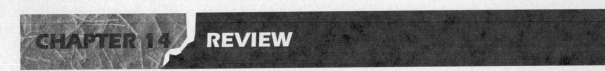

CHAPTER 14 / REVIEW

SUMMARY

- Teaching keeps children safe and healthy in the present and gives them tools to keep themselves safe and healthy for the rest of their lives.
- The goals of nutrition, health, and safety education for young children are to promote healthful behavior during the preschool years and to motivate children to develop good nutrition, health, and safety habits for the rest of their lives.
- The early childhood years are the best starting point for teaching children about nutrition, health, and safety.
- Preschool curricula help children develop a positive self-concept as they master skills, make choices, and initiate actions.
- Teachers should provide children with opportunities to practice many different types of skills and to master new ones.
- Teachers should provide children with specific, accurate information that is relevant to their developmental age.
- Preschool curricula should encourage children to form positive attitudes about others.
- Five basic guidelines for teaching young children involve offering a variety of experiences, planning developmentally appropriate material, keeping ideas simple, using repetition to provide practice for new skills and predictability to reassure children, and including all children in activities.
- Preparing lesson plans involves the following five steps: choosing a concept, choosing a topic, preparing instructional objectives, translating those objectives into activities, and evaluating plans after they have been carried out.
- When planning lessons, teachers need to maintain a balance between activity types, make connections with other subject areas, consider timing factors, and remain flexible.

ACQUIRING KNOWLEDGE

1. Summarize the goals of nutrition, health, and safety education.
2. Identify the four basic elements of a preschool curriculum.
3. Explain why teachers should help children develop a positive self-concept.
4. Identify three ways a nutrition, health, and safety curriculum can promote racial and cultural diversity.
5. Explain why it is important for a nutrition, health, and safety curriculum to offer variety in the way information is presented.
6. Describe a teacher-directed approach.
7. Describe a child-initiated approach.
8. Explain why it is important for teachers to use developmentally appropriate material.
9. Identify four points to remember that will help keep lessons simple.
10. Explain why repetition and predictability are important elements of curriculum planning.
11. Explain the importance of consistency in working with children.
12. Explain how teachers can be inclusive when planning activities.
13. List the five steps of preparing a lesson plan.
14. Identify five points that planners should take into consideration when choosing a topic for a lesson plan.
15. What is an instructional objective?
16. Once instructional objectives have been prepared, what is the next step in lesson planning?
17. What is the purpose of evaluating the lesson plan?
18. Why should lesson plans be reviewed at the end of each day?
19. What is the purpose of monthly or quarterly reviews of lesson plans?
20. What is the purpose of a follow-up activity?
21. Identify three guidelines to follow to maintain balance in curriculum planning.
22. Explain what it means to make connections in planning lessons.
23. What role does timing play in lesson planning?
24. Why is it important for teachers to keep transition times in mind when developing lesson plans?
25. Explain why teachers need to remain flexible.

THINKING CRITICALLY

1. Discuss ways in which teachers meet children's needs for the present and help prepare them for the future.
2. Explain why the instructional objective "enjoys nutritious food" is a poor objective. Then rewrite it.
3. Why is it important for teachers to plan lessons? What is wrong with simply deciding what to do each day when you arrive?
4. How can teachers achieve a balance between completing planned activities and remaining flexible? What are some reasons why teachers may need to adjust or change planned activities?

5. To be useful, information should be presented to children in ways that are appropriate to their developmental age. How can teachers judge what is appropriate for the developmental age of the children in their care?

OBSERVATIONS AND APPLICATIONS

1. Observe a preschool class during a lesson on nutrition, health, or safety. Write a brief description of the lesson. Note what the teacher does. Does the teacher present the material while the children listen? Do the children participate in the lesson? Describe parts of the lesson that are teacher-directed and what, if any, parts of the lesson or follow-up activities are child-initiated. Did the lesson hold the children's attention? What did the teacher do about children who appeared distracted or who had difficulty understanding what to do?

2. Observe an activity related to nutrition, health, or safety. Write a brief description of the activity. Note which skills were involved in completing the activity. Does this activity incorporate physical, emotional, intellectual, social, and creative skills? Is the instructional objective of the activity clear to you or do you need to ask the teacher to explain the purpose of the activity?

3. Suppose that several of the children in your preschool class are Asian Americans. One of the mothers asks if you would be interested in having her come to class to help celebrate the Chinese New Year in February. What are some ways that you can incorporate the celebration of the Chinese New Year into the nutrition, health, and safety curriculum? How would you respond to this mother's request?

4. Choose a nutrition, health, or safety concept. Write a brief lesson plan on the concept, making sure to incorporate the five steps of lesson planning.

FOR FURTHER INFORMATION

American Association of School Administrators. (1990). *Healthy kids for the year 2000: An action plan for schools*. Arlington, VA: Author.

Anspaugh, D. J., & Ezell, G. O. (1990). *Teaching today's health* (3rd ed.). Columbus, OH: Merrill.

Creswell, W. H., & Newman, I. M. (1993). *School health practice* (10th ed.). St. Louis: C. V. Mosby.

Fodor, J. T., & Dalis, G. T. (1989). *Health instruction: Theory and application* (4th ed.). Malvern, PA: Lea & Febiger.

McNeil, J. D. (1990). *Curriculum: A comprehensive introduction* (4th ed.). Boston: Little, Brown.

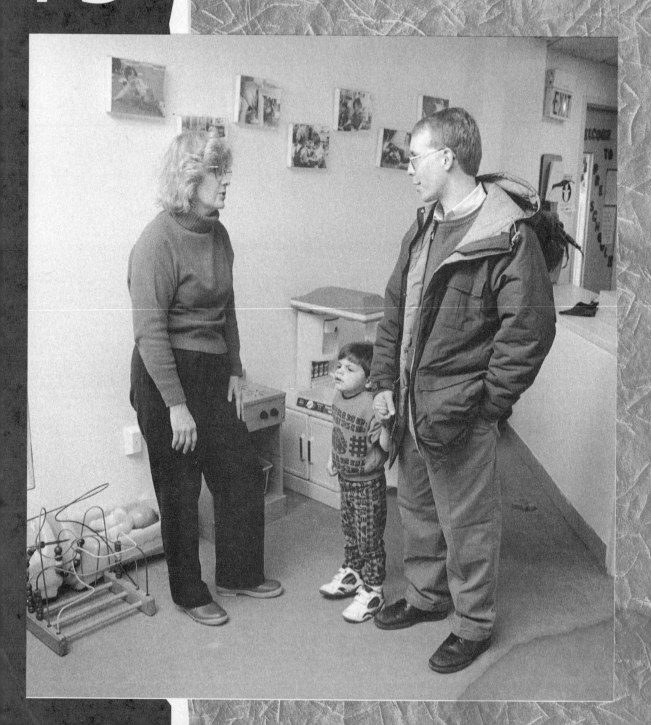

OBJECTIVES

Studying this chapter
will enable you to

- Describe how parents and the
  child care staff can work together
  to develop good nutrition, health,
  and safety habits in children
- List and explain ways in which
  caregivers can communicate
  effectively with parents
- Describe several ways parents can
  become involved in classroom
  activities
- Explain how teachers can organize
  and evaluate parent involvement
  and thereby improve their
  curricula and activities

CHAPTER TERMS

communication
cooperative
listening skills
observation
reflective statements

ROGER HARRIS, a city fire fighter,
arrived a little early at the James
Road Preschool to pick up his son
Seth. Joan Tucker, Seth's teacher, asked to
speak to him.

"Mr. Harris, I wanted to let you know
that Seth just hasn't been himself today.
His appetite was unusually poor. He only
ate a couple of bites of his lunch even
though we had spaghetti, his favorite
food. He didn't touch his afternoon snack
at all." Joan looked concerned. "Then he
slept nearly three-quarters of an hour
longer than usual during nap time," she
continued. "I wonder if he's coming down
with another ear infection or some other
illness."

"It sounds that way," Roger replied. "I
really appreciate your telling me. You
know, Seth wouldn't finish his orange juice
this morning. Maybe it hurts him to
swallow. He could be developing another
ear infection. Anyway, it sounds as if there's
a good chance you won't be seeing him at
school tomorrow."

"A lot of things are going around right
now," Joan said. "We've had some cases of
chicken pox and there's a flu bug starting

too." Joan handed Seth's backpack to Roger. "By the way, Seth's classmates are really looking forward to their visit to your firehouse next week. We've been reading about fire engines and building firehouses out of blocks all day."

"That's great!" replied Roger. "We're happy to have you visit. I've arranged for some of the other fire fighters to give safety demonstrations. If it isn't busy that day, we'll be able to take the kids for a short ride on the fire truck."

"The children will love that," said Joan. "Well, see you tomorrow—unless Seth is sick."

"Right," said Roger. He took Seth's hand and went out the door.

The Importance of Parent Involvement

Parents are a child's first caregivers and teachers. Even before children are born, parents begin caring for their nutrition, health, and safety needs. As children grow, they learn by observing and imitating what they see going on around them in their homes. Parents continue to be the primary decision-makers about nutrition, health, and safety issues throughout their children's school years. The relationship between parents and teachers can and should be mutually supportive and beneficial. It makes sense, therefore, for parents to be involved in the child care setting.

Working Together

Long before most children are enrolled in preschool, they have absorbed information and attitudes about their world. The family's cultural background and level of education, the amount of money available for food, and the personal preferences of family members all have an influence on ideas about nutrition. Attitudes about health and safety matters—for example ideas about the importance of exercise and the use of seat belts—are acquired in the family as well.

It is important for teachers to work with parents to build effective education programs. This means first understanding what each child brings to the classroom from his family situation. It also means acting in nonjudgmental ways to share information about nutrition, health, and safety. Most parents are eager for any information that will benefit their children. They are likely to be grateful for teachers' expertise in these matters as long as it is offered in a sensitive way. By sharing information with families, knowledge gained in school can be reinforced in the home environment.

Parents as a Resource

Working together with parents also involves understanding the importance of families as a resource. Caregivers cannot depend entirely on their own observations of children for information. They gain much valuable knowledge about the child's health as well as her special characteristics and needs from

Sample Preenrollment Questions

1. Does your child have any food sensitivities (allergies or intolerances)?

2. Does your child have any dietary restrictions for nonmedical reasons?

3. Are there any specific ethnic foods or other foods (not included on the center's monthly menu) that your child is accustomed to eating on a regular basis?

4. Does your child have allergies to dust, animals, insect stings, etc.?

5. Has your child had any major illnesses, or does your child have a history of repeated infections?

6. Is your child taking any medications?

7. Does your child have any physical or mental disabilities?

8. Do you have any special interests, resources, or talents that could help us improve our nutrition, health, and safety curriculum here at the center?

FIGURE 15.1 Sample Preenrollment Questions. Information about children's diet and health and the potential for parent involvement help preschool teachers plan effectively for children's care and instruction.

parents. Typically, the child care facility begins collecting information about children as soon as their parents express an interest in the center. There are several ways to gather information about children who are entering the program, including registration forms, preenrollment questionnaires (see Figure 15.1), conferences with parents, and orientation programs. The information that parents provide about their children can affect care and curriculum decisions in many ways.

The center should have a complete medical history of each child so care-givers can respond adequately to illnesses or accidents that occur during the day (see Chapter 13). If, for example, a child allergic to bee stings should be stung, caregivers can obtain emergency treatment to minimize complica-tions. Schools collect information about health care providers and dentists to call in an emergency as well as how parents or guardians can be reached.

Parents are also a source of nonmedical information. They know best what frightens their child, what comforts her, and what they view as her strengths and weaknesses. Parents know which foods are most familiar and best accepted by their child because of ethnic background, religious con-straints, or strong family preferences. They know how the child behaves when he is tired or coming down with an illness, and they know what may cause their child to become angry or frustrated. Some children may also need medication or special diets. Preschools that have advance information about children's needs and special characteristics can build a program that makes each child feel welcome and comfortable in the preschool setting. Parent information, coupled with teacher observation, can be extremely valuable. Joan knew from Seth's parents that he had a history of ear infec-tions. She had observed his food preferences and knew his typical eating patterns and behaviors. All these factors allowed her to spot his lack of ap-petite and lack of energy as possible signs of illness.

Parents are a valuable resource for more than information about their children, however. They can also enhance a program through their personal contributions. Some parents may be experts in specific nutrition, health, or safety areas. They may be fire fighters like Roger Harris, or they may be physicians, dentists, nurses, farmers, dietitians, safety engineers, or police officers. Parents may have special talents, such as a flair for using puppets to dramatize safe playground behavior or a trip to the dentist, or interesting hobbies such as backyard gardening. One parent may know a dairy farmer and be able to arrange a tour. Another parent may work at a newspaper and be able to supply leftover newsprint paper for the children's artwork. Most parents are willing to donate their time and expertise to the school; they wait only to be asked.

Communicating with Parents

Communicating with parents is an essential part of caring for and teaching their children. *Communication* is simply the exchange of messages between people. Whenever caregivers communicate with parents, they all should re-member that they are seeking an answer to the same question: "How can we help each other do what is best for the child?" Effective communication, however, takes time and effort.

Inviting Parents into an Information Exchange

The exchange of information between caregiver and parent begins with the parent's first visit to the center. Over a period of time, a sense of mutual trust

FOCUS ON Communicating with Parents

Nutritious Meals and Snacks

It is snack time at the Warner Community Preschool. Two parents, Ms. Martelli and Mr. Randall, have come to observe the class. As the children eat, the parents talk to the teacher, Colleen.

MS. MARTELLI: Is that an apple Laurie is eating? I've never been able to get her to eat fruit.

COLLEEN: Well, Ms. Martelli, I'll admit that it took some doing. But now Laurie loves apples. She even asks for one at snack time.

MS. MARTELLI: How did you do it?

COLLEEN: We try to encourage the children to eat well by offering them only healthful foods for meals and snacks. They often resist at first, but soon they try the new food—especially if they see me and some of the other children enjoying it.

MS. MARTELLI: But at home Laurie insists on cookies or chips for a snack. And she won't touch her vegetables at dinner.

COLLEEN: One thing you can do is keep a variety of wholesome snacks around for Laurie to choose from—like fresh fruits, dried fruits, granola bars, and so on. If she's hungry, she'll try something and then realize she likes it. But be sure to get rid of the snacks you don't want her to eat.

MS. MARTELLI: What about dinner?

COLLEEN: Try preparing the vegetables—different ones every day—in new ways. Show Laurie how much you like them.

MR. RANDALL: I wish vegetables were the only problem we had. My wife and I work such long hours that we often just order take-out food or heat up frozen dinners. There's no time to cook.

COLLEEN: Some people solve that problem by cooking several nutritious meals on the weekend. Then they refrigerate or freeze them. All they have to do at night is heat the food up. You might also try steaming a fresh or frozen vegetable to add to a take-out meal—it doesn't take very long.

MR. RANDALL: I guess that wouldn't be hard to do. It would just take some planning on our part.

COLLEEN: I know how hard it is. I have kids too, and both my husband and I work. But good nutrition is important for growing children.

MS. MARTELLI: Well, you've given us both some great ideas. I'm glad I came by today.

How well do you think Colleen responded to the problems of each of these parents? How would you have responded? What other suggestions might help these parents?

is established. Parents and caregivers begin to participate in the day-to-day dialogue that allows them to share the information they all need to provide the best care for the child.

Roger Harris and Joan exchanged a great deal of information in their brief conversation. She told him that Seth had behaved differently during the school day, and she offered an opinion that Seth might be coming down with an illness. In response, Roger told Joan how he intended to deal with the situation. If they had not exchanged this information, Roger might have resented not being told about Seth's condition and Joan might have worried that Seth's parents wouldn't recognize his symptoms and seek necessary medical help.

Trust and understanding will be built most effectively, however, if an information exchange deals with more than just child-centered issues. Parents like to know that teachers are interested in and concerned about the whole family. Teachers can ask questions about the parents' backgrounds and hobbies and can keep track of what is going on in the family. Is a new baby on the way? Is the family taking a special vacation or getting a new pet? When teachers remember and ask about these interwoven strands of family life—without intruding on the family's privacy—parents feel valued as people. Free exchange may also involve negative information. A parent may have lost a job or been in an automobile accident. Teachers should express genuine sympathy and support for parents who are coping with difficult situations. Perhaps the child is having nightmares or has shown uncharacteristic aggression. Communication about such matters helps the teacher understand and cope with the child's behavior during the school day. A continuing pattern of open communication builds a good relationship between home and school that pays off in many ways (Hendrick, 1990).

The teacher must develop good listening skills in order to communicate effectively. These skills are especially important when there is a conflict or problem to be resolved. *Listening skills* involve more than hearing; they require concentration on what is being said and active participation in the communication process. One useful listening technique involves *reflective statements*. A reflective statement is a statement in which the teacher restates the parent's feelings or concerns in order to show that he understands them and considers them important. For example, if a parent says, "The other children don't include Jenny in their games," the teacher might reply, "You're saying that Jenny feels as if she isn't part of the group." Making a reflective statement assures the parent that the teacher has heard and accepted the parent's remarks. The parent then feels willing to open up and share additional information. From this point, the teacher can move on to put the problem in a larger perspective and work toward a solution. In this case, the teacher might point out that because of shifting play patterns most children feel left out at one time or another. She could, however, suggest specific solutions to Jenny's mother, such as inviting other children from the class over individually for play dates. By reviewing the solution at the end of the conversation, the parent can be reassured that she has been heard and that the problem is being addressed (Fenwick, 1993).

Keeping Parents Informed

How do caregivers establish and continue an information exchange? The child care setting provides a number of excellent avenues for communication. They include drop-off and pickup times, parent conferences, newsletters and other informal exchanges, special events, and home visits. Caregivers should

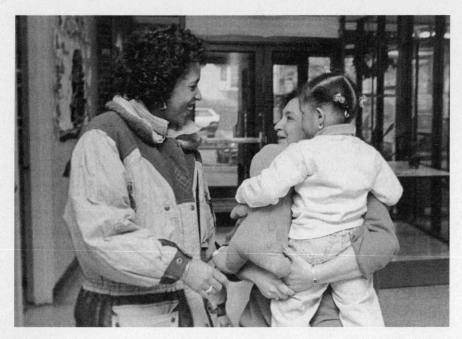

Effective communication with parents is an essential part of providing quality child care. Pickup and drop-off times are good opportunities for a quick conversation with a parent.

make use of as many opportunities as possible to keep parents informed about the child care facility and about parenting issues as a whole.

Drop-Off and Pickup Times.   One of the best ways to begin building trust and exchanging information is to make a point of being available to parents at the beginning and end of the day. This is a time when parents share specific information about their children that caregivers will want or need to know. Statements such as "Rachel wouldn't eat breakfast this morning so she'll probably be pretty hungry by snack time" or "Timmy won't be in tomorrow because he's spending the day with his grandfather" give information that the caregiver can use throughout the day. This is also a good time to encourage parents to share personal and family news. Caregivers should always be sensitive to the time constraints of parents who work outside the home, however. The end of the day may be a much better time than the beginning to talk to those parents.

Caregivers can also use this time to share information about the children and about the center's plans and activities. "Ellen helped us make muffins today" or "Remember to send a warm jacket along with Ming-Mei tomorrow for the zoo field trip" convey important information. When communicating at drop-off and pickup times, caregivers should show genuine interest and concentrate on the positive. Parents like to know who their children enjoy playing with and how skilled they are becoming at cutting with scissors or climbing the jungle gym. Caregivers should get into the habit of mentally filing away interesting tidbits to share with parents at pickup time. Of course, parents also need to know about the sort of information that Joan shared about Seth. Information about injuries or apparent illness must be conveyed. Other information, such as reports of serious behavioral problems, are best discussed in a more private setting.

Private Information.   Some information must be exchanged privately between a parent and a caregiver. Such communication may be in the form of notes, letters, and telephone calls, if necessary. A note can ask for some item of information, express praise for an accomplishment, or bring up a problem or concern. In many cases, the caregiver may write a note asking a parent to call so they can discuss the matter in an unhurried, private conversation. Centers should make a copy of any written communication that goes home. This avoids questions or misunderstandings about what was communicated.

Some child care centers maintain standard forms on which they record such daily occurrences as an infant's length of naps, the number of times the diaper was changed, the kind and amount of food eaten, activities, and any particular difficulties or accomplishments that were noted during the day. The school then provides the completed form to the infant's parents at the end of the day so the parents can have a record of what occurred.

This type of form helps parents in many ways. It can give parents information about their child's health and highlight symptoms of an oncoming illness. This information also helps parents to keep track of their children's normal growth and development (see Figure 15.2).

The most common way that preschools provide information privately is through meetings, or conferences, between parents and teachers. A conference gives teachers and parents an opportunity to discuss the child in private, without interruption. Conference times are sometimes viewed as times when a child's problems and deficiencies are discussed. Anticipating such a discussion can arouse great feelings of anxiety, shame, and guilt in parents and can discourage rather than promote communication between parent and caregiver. Teachers should try to present conferences in a more positive way. The teacher can begin with a description of the child's general adjustment to the program and daily experience. Progress in various developmental areas, new accomplishments and positive changes, and examples of how the curriculum can meet the child's developmental needs are also important (Bjorklund & Berger, 1987). In addition, parent-teacher conferences should always emphasize the friendly partnership between the teacher and the family. Teachers can suggest activities that parents can do at home to reinforce learning and can ask questions that allow parents to offer opinions and suggestions. When problems and concerns need to be discussed, the parent and teacher should formulate solutions together. In fact, the conference is the ideal place for the teacher to utilize the reflective statement technique to show understanding and acceptance of the parent's concerns and a willingness to work with the parent to try to solve problems.

Conferences usually cover the school's overall program as well as the range of a child's physical, intellectual, and social development. If, however, the teacher has specific concerns about the child, those issues can also be raised at the conference. The teacher may want to know whether the child is

Sample Infant Daily Report

Date: _____

PARENT INFORMATION

Child's Name _____

Time Dropped Off _____

Time of Last Feeding _____

Medications Needed? ☐ Yes   ☐ No If yes, specify amounts and times below.

Special Emergency Contact or Pickup Instructions:

Any other instructions?

Parent Signature _____

CENTER INFORMATION

Feedings: Naps:

Time	Type of Food/Amount Eaten	Slept from	To
_____	_____	_____	_____
_____	_____	_____	_____
_____	_____	_____	_____
_____	_____	_____	_____

Diapering:

Time	Description/Special Notes
_____	_____
_____	_____
_____	_____
_____	_____
_____	_____
_____	_____
_____	_____

☐ Injury report attached

☐ Please see caregiver

FIGURE 15.2 Sample Infant Daily Report. Completing a standard form for infants each day is especially useful because even minor alterations in routine patterns can signal changes in an infant's growth or health status.

sleeping well or getting plenty of exercise at home, for example, or the parent may want to discuss why the child refuses to eat dinner on most school days. Whatever the scope of the discussion, it is crucial for the teacher to maintain a written record of any decisions that the parents and teacher have made and to follow up promptly on any actions that need to be taken. Also, teachers should remember that all information about the child or family revealed in a conference should remain confidential (Hendrick, 1992). Such information should never be shared with or discussed around other parents or anyone outside the center.

Public Information.   Child care facilities share many kinds of general information with parents. Parent input can help a center focus this information clearly for their particular group of parents. It is important for caregivers to invite questions from parents and to take as much time as necessary to answer those questions fully and completely. At the beginning of their relationship with parents, the child care center staff should provide parents with a handbook that contains clear, brief summaries of the facility's rules and policies, hours of operation, and fee schedules so parents can have them on hand when questions arise.

There are, however, other ways to convey public information. Fliers and newsletters are two good ways to keep parents informed of the school's activities, projects, and upcoming events, as well as to share other useful material. One flier could give information about an end-of-year picnic. Another could remind parents about the symptoms of Reye's syndrome or alert them to product recalls on pacifiers or infant car seats. This type of information is usually available through public health or consumer safety organizations.

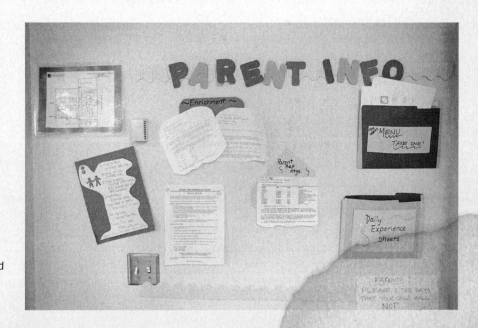

A bulletin board is a good place for a child care center to provide information to parents.

Newsletters are more comprehensive documents generated by the facility staff. Newsletters may include:

- Weekly menus and activity schedules
- Snack suggestions
- Lists of materials parents can provide (for example, yarn or old magazines) for projects
- Anecdotes about the children's activities
- Recipes for foods prepared at the center and recipes submitted by parents
- General nutrition, health, and safety information
- Lists of resources such as agencies and programs that promote nutrition, health, and safety education
- Information for and suggestions from parents on child care topics

In addition to menus and activity schedules, a sample newsletter might include quotations from children about their last field trip, suggestions for involving children in selecting and cooking foods at home, a home fire safety checklist, and a recipe for vegetable soup. Putting the daily menu on its own sheet allows parents to place it on the refrigerator or memo board so they can tell their children what is being served each day. This may also give families an opportunity to talk about foods and nutrition. Newsletter topics could also be handled through a bulletin board placed where parents will see it as they come into the center.

Some schools maintain a parents' resource center, a room or corner stocked with pamphlets, magazines, and books on nutrition, health, safety, and parenting issues. Parents can borrow these materials to answer questions or address specific problems. Resource centers can be expanded to meet the needs of the parents at the facility. For example, the area might include a clothing or toy exchange or a "business card" bulletin board advertising parents' skills such as home remodeling or massage therapy.

Special Events. Many preschools sponsor special programs for parents. An open house in which the school's curriculum is explained, a parenting workshop, or a presentation by a nutritionist are examples of special events that could both enhance communication between school and home and benefit parents. These special events are a good way to share information and form close ties with parents.

Workshops or seminars require a great deal of preparation on the part of the school's staff. Preplanning activities, for example, might include circulating a survey of parent concerns, selecting a meeting place, making child care arrangements, lining up speakers, and purchasing materials and supplies. These types of events, however, can be very rewarding when they are handled well.

Some special events may be primarily social occasions. A center might hold an annual potluck dinner, for example, in which each family could bring a special food from its own ethnic tradition. This is a good way for

FOCUS ON / Cultural Diversity

An Ethnic Snack Fair

A good way to both teach children about other cultures and invite parent involvement in the program is to put on an ethnic snack fair. Preschoolers can bring in ingredients from home, and teachers can help with the food preparation and setup.

The first step is to decide which countries or ethnic groups will be featured. If a class or school has many children with a common ethnic background—Native American or Hispanic, for example—several of the snacks should be from that ethnic tradition. Students and their parents may provide other suggestions.

Set up one table per country or ethnic group. Identify the tables with flags or posters taped to the front of the table.

Many different foods might be offered. Preschoolers will have fun putting together tacos by filling shells with meat, cheese, and vegetables. A Mexican table might also feature guacamole. Even the youngest children can help mash ripe avocados and stir in other ingredients.

For a Middle Eastern table, hummus is a good choice. A teacher can puree the chick peas, the main ingredient in hummus. Preschoolers can mix the chick peas with onion, garlic, and tahini (a sesame seed paste), and serve the hummus with wedges of pita bread.

A French table might feature small slices of toasted French bread spread with soft cheeses. The children can also arrange apples over prepared pastry for a French apple tart.

For Caribbean-inspired treats, children can skewer chunks of tropical fruits. Fruit nectars might be served as a beverage at a Caribbean table.

To set the atmosphere for the ethnic food fair, play taped music from the countries or ethnic groups featured. Children who have helped to plan, prepare, and serve the foods may even be tempted to eat something that is "different" from what they eat every day.

families to get to know each other and learn to appreciate other cultures and traditions.

Home Visits. Home visits can be a very effective way for caregivers to communicate with children and their parents. Seeing a child in his home setting can provide a caregiver with many insights about the child and his family. Children greatly enjoy a home visit because it demonstrates their caregiver's interest in them and in their family (Hildebrand, 1990).

Caregivers should visit a home only by prior arrangement and only when it is clear that the visit is welcomed. Home visits can make parents nervous if they feel that they or their home are being judged. To put them at ease, the caregiver should show sincere interest in the child and the family and build the conversation around the parents' concerns. Some parents, on the other hand, will feel more at ease talking in their own homes and may be encouraged to offer helpful information and suggestions.

Keeping the Lines of Communication Open

Caregivers should always remember that communication is a two-way street. Caregivers need to provide a great deal of information to parents and children, but they must be open to receiving information from parents as well.

Parents enjoy making contributions to the information exchange if the school welcomes and respects their efforts. To make newsletters more personal, many schools solicit items of interest from parents, such as dates of children's birthdays, birth and job announcements, and family vacation reports. Bulletin boards can be another form of two-way communication if parents feel free to post photographs, announcements, articles about parenting, and other items of interest.

Parent contributions to newsletters and bulletin boards fulfill another important role because they allow parents to get to know and share information with one another as well as with the school. Special events serve this same purpose. Any special event should include a refreshment and socializing time that allows parents to talk to one another. Special events are especially beneficial to parents who feel isolated at home. Such events give these parents a chance to meet others with similar interests and to discover that they share common problems and concerns (Hendrick, 1990).

When caregivers and parents share information with each other, they also have the opportunity to share a wide variety of values and parenting skills. This sharing can affect parents in subtle but important ways. One parent, for example, may think that spanking is the only way to discipline a child. But when that parent hears caregivers or other parents talk about giving disruptive children a "time-out," the first parent may decide to try the time-out technique of disciplining. In the same way, parents with limited knowledge of nutrition will be exposed to good nutritional practices in the fliers, menus, and recipes provided by the facility and in conversations with other parents during special events. Over time, they may begin to provide more nutritious meals and snacks at home. One of the benefits of this kind of casual and incidental sharing of values and skills is that it helps people become better parents without singling out anyone for criticism or blame.

Barriers to Communication

Communication between caregivers and parents is vitally important, and yet barriers to communication can arise. When parents bring their children to the child care center, they may bring anxieties and other negative emotions as well. Working parents may feel guilty about leaving their children in the care of others. Parental stress and fatigue can also be powerful barriers to communication. Some parents may worry that they will be replaced by the caregiver in the child's affections (Hendrick, 1992). Or they may be very defensive, reading into almost any conversation a criticism of their parenting skills. Another barrier to communication from the parents' side is the fear that by speaking openly about a problem they will turn the caregiver against their child (Hendrick, 1992). This, of course, should never be the case in any child care setting.

Caregivers' emotions also can be a factor in erecting communication barriers. They may enter a dialogue with a parent, expecting to be disapproved of or criticized, and fail to hear the concern about the child that the parent is expressing. Some caregivers find themselves blaming parents for their children's difficulties (Hendrick, 1992) or disapproving of parents whose parenting skills and knowledge seem limited. These feelings, no matter how well hidden, will be communicated to the parent. In such cases, an atmosphere of trust and cooperation will be difficult.

Caregivers can overcome these emotional barriers to communication by making an effort to understand, accept, and respect all parents and children. When practices at home and the school's policies conflict and cannot be reconciled, it can be made clear to the child (and parent) that each place has its own set of rules to follow (Hendrick, 1990).

The most important thing that caregivers can do, however, to encourage trust is to show parents that they like and appreciate their children. All parents think that their children are special and want to know that other people like their children as well. When parents realize that caregivers are primarily concerned with the welfare of their children, trust and openness can take root and grow in the relationship.

Parents in the Classroom

One of the most direct ways to interest parents in their children's preschool facility is to invite parents into the classroom. Many nutrition, health, and safety activities are perfect vehicles for parent involvement. Different parents will be able to participate in different ways. Some will want to and have time to work directly with the children, others will work with materials and supplies (helping to maintain playground equipment, for example), and still others can help out by doing tasks at home. There are an almost endless number of ways to involve parents in the facility's activities.

Observation

Most child care facilities have an open-door policy in which parents are invited to observe the classroom at any time during the school's hours of operation. *Observation* involves watching and listening to classroom activities, usually without direct participation. Such visits help parents become familiar with what goes on in the facility and lets caregivers know that parents are concerned and interested participants.

One way to allow parents to observe the facility is to invite them to join their children at lunch. If the center is close to their workplace, even parents who hold full-time jobs can sometimes enjoy a lunch break with their child. This practice helps parents to see how their child interacts with peers and caregivers in the facility. Caregivers can also use this opportunity to display effective methods for offering nutritious foods. Parents are sometimes

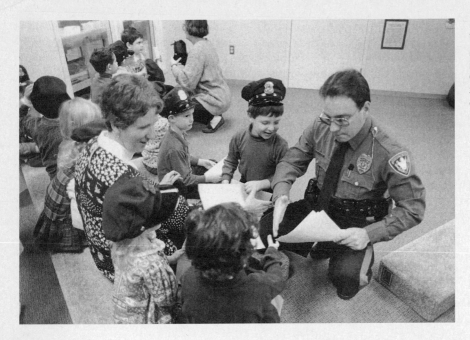

Preschools can benefit from the expertise of parents who are professionals. This police officer parent is presenting safety information to the children.

astounded but pleased at the variety and amounts of food their children eat at the facility (Whitener & Keeling, 1984).

Presentations and Activities

Parents can be valuable resources for presenting many types of information to children. When Joan discovered that Seth's father was a fire fighter, she asked him to arrange a tour of his firehouse for her class. Roger Harris was glad to help. The preschool can benefit from the expertise of parents in a variety of professions. Parents who are chefs, dental hygienists, or police officers, for example, could share information about nutrition, health, and safety. Of course, parents' contributions will not always relate directly to nutrition, health, or safety, but they should always be welcomed. A printer could show how books are made, a hairdresser can demonstrate a haircut, or a chemist can perform a simple experiment. The school can also invite parents who come from different ethnic backgrounds to supervise or assist at the preparation of an ethnic or religious holiday meal to serve to the children. A Chinese parent might help prepare a meal for Chinese New Year, or a Jewish parent could prepare and explain foods for a Passover dinner.

Volunteering

Many preschools invite parents to work directly with children in assisting the caregivers. Parents can help children prepare foods or plant a garden. They may also help chaperone them on a field trip to a farm, store, or factory. Parents can also aid caregivers in general ways, such as supervising

WHOLESOME SNACKS

Layered Fruit Dessert

Ingredients:

¾ cup low-fat cottage cheese

1 tablespoon honey

⅛ teaspoon ground nutmeg

1⅓ cups cantaloupe cubes

1⅓ cups honeydew melon cubes

1 teaspoon unsweetened wheat germ

Directions:

1. Blend cottage cheese, honey, and nutmeg in a blender until smooth.
2. Mix melon cubes and place ⅓ cup fruit in each serving dish.
3. Top with about 1½ tablespoons cheese mixture. Repeat layers.
4. Sprinkle ¼ teaspoon wheat germ on each serving, if desired.

Yield: 4 servings

Each serving contains:

Calories: 85
Protein: 7 g
Fat: 1 g
Carbohydrates: 17 g

Source: USDA. *Dietary guidelines for Americans: Avoid too much sugar.* HG-232-9. Washington, DC: Human Nutrition Information Service.

children as they wash their hands, eat, and clean up at mealtimes. In addition, parents can be asked to help decorate rooms, serve snacks, or assist with activities at school holiday parties and birthday parties.

Parents can also volunteer by performing various activities on their own time or at home. Parents with home computers and desktop publishing skills can be recruited to produce the center's newsletters and other publications. On birthdays and holidays, parents can prepare nutritious party foods and snacks as a special treat for the children. Parents can also help the school staff by calling other parents to notify them when the school is closed because of inclement weather.

Many schools request donations from parents who have access to special materials, such as newsprint, buttons, fabric, cardboard, or scrap lumber. Unusual items such as large appliance cartons are also appreciated from time to time. Donating materials is a form of volunteerism that should be recognized and acknowledged.

Some preschools are parent cooperatives. In a *cooperative*, parent governing boards make policy decisions and hire teachers and other staff members. Parents act as assistants for teachers, often in exchange for a lower tuition fee for the child. Parents may also serve on the policy-making board or on any of its committees, such as the committee for menu planning or fundraising. Many cooperatives sponsor periodic weekend or evening work parties to clean up, fix, and repaint school equipment, and they may also offer parent education classes. Many parents find these events an enjoyable way to get to know teachers and other parents better (Hildebrand, 1990).

Organizing and Evaluating Parent Involvement

Parents are most likely to become involved in the classroom when they are made to feel welcome and when they feel that their ideas and suggestions are taken seriously. Caregivers can help to do this by organizing parent involvement properly from the beginning and by evaluating in an ongoing way to allow for constant improvement.

Organization

When parents volunteer to work with children, they should be asked to do things that are fun for both them and the children. Staff members should avoid giving parents unpleasant chores or overwhelming them with duties and tasks that are beyond their abilities. A parent volunteer is not a trained teacher and should not be expected to supervise a large group or deal with difficult discipline problems. Teachers need to pay attention to parent volunteers and make sure they know ahead of time exactly what is expected of them. Whenever possible, teachers should show parents that they appreciate their comments, suggestions, and ideas either by putting them into practice

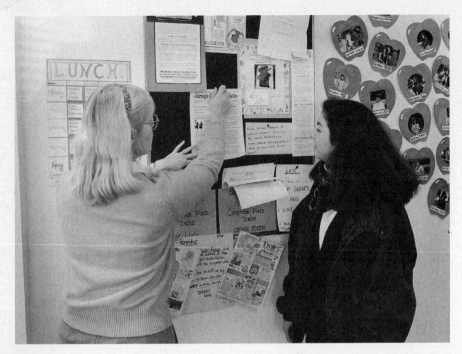

Some parents may bring in helpful information, such as an article on parenting or a favorite snack recipe. One way of recognizing these contributions is to include them in the center's newsletter.

or by sharing them with others. If a parent submits recipes for nutritious snacks or brings in a helpful article on parenting, include the material in the next newsletter or tack it up on the bulletin board.

Always recognize the contributions of parent volunteers with a heartfelt "thank you" at the time the contribution is made and later in newsletters, at public meetings, and in individual thank-you notes. Such recognition gives parent volunteers a feeling of satisfaction and invites the participation of other parents in activities. When appropriate, the school can even organize an awards ceremony and present parent volunteers with certificates of appreciation, small gifts, or some other token of recognition.

Evaluation

It is important for teachers to evaluate parent involvement in the child care center. A number of questions are appropriate. How well are parents and teachers communicating with one another? Is the facility adequately addressing the needs of parents? How well is the facility conforming to the parents' expectations? Is the facility making the best use of the time and talents of parent volunteers? What can be done to improve the program?

There are several ways to answer these questions. It is important, however, that both parents and teachers participate in the evaluation process.

Parents Evaluate the Program. Parents should be given many opportunities to express their feelings about their involvement in the programs

FOCUS ON Promoting Healthful Habits

Inviting a Parent to Speak to the Class

Jackie teaches a prekindergarten class at the Carter Road Preschool. Today the class has a special visitor.

"Ravi," Jackie says, "why don't you introduce our visitor to the class?"

Ravi looks a little sheepish, but as he nears the guest, he looks up and smiles proudly. He takes the hand of the woman in the blue dress and says proudly, "This is my mom. She's a doctor." Then he hurries back to his seat.

Ravi's mother starts to talk. She tells the class that she is a pediatrician—a doctor who takes care of children. She tells them that she became a children's doctor because she loves children and wants them to be healthy and strong. She tells the children some of the things she does each day and asks if they have questions.

"Why do I have to cover my mouth when I sneeze?" asks Scott, who is just getting over a cold.

"When you sneeze, germs that cause colds come out of your mouth as well as your nose. If you don't cover your mouth, the germs may get into someone else and give them a cold

too," answers Ravi's mother. "You should also wash your hands after you sneeze or blow your nose. That way your hands don't leave germs on the things you touch."

"Do you give people shots?" asks Robbie.

"Yes, I do," Ravi's mother says. "I know getting a shot may hurt, but sometimes shots are necessary. Some shots you get from the doctor keep you from getting diseases. Other shots help you get well once you are sick. Doctors don't like hurting people with shots, but sometimes the littler hurt of a shot is better than the bigger hurt of a bad sickness."

When the children have no more questions, Ravi's mother brings out several stethoscopes and lets the children listen to each other's heartbeats. The children are fascinated. As Ravi's mother leaves, Jackie thanks her for her time and interest.

Do you think Jackie should have taken a more active role in the presentation? How would you have prepared children for such a visit? What would you ask the visitor to talk about?

and activities of the facility. If communication between parents and teachers is good, it may be enough merely to talk to parents after an activity to discover their reactions. Often, however, a more formal evaluation is needed. Short surveys can be distributed after workshops, other special events, and any activities that parents participate in. Parents can be asked questions like the following:

- Was this activity helpful and enjoyable?
- What did you like most about the activity?
- How could this activity be improved?
- Was advance planning adequate?
- Did you feel that your contributions were valued?
- What would you have added to this activity or done differently?

Some parents will be more frank if they know that their criticism will not be held against them. Devising a questionnaire in which statements can be rated on a scale of 1 to 5 (1 = disagree strongly and 5 = agree strongly) can work well if the anonymity of the respondent is assured. Both positive and negative reactions can be very valuable for future planning.

Teachers Evaluate the Program.   Evaluation by teachers occurs in several ways. One way to judge effectiveness is to note whether parents are responding. Teachers should keep track of attendance at special events and note whether parents are taking newsletters, tips, recipes, and other distributed material. Teachers should also note whether parents are contributing their own materials and information, volunteering their time, using parents' bulletin boards, or submitting items to the newsletter.

Teachers should read all evaluation forms, questionnaires, and surveys very carefully to find out what parents like and dislike about the center's staff and programs. Just as parents should not be afraid to criticize the facility or its teachers, teachers should not be afraid to receive constructive criticism and to make changes when the criticism is valid.

Teachers must perform their own evaluation of activities involving parents. Did the children seem to enjoy the last activity with Mrs. Larson and do they look forward to another one? Did the trip to the dentist's office fit in with the school curriculum and build on already acquired skills? Is the newsletter free of typographical errors and is it distributed on time? Do volunteers generally show up when they are scheduled and are they prepared to carry out their activities?

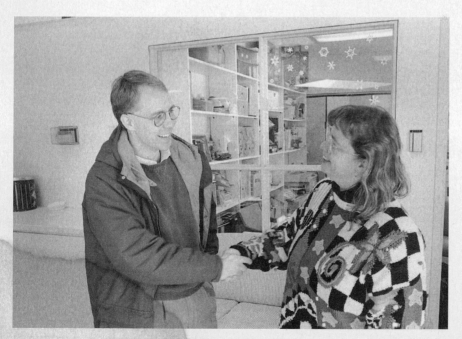

One good means of establishing an effective partnership with parents is to greet their contributions and ideas with respect and open-mindedness.

Teachers should ask themselves if they are making the best use of parent volunteers. Have they checked parents' occupations to see if any of them could make a presentation, donate materials, or arrange a field trip?

Finally, teachers need to monitor their responses to the contributions of all parents. Do they greet the ideas and suggestions of all the parents with respect and open-mindedness? Do they recognize and thank volunteers for their efforts every time? Taking the contributions and volunteer efforts of parents for granted is one sure way to alienate parents and make certain that their contributions of ideas, time, and support will disappear. On the other hand, with careful attention, an effective partnership can flourish.

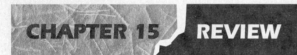

CHAPTER 15 / REVIEW

SUMMARY

- It is important to work together with parents to meet children's nutrition, health, and safety needs. Parents are a valuable resource for preschool programs.
- Child care centers gather information about children to assure their safety and to adjust the school curriculum and procedures to meet the special needs of the children.
- Building trust and understanding requires a personal interest in parents and children and the development of good listening skills. When teachers make reflective statements, they show parents that they understand and empathize with their concerns.
- Teachers can use drop-off and pickup times to exchange information with parents and to help build mutual trust.
- Private information can be exchanged through notes, letters, telephone calls, or conferences. Conferences should emphasize the child's accomplishments and progress and encourage cooperation between parents and teachers in solving any problems.
- Child care facilities can provide parents with general information through a parent handbook, fliers, newsletters, and parents' resource centers stocked with pamphlets, magazines, and books on relevant topics.
- Special events such as open houses, workshops, or presentations by experts can be valuable ways to convey information.
- Home visits can be an effective method of communication between parents and caregivers. They show the caregiver's interest in both the child and the family.
- Communication lines can be kept open if parents are encouraged to share information with the facility and with one another. This sharing of information benefits both the center and the parents themselves.

- Communicating effectively with parents is crucial and may require caregivers to overcome barriers such as guilt and anxiety on the part of the parents or the caregiver's own feelings of disapproval toward parents. Caregivers should show acceptance and respect for parents and appreciation of the children in their care.

- Parents can come into the classroom to observe classes, eat lunch with their children, make presentations, or work as volunteers in the facility.

- Teachers should organize parent involvement carefully, making sure that parents are comfortable and that they feel appreciated.

- Evaluation of parent involvement is crucial for program improvement. Parents can evaluate the program through informal comments or formal questionnaires.

- Teachers can evaluate the program for parent involvement by obtaining and reviewing parents' informal and formal responses, considering the quality of volunteer participation, determining if the best use has been made of the volunteers available, and monitoring their own responses to the contributions that all parents make to the program.

ACQUIRING KNOWLEDGE

1. List two ways caregivers can work together with parents to build an effective education program.
2. Define communication.
3. Describe the types of information teachers should seek out during conversations with parents, other than information that is directly child-centered.
4. Define listening skills.
5. Explain why reflective statements are an important communication tool for teachers.
6. List four opportunities the child care setting provides for information exchange with parents.
7. What is the difference between the type of information that is appropriately exchanged in public and that which needs to be exchanged in private settings?
8. Identify three types of everyday information that caregivers can effectively communicate to parents of infants using standard forms.
9. What is the most common way that preschools provide information privately?
10. Describe three ways that teachers can make conferences a time for promoting rather than discouraging communication.
11. What information should be included in a parent handbook?
12. Identify five types of information that could be included in child care center newsletters.
13. What is a parents' resource center?
14. Identify three ways that parents' emotions may interfere with communication.

15. Identify three ways that caregivers' emotions may interfere with communication.
16. Explain how caregivers can overcome various emotional barriers to communication.
17. When practices at home and school policies cannot be reconciled, what should caregivers do?
18. What are the benefits of having parents observe a child's class?
19. Explain how parents can be valuable resources for presenting information to children in the child care center.
20. Identify four ways parents can work directly with children in the classroom and assist the caregivers.
21. List two ways that parents can help the school without coming into the classroom.
22. Explain the role parents play in a cooperative preschool.
23. What are three guidelines for organizing the volunteer efforts of parents?
24. Identify two ways to solicit parents' evaluation of the center's efforts at involving them in activities.
25. Identify three ways teachers can evaluate the effectiveness of their efforts at involving parents.

THINKING CRITICALLY

1. Explain why it is important for teachers to work together with parents.
2. Explain why good listening skills are important for teachers.
3. Explain the role that special events such as speakers and family dinners play in communication between the home and the school.
4. What might a caregiver learn from a home visit that might not be learned from a conference held in the school?
5. Why is communication among parents important?

OBSERVATIONS AND APPLICATIONS

1. Observe the interactions between parents and caregivers at the beginning and/or end of the school day. Do caregivers make a point of talking to certain parents? About what? Do caregivers ask questions about family members other than the child in their care? Do you observe any parents telling caregivers about situations at home or about health concerns?
2. Observe a special event held at a preschool. Note what kind of special event it is. Who organized this event—the center's staff or a parent group? Is the event for one class or for the whole school? Note the interactions between parents at this event.
3. Ahmed Shah is in your preschool class. His mother asks to come and observe your class. Although you normally welcome parent observation, there are several children in the class who still cry every morning when they are dropped off. You are afraid that having a parent in the class at this time will be upsetting for these few children. What would you suggest to Mrs. Shah?

4. Suppose you work in a child care center. You feel that the parents of the children who attend do not feel comfortable at the center. They usually drop off and pick up their children without saying very much to you. When the center sponsors activities for the parents or families, the attendance is poor. In addition, few parents volunteer to help out with activities in the class. How could you improve relations between the school and the parents and increase the amount of parent participation?

FOR FURTHER INFORMATION

Aronson, S., & Smith, H. (1993). *Model child care health policies*, Publication 716. Washington, DC: National Association for the Education of Young Children.

Bjorklund, G., & Berger, C. (1987). Making conferences work for parents, teachers, and children. *Young Children, 41*(2), 26–31.

Bredekamp, S., & Rosegrant, T. (Eds.). (1992). *Reaching potentials: Appropriate curriculum and assessment for young children, 1.* Washington, DC: National Association for the Education of Young Children.

Fenwick, K. (1993, September). Diffusing conflict with parents: A model for communication. *Exchange*, pp. 59–60.

Hendrick, J. (1990). *Total learning: Developmental curriculum for the young child* (3rd ed.). Columbus, OH: Merrill.

Hendrick, J. (1992). *The whole child: Developmental education for the early years* (5th ed.). New York: Macmillan.

Hildebrand, V. (1990). *Guiding young children* (4th ed.). New York: Macmillan.

National Association for the Education of Young Children. (1991). *Accreditation criteria and procedures* (rev. ed.), Publication 920. Washington, DC: Author.

Powell, D. R. (1989). *Families and early childhood programs.* Washington, DC: National Association for the Education of Young Children.

Whitener, C. B., & Keeling, M. H. (1984). *Nutrition education for young children: Strategies and activities.* Englewood Cliffs, NJ: Prentice-Hall.

Appendix A
Recommended Dietary Allowances[1]

Nutrient	Infants[2] Birth to 6 months	Infants[2] 6 months to 1 year	Children[2] 1 to 3 years	Children[2] 4 to 6 years
Protein (gm)	13	14	16	24
Vitamin A (mcg RE)	375	375	400	500
Vitamin D (mcg)	7.5	10	10	10
Vitamin E (mg α-TE)	3	4	6	7
Vitamin K (mcg)	5	10	15	20
Vitamin C (mg)	30	35	40	45
Thiamin (mg)	0.3	0.4	0.7	0.9
Riboflavin (mg)	0.4	0.5	0.8	1.1
Niacin (mg NE)	5	6	9	12
Vitamin B_6 (mg)	0.3	0.6	1.0	1.1
Folacin (mcg)	25	35	50	75
Vitamin B_{12} (mcg)	0.3	0.5	0.7	1.0
Calcium (mg)	400	600	800	800
Phosphorus (mg)	300	500	800	800
Magnesium (mg)	40	60	80	120
Iron (mg)	6	10	10	10
Zinc (mg)	5	5	10	10
Iodine (mcg)	40	50	70	90
Selenium (mcg)	10	15	20	20

KEY: gm = grams, mg = milligrams, mcg = micrograms, RE = retinol equivalents, α-TE = alpha-tocopherol equivalents, NE = niacin equivalents. The equivalents are technical terms for measures of vitamin activity in the body.

[1] The allowances, expressed as average daily intakes over time, are intended to provide for individual variations among most normal persons as they live in the United States under usual environmental stresses. Diets should be based on a variety of common foods in order to provide other nutrients for which human requirements have been less well defined.

[2] The allowances are based on a median weight of 13 pounds and a median height of 24 inches for infants from birth to 6 months; a weight of 20 pounds and a height of 28 inches for infants from 6 months to 1 year; a weight of 29 pounds and a height of 35 inches for children from 1 to 3 years; and a weight of 44 pounds and a height of 44 inches for children from 4 to 6 years. The use of these figures does not imply that the height-to-weight ratios are ideal.

Table adapted from: National Research Council. (1989). *Recommended dietary allowances*. Washington, DC: National Academy Press.

Appendix B
Nutritive Value of Selected Foods

Foods — approximate measures, units, and weight (of edible portion only)	Food energy (Calories)	Protein (Grams)	Fat (Grams)	Saturated fat (Grams)	Cholesterol (Milligrams)	Carbohydrate (Grams)	Calcium (Milligrams)	Iron (Milligrams)	Sodium (Milligrams)	Vitamin A value (IU) (International units)	Thiamin (Milligrams)	Riboflavin (Milligrams)	Niacin (Milligrams)	Ascorbic acid (Milligrams)
Dairy Products														
Cheese:														
Natural:														
Cheddar:														
Cut piece...............1 in³	70	4	6	3.6	18	Tr	123	0.1	105	180	Tr	0.06	Tr	0
Shredded...............1 cup	455	28	37	23.8	119	1	815	0.8	701	1,200	0.03	0.42	0.1	0
Cottage (curd not pressed down):														
Creamed (cottage cheese, 4% fat):														
Large curd...............1 cup	235	28	10	6.4	34	6	135	0.3	911	370	0.05	0.37	0.3	Tr
Small curd...............1 cup	215	26	9	6.0	31	6	126	0.3	850	340	0.04	0.34	0.3	Tr
With fruit...............1 cup	280	22	8	4.9	25	30	108	0.2	915	280	0.04	0.29	0.2	Tr
Lowfat (2%)...............1 cup	205	31	4	2.8	19	8	155	0.4	918	160	0.05	0.42	0.3	Tr
Cream...............1 oz	100	2	10	6.2	31	1	23	0.3	84	400	Tr	0.06	Tr	0
Feta...............1 oz	75	4	6	4.2	25	1	140	0.2	316	130	0.04	0.24	0.3	0
Mozzarella, made with:														
Whole milk...............1 oz	80	6	6	3.7	22	1	147	0.1	106	220	Tr	0.07	Tr	0
Part skim milk (low moisture)...............1 oz	80	8	5	3.1	15	1	207	0.1	150	180	0.01	0.10	Tr	0
Muenster...............1 oz	105	7	9	5.4	27	Tr	203	0.1	178	320	Tr	0.09	Tr	0
Parmesan, grated:														
Cup, not pressed down...............1 cup	455	42	30	19.1	79	4	1,376	1.0	1,861	700	0.05	0.39	0.3	0
Tablespoon...............1 tbsp	25	2	2	1.0	4	Tr	69	Tr	93	40	Tr	0.02	Tr	0
Ounce...............1 oz	130	12	9	5.4	22	1	390	0.3	528	200	0.01	0.11	0.1	0
Ricotta, made with:														
Whole milk...............1 cup	430	28	32	20.4	124	7	509	0.9	207	1,210	0.03	0.48	0.3	0
Part skim milk...............1 cup	340	28	19	12.1	76	13	669	1.1	307	1,060	0.05	0.46	0.2	0
Swiss...............1 oz	105	8	8	5.0	26	1	272	Tr	74	240	0.01	0.10	Tr	0

Nutrients in Indicated Quantity

Foods

Foods approximate measures, units, and weight (of edible portion only)	Nutrients in Indicated Quantity													
	Food energy	Protein	Fat	Saturated fat	Cholesterol	Carbohydrate	Calcium	Iron	Sodium	Vitamin A value (IU)	Thiamin	Riboflavin	Niacin	Ascorbic acid
	Calories	Grams	Grams	Grams	Milligrams	Grams	Milligrams	Milligrams	Milligrams	International units	Milligrams	Milligrams	Milligrams	Milligrams
Pasteurized process cheese:														
American.............1 oz.........	105	6	9	5.6	27	Tr	174	0.1	406	340	0.01	0.10	Tr	0
Milk:														
Fluid:														
Whole (3.3% fat).......1 cup......	150	8	8	5.1	33	11	291	0.1	120	310	0.09	0.40	0.2	2
Lowfat (2%):														
No milk solids added......1 cup......	120	8	5	2.9	18	12	297	0.1	122	500	0.10	0.40	0.2	2
Lowfat (1%):														
No milk solids added......1 cup......	100	8	3	1.6	10	12	300	0.1	123	500	0.10	0.41	0.2	2
Nonfat (skim):														
No milk solids added......1 cup......	85	8	Tr	0.3	4	12	302	0.1	126	500	0.09	0.34	0.2	2
Buttermilk.............1 cup......	100	8	2	1.3	9	12	285	0.1	257	80	0.08	0.38	0.1	2
Canned:														
Condensed, sweetened......1 cup......	980	24	27	16.8	104	166	868	0.6	389	1,000	0.28	1.27	0.6	8
Evaporated:														
Whole milk..............1 cup......	340	17	19	11.6	74	25	657	0.5	267	610	0.12	0.80	0.5	5
Skim milk..............1 cup......	200	19	1	0.3	9	29	738	0.7	293	1,000	0.11	0.79	0.4	3
Chocolate milk (commercial):														
Regular...............1 cup......	210	8	8	5.3	31	26	280	0.6	149	300	0.09	0.41	0.3	2
Lowfat (2%)...........1 cup......	180	8	5	3.1	17	26	284	0.6	151	500	0.09	0.41	0.3	2
Lowfat (1%)...........1 cup......	160	8	3	1.5	7	26	287	0.6	152	500	0.10	0.42	0.3	2
Milk desserts, frozen:														
Ice cream, vanilla:														
Regular (about 11% fat):														
Hardened............1 cup......	270	5	14	8.9	59	32	176	0.1	116	540	0.05	0.33	0.1	1
Soft serve (frozen custard) 1 cup	375	7	23	13.5	153	38	236	0.4	153	790	0.08	0.45	0.2	1
Rich (about 16% fat), hardened......1 cup......	350	4	24	14.7	88	32	151	0.1	108	900	0.04	0.28	0.1	1
Ice milk, vanilla:														
Hardened (about 4% fat).....1 cup......	185	5	6	3.5	18	29	176	0.2	105	210	0.08	0.35	0.1	1
Soft serve (about 3% fat)......1 cup......	225	8	5	2.9	13	38	274	0.3	163	175	0.12	0.54	0.2	1
Sherbert (about 2% fat)..........1 cup......	270	2	4	2.4	14	59	103	0.3	88	190	0.03	0.09	0.1	4

Nutrients in Indicated Quantity

Foods — approximate measures, units, and weight (of edible portion only)	Food energy Calories	Protein Grams	Fat Grams	Saturated fat Grams	Cholesterol Milligrams	Carbohydrate Grams	Calcium Milligrams	Iron Milligrams	Sodium Milligrams	Vitamin A value (IU) International units	Thiamin Milligrams	Riboflavin Milligrams	Niacin Milligrams	Ascorbic acid Milligrams
Yogurt:														
With added milk solids:														
Made with lowfat milk:														
Fruit-flavored[1] ....8-oz container ...	230	10	2	1.6	10	43	345	0.2	133	100	0.08	0.40	0.2	1
Plain...........8-oz container ...	145	12	4	2.3	14	16	415	0.2	159	150	0.10	0.49	0.3	2
Made with nonfat milk ......8-oz container ...	125	13	Tr	0.3	4	17	452	0.2	174	20	0.11	0.53	0.3	2
Eggs														
Eggs, large (24 oz per dozen):														
Cooked:														
Fried in margarine ......1 egg	90	6	7	1.9	211	1	25	0.7	162	390	0.03	0.24	Tr	0
Scrambled (milk added) in margarine..............1 egg	100	7	7	2.2	215	1	44	0.7	171	420	0.03	0.27	Tr	Tr
Fats and Oils														
Butter:														
Pat (1 in square, ⅓ in high; 90 per lb)......1 pat......	35	Tr	4	2.5	11	Tr	1	Tr	41[2]	150[3]	Tr	Tr	Tr	0
Fats, cooking (vegetable shortenings) ....1 tbsp......	115	0	13	3.3	0	0	0	0.0	0	0	0.00	0.00	0.0	0
Lard ....1 tbsp......	115	0	13	5.1	12	0	0	0.0	0	0	0.00	0.00	0.0	0
Margarine:														
Imitation (about 40% fat) soft..1 tbsp........	50	Tr	5	1.1	0	Tr	2	0.0	134[4]	460[5]	Tr	Tr	Tr	Tr

Nutrients in Indicated Quantity

Foods — approximate measures, units, and weight (of edible portion only)	Food energy (Calories)	Protein (Grams)	Fat (Grams)	Saturated fat (Grams)	Cholesterol (Milligrams)	Carbohydrate (Grams)	Calcium (Milligrams)	Iron (Milligrams)	Sodium (Milligrams)	Vitamin A value (IU) (International units)	Thiamin (Milligrams)	Riboflavin (Milligrams)	Niacin (Milligrams)	Ascorbic acid (Milligrams)
Regular (about 80% fat):														
Hard (4 sticks per lb):														
Pat (1 in square, ⅓ in high; 90 per lb) ...... 1 pat	35	Tr	4	0.8	0	Tr	1	Tr	47	170[5]	Tr	Tr	Tr	Tr
Soft ...... 1 tbsp	100	Tr	11	1.9	0	Tr	4	0.0	151[11]	460[12]	Tr	Tr	Tr	Tr
Spread (about 60% fat):														
Hard (4 sticks per lb):														
Pat (1 in square, ⅓ in high; 90 per lb) ...... 1 pat	25	Tr	3	0.7	0	0	1	0.0	50[4]	170[5]	Tr	Tr	Tr	Tr
Soft ...... 1 tbsp	75	Tr	9	1.8	0	0	3	0.0	139[4]	460[5]	Tr	Tr	Tr	Tr
Oils, salad or cooking:														
Corn ...... 1 tbsp	125	0	14	1.8	0	0	0	0.0	0	0	0.00	0.00	0.00	0
Olive ...... 1 tbsp	125	0	14	1.9	0	0	0	0.0	0	0	0.00	0.00	0.00	0
Peanut ...... 1 tbsp	125	0	14	2.4	0	0	0	0.0	0	0	0.00	0.00	0.00	0
Soybean oil, hydrogenated (partially hardened) ...... 1 tbsp	125	0	14	2.1	0	0	0	0.0	0	0	0.00	0.00	0.00	0
Salad dressings:														
Commercial:														
Blue cheese ...... 1 tbsp	75	1	8	1.5	3	1	12	Tr	164	30	Tr	0.02	Tr	Tr
French:														
Regular ...... 1 tbsp	85	Tr	9	1.4	0	1	2	Tr	188	Tr	Tr	Tr	Tr	Tr
Low calorie ...... 1 tbsp	25	Tr	2	0.2	0	2	6	Tr	306	Tr	Tr	Tr	Tr	Tr
Italian:														
Regular ...... 1 tbsp	80	Tr	9	1.3	0	1	1	Tr	162	30	Tr	Tr	Tr	Tr
Low calorie ...... 1 tbsp	5	Tr	Tr	Tr	0	2	1	Tr	136	Tr	Tr	Tr	Tr	Tr
Mayonnaise:														
Regular ...... 1 tbsp	100	Tr	11	1.7	8	Tr	3	0.1	80	40	0.00	0.00	Tr	0
Imitation ...... 1 tbsp	35	Tr	3	0.5	4	2	Tr	0.0	75	0	0.00	0.00	0.0	0
Thousand island:														
Regular ...... 1 tbsp	60	Tr	6	1.0	4	2	2	0.1	112	50	Tr	Tr	Tr	0
Low calorie ...... 1 tbsp	25	Tr	2	0.2	2	2	2	0.1	150	50	Tr	Tr	Tr	0

Foods: approximate measures, units, and weight (of edible portion only)	Nutrients in Indicated Quantity													
	Food energy (Calories)	Protein (Grams)	Fat (Grams)	Saturated fat (Grams)	Cholesterol (Milligrams)	Carbohydrate (Grams)	Calcium (Milligrams)	Iron (Milligrams)	Sodium (Milligrams)	Vitamin A value (IU) (International units)	Thiamin (Milligrams)	Riboflavin (Milligrams)	Niacin (Milligrams)	Ascorbic acid (Milligrams)
Salad dressings:														
Prepared from home recipe:														
Vinegar and oil........1 tbsp	70	0	8	1.5	0	Tr	0	0.0	Tr	0	0.00	0.00	0.0	0
Fish and Shellfish														
Fish sticks, frozen, reheated, (stick, 4 by 1 by ½ in)........1 fish stick	70	6	3	0.8	26	4	11	0.3	53	20	0.03	0.05	0.6	0
Haddock, breaded, fried[6] ....3 oz	175	17	9	2.4	75	7	34	1.0	123	70	0.06	0.10	2.9	0
Salmon:														
Canned (pink), solids and liquid........3 oz	120	17	5	0.9	34	0	167[7]	0.7	443	60	0.03	0.15	6.8	0
Baked (red)........3 oz	140	21	5	1.2	60	0	26	0.5	55	290	0.18	0.14	5.5	0
Sardines, Atlantic, canned in oil, drained solids........3 oz	175	20	9	2.1	85	0	371[7]	2.6	425	190	0.03	0.17	4.6	0
Scallops, breaded, frozen, reheated........6 scallops.	195	15	10	2.5	70	10	39	2.0	298	70	0.11	0.11	1.6	0
Shrimp:														
Canned, drained solids........3 oz	100	21	1	0.2	128	1	98	1.4	1,955	50	0.01	0.03	1.5	0
French fried (7 medium)[8] ....3 oz	200	16	10	2.5	168	11	61	2.0	384	90	0.06	0.09	2.8	0
Tuna, canned, drained solids:														
Oil pack, chunk light........3 oz	165	24	7	1.4	55	0	7	1.6	303	70	0.04	0.09	10.1	0
Water pack, solid white........3 oz	135	30	1	0.3	48	0	17	0.6	468	110	0.03	0.10	13.4	0
Tuna salad[9] ....1 cup	375	33	19	3.3	80	19	31	2.5	877	230	0.06	0.14	13.3	6

Foods

Foods — approximate measures, units, and weight (of edible portion only)	Food energy — Calories	Protein — Grams	Fat — Grams	Saturated fat — Grams	Cholesterol — Milligrams	Carbohydrate — Grams	Calcium — Milligrams	Iron — Milligrams	Sodium — Milligrams	Vitamin A value (IU) — International units	Thiamin — Milligrams	Riboflavin — Milligrams	Niacin — Milligrams	Ascorbic acid — Milligrams
Fruits and Fruit Juices														
Apples:														
Raw:														
Unpeeled, without cores:														
2¾-in diam. (about 3 per lb with cores) ....1 apple	80	Tr	Tr	0.1	0	21	10	0.2	Tr	70	0.02	0.02	0.1	8
Peeled, sliced ....1 cup	65	Tr	Tr	0.1	0	16	4	0.1	Tr	50	0.02	0.01	0.1	4
Apple juice, bottled or canned[10] ....1 cup	115	Tr	Tr	Tr	0	29	17	0.9	7	Tr	0.05	0.04	0.2	2[11]
Applesauce, canned:														
Sweetened ....1 cup	195	Tr	Tr	0.1	0	51	10	0.9	8	30	0.03	0.07	0.5	4[11]
Unsweetened ....1 cup	105	Tr	Tr	Tr	0	28	7	0.3	5	70	0.03	0.06	0.5	3[11]
Apricots:														
Raw, without pits (about 12 per lb with pits) ....3 apricots	50	1	Tr	Tr	0	12	15	0.6	1	2,770	0.03	0.04	0.6	11
Canned (fruit and liquid):														
Heavy syrup pack ....3 halves	70	Tr	Tr	Tr	0	18	8	0.3	3	1,050	0.02	0.02	0.3	3
Juice pack ....3 halves	40	1	Tr	Tr	0	10	10	0.3	3	1,420	0.02	0.02	0.3	4
Dried:														
Uncooked (28 large or 37 medium halves per cup) ....1 cup	310	5	1	Tr	0	80	59	6.1	13	9,410	0.01	0.20	3.9	3
Bananas, raw, without peel:														
Whole (about 2½ per lb with peel) ....1 banana	105	1	1	0.2	0	27	7	0.4	1	90	0.05	0.11	0.6	10
Sliced ....1 cup	140	2	1	0.3	0	35	9	0.5	2	120	0.07	0.15	0.8	14
Blueberries:														
Raw ....1 cup	80	1	1	Tr	0	20	9	0.2	9	150	0.07	0.07	0.5	19
Frozen, sweetened ....1 cup	185	1	Tr	Tr	0	50	14	0.9	2	100	0.05	0.12	0.6	2

Foods approximate measures, units, and weight (of edible portion only)	Nutrients in Indicated Quantity													
	Food energy	Protein	Fat	Saturated fat	Cholesterol	Carbohydrate	Calcium	Iron	Sodium	Vitamin A value (IU)	Thiamin	Riboflavin	Niacin	Ascorbic acid
	Calories	Grams	Grams	Grams	Milligrams	Grams	Milligrams	Milligrams	Milligrams	International units	Milligrams	Milligrams	Milligrams	Milligrams
Cranberry juice cocktail, bottled, sweetened............1 cup......	145	Tr	Tr	Tr	0	38	8	0.4	10	10	0.01	0.04	0.1	108[12]
Cranberry sauce, sweetened, canned, strained......1 cup......	420	1	Tr	Tr	0	108	11	0.6	80	60	0.04	0.06	0.3	6
Fruit cocktail, canned, fruit and liquid:														
Heavy syrup pack...........1 cup........	185	1	Tr	Tr	0	48	15	0.7	15	520	0.05	0.05	1.0	5
Juice pack.............1 cup........	115	1	Tr	Tr	0	29	20	0.5	10	760	0.03	0.04	1.0	7
Grapefruit:														
Raw, without peel, membrane and seeds (3¾-in diam., 1 lb 1 oz, whole, with refuse)......½ grapefruit	40	1	Tr	Tr	0	10	14	0.1	Tr	10[13]	0.04	0.02	0.3	41
Canned, sections with syrup ...1 cup......	150	1	Tr	Tr	0	39	36	1.0	5	Tr	0.10	0.05	0.6	54
Grapefruit juice:														
Raw.............1 cup............	95	1	Tr	Tr	0	23	22	0.5	2	20	0.10	0.05	0.5	94
Canned:														
Unsweetened.............1 cup............	95	1	Tr	Tr	0	22	17	0.5	2	20	0.10	0.05	0.6	72
Sweetened ....1 cup......	115	1	Tr	Tr	0	28	20	0.9	5	20	0.10	0.06	0.8	67
Grapes, European type (adherent skin), raw:														
Thompson Seedless..............10 grapes..	35	Tr	Tr	0.1	0	9	6	0.1	1	40	0.05	0.03	0.2	5
Grape juice:														
Canned or bottled.................1 cup......	155	1	Tr	0.1	0	38	23	0.6	8	20	0.07	0.09	0.7	Tr[14]

Nutrients in Indicated Quantity

Foods: approximate measures, units, and weight (of edible portion only)	Food energy Calories	Protein Grams	Fat Grams	Saturated fat Grams	Cholesterol Milligrams	Carbohydrate Grams	Calcium Milligrams	Iron Milligrams	Sodium Milligrams	Vitamin A value (IU) International units	Thiamin Milligrams	Riboflavin Milligrams	Niacin Milligrams	Ascorbic acid Milligrams
Lemonade concentrate:														
Diluted with 4⅓ parts water by volume..........6 oz..........	80	Tr	Tr	Tr	0	21	2	0.1	1	10	0.01	0.02	0.2	13
Melons, raw, without rind and cavity contents:														
Cantaloupe, orange-fleshed (5-in diam., 2⅓ lb, whole, with rind and cavity contents)......½ melon......	95	2	1	0.1	0	22	29	0.6	24	8,610	0.10	0.06	1.5	113
Honeydew (6½-in diam., 5¼ lb, whole, with rind and cavity contents)..........⅒ melon....	45	1	Tr	Tr	0	12	8	0.1	13	50	0.10	0.02	0.8	32
Nectarines, raw, without pits (about 3 per lb with pits)..................1 nectarine	65	1	1	0.1	0	16	7	0.2	Tr	1,000	0.02	0.06	1.3	7
Oranges, raw:														
Whole, without peel and seeds (2⅝-in diam., about 2½ per lb, with peel and seeds)......1 orange ...	60	1	Tr	Tr	0	15	52	0.1	Tr	270	0.11	0.05	0.4	70
Sections without membranes...1 cup..........	85	2	Tr	Tr	0	21	72	0.2	Tr	370	0.16	0.07	0.5	96
Orange juice:														
Raw, al l varieties..............1 cup..........	110	2	Tr	0.1	0	26	27	0.5	2	500	0.22	0.07	1.0	124
Frozen concentrate:														
Diluted with 3 parts water by volume..........1 cup..........	110	2	Tr	Tr	0	27	22	0.2	2	190	0.20	0.04	0.5	97
Peaches:														
Raw:														
Whole, 2½-in diam., peeled, pitted (about 4 per lb with peels and pits).........1 peach....	35	1	Tr	Tr	0	10	4	0.1	Tr	470	0.01	0.04	0.9	6
Sliced...............1 cup....	75	1	Tr	Tr	0	19	9	0.2	Tr	910	0.03	0.07	1.7	11
Canned, fruit and liquid:														
Heavy syrup pack.............1 cup..........	190	1	Tr	Tr	0	51	8	0.7	15	850	0.03	0.06	1.6	7

Foods	Nutrients in Indicated Quantity													
approximate measures, units, and weight (of edible portion only)	Food energy	Protein	Fat	Saturated fat	Cholesterol	Carbohydrate	Calcium	Iron	Sodium	Vitamin A value (IU)	Thiamin	Riboflavin	Niacin	Ascorbic acid
	Calories	Grams	Grams	Grams	Milligrams	Grams	Milligrams	Milligrams	Milligrams	International units	Milligrams	Milligrams	Milligrams	Milligrams
Juice pack..............1 cup	110	2	Tr	Tr	0	29	15	0.7	10	940	0.02	0.04	1.4	9
Frozen, sliced, sweetened ....1 cup	235	2	Tr	Tr	0	60	8	0.9	15	710	0.03	0.09	1.6	236[15]
Pears:														
Raw, with skin, cored:														
Bartlett, 2½-in diam. (about 2½ per lb with cores and stems) ....1 pear	100	1	1	Tr	0	25	18	0.4	Tr	30	0.03	0.07	0.2	7
Canned, fruit and liquid:														
Heavy syrup pack..........1 cup	190	1	Tr	Tr	0	49	13	0.6	13	10	0.03	0.06	0.6	3
Juice pack..............1 cup	125	1	Tr	Tr	0	32	22	0.7	10	10	0.03	0.03	0.5	4
Pineapple:														
Raw, diced..............1 cup	75	1	1	Tr	0	19	11	0.6	2	40	0.14	0.06	0.7	24
Canned, fruit and liquid:														
Heavy syrup pack:														
Crushed, chunks, tidbits...1 cup	200	1	Tr	Tr	0	52	36	1.0	3	40	0.23	0.06	0.7	19
Juice pack:														
Chunks or tidbits..........1 cup	150	1	Tr	Tr	0	39	35	0.7	3	100	0.24	0.05	0.7	24
Pineapple juice, unsweetened, canned ....1 cup	140	1	Tr	Tr	0	34	43	0.7	3	10	0.14	0.06	0.6	27
Prunes, dried:														
Uncooked ....4 extra large 5 large	115	1	Tr	Tr	0	31	25	1.2	2	970	0.04	0.08	1.0	2
Prune juice, canned or bottled..............1 cup	180	2	Tr	Tr	0	45	31	3.0	10	10	0.04	0.18	2.0	10
Raisins, seedless:														
Cup, not pressed down..........1 cup	435	5	1	0.2	0	115	71	3.0	17	10	0.23	0.13	1.2	5

Foods

approximate measures, units, and weight (of edible portion only)	Nutrients in Indicated Quantity													
	Food energy	Protein	Fat	Saturated fat	Cholesterol	Carbohydrate	Calcium	Iron	Sodium	Vitamin A value (IU)	Thiamin	Riboflavin	Niacin	Ascorbic acid
	Calories	Grams	Grams	Grams	Milligrams	Grams	Milligrams	Milligrams	Milligrams	International units	Milligrams	Milligrams	Milligrams	Milligrams
Raspberries:														
Raw .... 1 cup	60	1	1	Tr	0	14	27	0.7	Tr	160	0.04	0.11	1.1	31
Frozen, sweetened ..... 1 cup...........	255	2	Tr	Tr	0	65	38	1.6	3	150	0.05	0.11	0.6	41
Strawberries:														
Raw, capped, whole .... 1 cup......	45	1	1	Tr	0	10	21	0.6	1	40	0.03	0.10	0.3	84
Frozen, sweetened, sliced ...... 1 cup..........	245	1	Tr	Tr	0	66	28	1.5	8	60	0.04	0.13	1.0	106
Watermelon, raw, without rind and seeds:														
Piece (4 by 8 in wedge with rind and seeds; 1/16 of 32⅔-lb melon, 10 by 16 in) .... 1 piece	155	3	2	0.3	0	35	39	0.8	10	1,760	0.39	0.10	1.0	46

Grain Products

Bagels, plain or water, enriched, 3½-in diam.[16] .... 1 bagel......	200	7	2	0.3	0	38	29	1.8	245	0	0.26	0.20	2.4	0
Biscuits. baking powder, 2-in diam. (enriched flour, vegetable shortening):														
From mix.[16] .... 1 biscuit........	95	2	3	0.8	Tr	14	58	0.7	262	20	0.12	0.11	0.8	Tr
From refrigerated dough........ 1 biscuit......	65	1	2	0.6	1	10	4	0.5	249	0	0.08	0.05	0.7	0
Breads:														
Italian bread, enriched:														
Slice, 4½ by 3¼ by ¾ in .... 1 slice	85	3	Tr	Tr	0	17	5	0.8	176	0	0.12	0.07	1.0	0
Pita bread, enriched, white, 6½-in diam. .... 1 pita...........	165	6	1	0.1	0	33	49	1.4	339	0	0.27	0.12	2.2	0
Rye bread, light (⅔ enriched wheat flour, ⅓ rye flour):[17]														
Slice, 4¾ by 3¾ by 7/16 in .... 1 slice	65	2	1	0.2	0	12	20	0.7	175	0	0.10	0.08	0.8	0

Appendix B: continued

Foods		Nutrients in Indicated Quantity													
approximate measures, units, and weight (of edible portion only)		Food energy	Protein	Fat	Saturated fat	Cholesterol	Carbohydrate	Calcium	Iron	Sodium	Vitamin A value (IU)	Thiamin	Riboflavin	Niacin	Ascorbic acid
		Calories	Grams	Grams	Grams	Milligrams	Grams	Milligrams	Milligrams	Milligrams	International units	Milligrams	Milligrams	Milligrams	Milligrams
White bread, enriched:[17]															
Slice (18 per loaf)	1 slice	65	2	1	0.3	0	12	32	0.7	129	Tr	0.12	0.08	0.9	Tr
Slice (22 per loaf)	1 slice	55	2	1	0.2	0	10	25	0.6	101	Tr	0.09	0.06	0.7	Tr
Whole-wheat bread:[17]															
Slice (16 per loaf)	1 slice	70	3	1	0.4	0	13	20	1.0	180	Tr	0.10	0.06	1.1	Tr
Breakfast cereals:															
Hot type, cooked:															
Corn (hominy) grits:															
Instant, plain	1 pkt.	80	2	Tr	Tr	0	18	7	1.0[18]	343	0	0.18[18]	0.08[18]	1.3[18]	0
Cream of Wheat®:															
Regular, quick, instant	1 cup	140	4	Tr	0.1	0	29	54[19]	10.9[19]	5[20][21]	0	0.24[19]	0.07[19]	1.5[19]	0
Mix'n Eat, plain	1 pkt.	100	3	Tr	Tr	0	21	20[19]	8.1[19]	241	1,250[19]	0.43[19]	0.28[19]	5.0[19]	0
Oatmeal or rolled oats:															
Regular, quick, instant, nonfortified	1 cup	145	6	2	0.4	0	25	19	1.6	2[22]	40	0.26	0.05	0.3	0
Instant, fortified:															
Plain	1 pkt.	105	4	2	0.3	0	18	163[18]	6.3[18]	285[18]	1,510[18]	0.53[18]	0.28[18]	5.5[18]	0
Flavored	1 pkt.	160	5	2	0.3	0	31	168[18]	6.7[18]	254[18]	1,530[18]	0.53[18]	0.38[18]	5.9[18]	Tr
Breakfast cereals:															
Ready to eat:															
Cheerios® (about 1¼ cup)	1 oz	110	4	2	0.3	0	20	48	4.5[23]	307	1,250[23]	0.37[23]	0.43[23]	5.0[23]	15[23]
Corn Flakes (about 1¼ cup):															
Kellogg's®	1 oz	110	2	Tr	Tr	0	24	1	1.8[23]	351	1,250[23]	0.37[23]	0.43[23]	5.0[23]	15[23]
100% Natural Cereal (about ¼ cup)	1 oz	135	3	6	4.1	Tr	18	49	0.8	12	20	0.09	0.15	0.6	0

Foods approximate measures, units, and weight (of edible portion only)	Nutrients in Indicated Quantity													
	Food energy	Protein	Fat	Saturated fat	Cholesterol	Carbohydrate	Calcium	Iron	Sodium	Vitamin A value (IU)	Thiamin	Riboflavin	Niacin	Ascorbic acid
	Calories	Grams	Grams	Grams	Milligrams	Grams	Milligrams	Milligrams	Milligrams	International units	Milligrams	Milligrams	Milligrams	Milligrams
Raisin Bran:														
Kellogg's® (about ¾ cup)..1 oz..........	90	3	1	0.1	0	21	10	3.5[23]	207	960[23]	0.28[23]	0.34[23]	3.9[23]	0
Post® (about ½ cup)........1 oz..........	85	3	1	0.1	0	21	13	4.5[23]	185	1,250[23]	0.37[23]	0.43[23]	5.0[23]	0
Rice Krispies® (about 1 cup) 1 oz..........	110	2	Tr	Tr	0	25	4	1.8[23]	340	1,250[23]	0.37[23]	0.43[23]	5.0[23]	15[23]
Shredded Wheat (about ⅔ cup) ....1 oz..........	100	3	1	0.1	0	23	11	1.2	3	0	0.07	0.08	1.5	0
Wheaties® (about 1 cup).....1 oz..........	100	3	Tr	0.1	0	23	43	4.5[23]	354	1,250[23]	0.37[23]	0.43[23]	5.0[23]	15[23]
Cakes prepared from cake mixes with enriched flour:[24]														
Angel food:														
Piece, 1/12 of cake ....1 piece	125	3	Tr	Tr	0	29	44	0.2	269	0	0.03	0.11	0.1	0
Coffeecake, crumb:														
Piece, ⅙ of cake...................1 piece	230	5	7	2.0	47	38	44	1.2	310	120	0.14	0.15	1.3	Tr
Devil's food with chocolate frosting:														
Piece, 1/16 of cake ....1 piece	235	3	8	3.5	37	40	41	1.4	181	100	0.07	0.10	0.6	Tr
Cupcake, 2½-in diam...........1 cupcake..	120	2	4	1.8	19	20	21	0.7	92	50	0.04	0.05	0.3	Tr
Yellow with chocolate frosting:														
Piece, 1/16 of cake ....1 piece	235	3	8	3.0	36	40	63	1.0	157	100	0.08	0.10	0.7	Tr
Cookies made with enriched flour:														
Brownies with nuts:														
From home recipe, 1¾ by 1¾ by ⅞ in[25] ....1 brownie..	95	1	6	1.4	18	11	9	0.4	51	20	0.05	0.05	0.3	Tr
Chocolate chip:														
Commercial, 2¼-in diam., ⅜ in thick..........................4 cookies ...	180	2	9	2.9	5	28	13	0.8	140	50	0.10	0.23	1.0	Tr
From home recipe, 2⅓-in diam.[26] ....4 cookies ...	185	2	11	3.9	18	26	13	1.0	82	20	0.06	0.06	0.6	0
From refrigerated dough, 2¼-in diam., ⅜ in thick........4 cookies ...	225	2	11	4.0	22	32	13	1.0	173	30	0.06	0.10	0.9	0

Foods — approximate measures, units, and weight (of edible portion only)	Nutrients in Indicated Quantity													
	Food energy	Protein	Fat	Saturated fat	Cholesterol	Carbohydrate	Calcium	Iron	Sodium	Vitamin A value (IU)	Thiamin	Riboflavin	Niacin	Ascorbic acid
	Calories	Grams	Grams	Grams	Milligrams	Grams	Milligrams	Milligrams	Milligrams	International units	Milligrams	Milligrams	Milligrams	Milligrams
Oatmeal with raisins, 2⅝-in diam., ¼ in thick............4 cookies ...	245	3	10	2.5	2	36	18	1.1	148	40	0.09	0.08	1.0	0
Peanut butter cookie, from home recipe, 2⅝-in diam.[26] ....4 cookies ...	245	4	14	4.0	22	28	21	1.1	142	20	0.07	0.07	1.9	C
Sandwich type (chocolate or vanilla), 1¾-in diam., ⅜ in thick ....4 cookies ...	195	2	8	2.0	0	29	12	1.4	189	0	0.09	0.07	0.8	0
Shortbread: Commercial ....4 small cookies	155	2	8	2.9	27	20	13	0.8	123	30	0.10	0.09	0.9	0
Sugar cookie, from refrigerated dough, 2½-in diam., ¼ in thick	235	2	12	2.3	29	31	50	0.9	261	40	0.09	0.06	1.1	0
Vanilla wafers, 1¾-in diam., ¼ in thick ....10 cookies ...	185	2	7	1.8	25	29	16	0.8	150	50	0.07	0.10	1.0	0
Corn chips ....1-oz package...	155	2	9	1.4	0	16	35	0.5	233	110	0.04	0.05	0.4	1
Crackers:[27]														
Cheese: Plain, 1 in square ....10 crackers	50	1	3	0.9	6	6	11	0.3	112	20	0.05	0.04	0.4	0
Sandwich type (peanut butter)...........1 sandwich	40	1	2	0.4	1	5	7	0.3	90	Tr	0.04	0.03	0.6	0
Graham, plain, 2½ in square....2 crackers ...	60	1	1	0.4	0	11	6	0.4	86	0	0.02	0.03	0.6	0
Melba toast, plain...........1 piece	20	1	Tr	0.1	0	4	6	0.1	44	0	0.01	0.01	0.1	0
Saltines[28] ....4 crackers ...	50	1	1	0.5	4	9	3	0.5	165	0	0.06	0.05	0.6	0
Snack-type, standard ....1 round cracker......	15	Tr	1	0.2	0	2	3	0.1	30	Tr	0.01	0.01	0.1	0
Wheat, thin.........4 crackers ..	35	1	1	0.5	0	5	3	0.3	69	Tr	0.04	0.03	0.4	0
French toast, from home recipe...........1 slice	155	6	7	1.6	112	17	72	1.3	257	110	0.12	0.16	1.0	Tr

Nutrients in Indicated Quantity

Foods — approximate measures, units, and weight (of edible portion only)	Food energy (Calories)	Protein (Grams)	Fat (Grams)	Saturated fat (Grams)	Cholesterol (Milligrams)	Carbohydrate (Grams)	Calcium (Milligrams)	Iron (Milligrams)	Sodium (Milligrams)	Vitamin A value (IU) (International units)	Thiamin (Milligrams)	Riboflavin (Milligrams)	Niacin (Milligrams)	Ascorbic acid (Milligrams)
Macaroni, enriched, cooked (cut lengths, elbows, shells):														
Firm stage (hot) .... 1 cup	190	7	1	0.1	0	39	14	2.1	1	0	0.23	0.13	1.8	0
Muffins made with enriched flour, 2½-in diam., 1½ in high:														
From home recipe:														
Blueberry[29] .... 1 muffin........	135	3	5	1.5	19	20	54	0.9	198	40	0.10	0.11	0.9	1
Bran[30] .... 1 muffin........	125	3	6	1.4	24	19	60	1.4	189	230	0.11	0.13	1.3	3
Corn (enriched, degermed cornmeal and flour)[30] .... 1 muffin......	145	3	5	1.5	23	21	66	0.9	169	80	0.11	0.11	0.9	Tr
From commercial mix (egg and water added):														
Blueberry................... 1 muffin........	140	3	5	1.4	45	22	15	0.9	225	50	0.10	0.17	1.1	Tr
Bran .... 1 muffin........	140	3	4	1.3	28	24	27	1.7	385	100	0.08	0.12	1.9	0
Corn...................... 1 muffin........	145	3	6	1.7	42	22	30	1.3	291	90	0.09	0.09	0.8	Tr
Noodles (egg noodles), enriched, cooked .... 1 cup	200	7	2	0.5	50	37	16	2.6	3	110	0.22	0.13	1.9	0
Pancakes, 4-in diam.:														
Plain:														
From home recipe using enriched flour .... 1 pancake..	60	2	2	0.5	16	9	27	0.5	115	30	0.06	0.07	0.5	Tr
From mix (with enriched flour), egg, milk, and oil added .... 1 pancake.	60	2	2	0.5	16	8	36	0.7	160	30	0.09	0.12	0.8	Tr
Piecrust, made with enriched flour and vegetable shortening, baked:														
From home recipe, 9-in diam. .... 1 pie shell..	900	11	60	14.8	0	79	25	4.5	1,100	0	0.54	0.40	5.0	0
From mix, 9-in diam. .... Piecrust for 2-crust pie..	1,485	20	93	22.7	0	141	131	9.3	2,602	0	1.06	0.80	9.9	0

Foods	Food energy	Protein	Fat	Saturated fat	Cholesterol	Carbohydrate	Calcium	Iron	Sodium	Vitamin A value (IU)	Thiamin	Riboflavin	Niacin	Ascorbic acid
approximate measures, units, and weight (of edible portion only)	Calories	Grams	Grams	Grams	Milli-grams	Grams	Milli-grams	Milli-grams	Milli-grams	Interna-tional units	Milli-grams	Milli-grams	Milli-grams	Milli-grams
Pies, piecrust made with enriched flour, vegetable shortening, 9-in diam.:														
Apple:														
Piece, ⅙ of pie ....1 piece	405	3	18	4.6	0	60	13	1.6	476	50	0.17	0.13	1.6	2
Blueberry:														
Piece, ⅙ of pie ....1 piece	380	4	17	4.3	0	55	17	2.1	423	140	0.17	0.14	1.7	6
Cherry:														
Piece, ⅙ of pie ....1 piece	410	4	18	4.7	0	61	22	1.6	480	700	0.19	0.14	1.6	0
Custard:														
Piece, ⅙ of pie ....1 piece	330	9	17	5.6	169	36	146	1.5	436	350	0.14	0.32	0.9	0
Lemon meringue:														
Piece, ⅙ of pie ....1 piece	355	5	14	4.3	143	53	20	1.4	395	240	0.10	0.14	0.8	4
Pumpkin:														
Piece, ⅙ of pie ....1 piece	320	6	17	6.4	109	37	78	1.4	325	3,750	0.14	0.21	1.2	0
Popcorn, popped:														
Air-popped, unsalted ....1 cup......	30	1	Tr	Tr	0	6	1	0.2	Tr	10	0.03	0.01	0.2	0
Popped in vegetable oil, salted.......1 cup......	55	1	3	0.5	0	6	3	0.3	86	20	0.01	0.02	0.1	0
Pretzels, made with enriched flour:														
Stick, 2¼ in long ....10 pretzels.	10	Tr	Tr	Tr	0	2	1	0.1	48	0	0.01	0.01	0.1	0
Rice:														
White, enriched:														
Commercial varieties, all types:														
Cooked, served hot........1 cup......	225	4	Tr	0.1	0	50	21	1.8	0	0	0.23	0.02	2.1	0
Instant, ready-to-serve, hot ..1 cup......	180	4	0	0.1	0	40	5	1.3	0	0	0.21	0.02	1.7	0

Nutrients in Indicated Quantity

Foods — approximate measures, units, and weight (of edible portion only)	Food energy	Protein	Fat	Saturated fat	Cholesterol	Carbohydrate	Calcium	Iron	Sodium	Vitamin A value (IU)	Thiamin	Riboflavin	Niacin	Ascorbic acid
	Calories	Grams	Grams	Grams	Milligrams	Grams	Milligrams	Milligrams	Milligrams	International units	Milligrams	Milligrams	Milligrams	Milligrams
Rolls, enriched:														
Commercial:														
Dinner, 2½-in diam., 2 in high......1 roll......	85	2	2	0.5	Tr	14	33	0.8	155	Tr	0.14	0.09	1.1	Tr
Frankfurter and hamburger (8 per 11½-oz pkg.)......1 roll......	115	3	2	0.5	Tr	20	54	1.2	241	Tr	0.20	0.13	1.6	Tr
Hard, 3¾-in diam., 2 in high......1 roll......	155	5	2	0.4	Tr	30	24	1.4	313	0	0.20	0.12	1.7	0
Spaghetti, enriched, cooked:														
Firm stage, "al dente," served hot......1 cup......	190	7	1	0.1	0	39	14	2.0	1	0	0.23	0.13	1.8	0
Tortillas, corn......1 tortilla...	65	2	1	0.1	0	13	42	0.6	1	80	0.05	0.03	0.4	0
Waffles, made with enriched flour, 7-n diam.:														
From home recipe......1 waffle...	245	7	13	4.0	102	26	154	1.5	445	140	0.18	0.24	1.5	Tr
From mix, egg and milk added......1 waffle...	205	7	8	2.7	59	27	179	1.2	515	170	0.14	0.23	0.9	Tr

Legumes, Nuts, and Seeds

Beans, dry:														
Cooked, drained:														
Black......1 cup......	225	15	1	0.1	0	41	47	2.9	1	Tr	0.43	0.05	0.9	0
Lima......1 cup......	260	16	1	0.2	0	49	55	5.9	4	0	0.25	0.11	1.3	0
Pea (navy)......1 cup......	225	15	1	0.1	0	40	95	5.1	13	0	0.27	0.13	1.3	0
Canned solids and liquid:														
Red kidney......1 cup......	230	15	1	0.1	0	42	74	4.6	968	10	0.13	0.10	1.5	0
Black-eyed peas, dry, cooked (with residual cooking liquid)......1 cup......	190	13	1	0.2	0	35	43	3.3	20	30	0.40	0.10	1.0	0

Foods	Nutrients in Indicated Quantity													
approximate measures, units, and weight (of edible portion only)	Food energy	Protein	Fat	Saturated fat	Cholesterol	Carbohydrate	Calcium	Iron	Sodium	Vitamin A value (IU)	Thiamin	Riboflavin	Niacin	Ascorbic acid
	Calories	Grams	Grams	Grams	Milligrams	Grams	Milligrams	Milligrams	Milligrams	International units	Milligrams	Milligrams	Milligrams	Milligrams
Coconut:														
Raw:														
Shredded or grated .... 1 cup	285	3	27	23.8	0	12	11	1.9	16	0	0.05	0.02	0.4	3
Peanut butter .... 1 tbsp	95	5	8	1.4	0	3	5	0.3	75	0	0.02	0.02	2.2	0
Peas, split, dry, cooked ..... 1 cup	230	16	1	0.1	0	42	22	3.4	26	80	0.30	0.18	1.8	0
Soy products:														
Miso .... 1 cup	470	29	13	1.8	0	65	188	4.7	8,142	110	0.17	0.28	0.8	0
Tofu, piece 2½ by 2¾ by 1 in .... 1 piece	85	9	5	0.7	0	3	108	2.3	8	0	0.07	0.04	0.1	0

Meat and Meat Products

Beef, cooked:														
Ground beef, broiled, patty, 3 by ⅝ in:														
Lean .... 3 oz	230	21	16	6.2	74	0	9	1.8	65	Tr	0.04	0.18	4.4	0
Regular .... 3 oz	245	20	18	6.9	76	0	9	2.1	70	Tr	0.03	0.16	4.9	0
Roast, oven cooked, no liquid added:														
Relatively fat, such as rib:														
Lean and fat, 2 pieces, 4⅛ by 2¼ by ¼ in .... 3 oz	315	19	26	10.8	72	0	8	2.0	54	Tr	0.06	0.16	3.1	0
Relatively lean, such as eye of round:														
Lean and fat, 2 pieces, 2½ by 2½ by ⅜ in .... 3 oz	205	23	12	4.9	62	0	5	1.6	50	Tr	0.07	0.14	3.0	0

Foods approximate measures, units, and weight (of edible portion only)	Food energy	Protein	Fat	Saturated fat	Cholesterol	Carbohydrate	Calcium	Iron	Sodium	Vitamin A value (IU)	Thiamin	Riboflavin	Niacin	Ascorbic acid
	Calories	Grams	Grams	Grams	Milligrams	Grams	Milligrams	Milligrams	Milligrams	International units	Milligrams	Milligrams	Milligrams	Milligrams
Steak:														
Sirloin, broiled:														
Lean and fat, piece, 2½ by 2½ by ¾ in. ...... 3 oz	240	23	15	6.4	77	0	9	2.6	53	Tr	0.10	0.23	3.3	0
Lamb, cooked:														
Chops, (3 per lb with bone):														
Arm, braised:														
Lean and fat ...... 2.2 oz	220	20	15	6.9	77	0	16	1.5	46	Tr	0.04	0.16	4.4	0
Lean only ...... 1.7 oz	135	17	7	2.9	59	0	12	1.3	36	Tr	0.03	0.13	3.0	0
Pork, cured, cooked:														
Bacon:														
Regular ...... 3 medium slices	110	6	9	3.3	16	Tr	2	0.3	303	0	0.13	0.05	1.4	6
Canadian-style ...... 2 slices	85	11	4	1.3	27	1	5	0.4	711	0	0.38	0.09	3.2	10
Ham, light cure, roasted:														
Lean and fat, 2 pieces, 4⅛ by 2¼ by ¼ in. ...... 3 oz	205	18	14	5.1	53	0	6	0.7	1,009	0	0.51	0.19	3.8	0
Cooked ham (8 slices per 8-oz pkg):														
Regular ...... 2 slices	105	10	6	1.9	32	2	4	0.6	751	0	0.49	0.14	3.0	16[31]
Pork, fresh, cooked:														
Ham (leg). roasted:														
Lean and fat, piece, 2½ by 2½ by ¾ in. ...... 3 oz	250	21	18	6.4	79	0	5	0.9	50	10	0.54	0.27	3.9	Tr
Rib, roasted:														
Lean and fat, piece, 2½ by ¾ in. ...... 3 oz	270	21	20	7.2	69	0	9	0.8	37	10	0.50	0.24	4.2	Tr
Sausages:														
Bologna, slice (8 per 8-oz pkg) ...... 2 slices	180	7	16	6.1	31	2	7	0.9	581	0	0.10	0.08	1.5	12[31]
Frankfurter (10 per 1-lb pkg). cooked (reheated) ...... 1 frankfurter	145	5	13	4.8	23	1	5	0.5	504	0	0.09	0.05	1.2	12[31]

Nutrients in Indicated Quantity

Foods	Nutrients in Indicated Quantity													
approximate measures, units, and weight (of edible portion only)	Food energy	Protein	Fat	Saturated fat	Cholesterol	Carbohydrate	Calcium	Iron	Sodium	Vitamin A value (IU)	Thiamin	Riboflavin	Niacin	Ascorbic acid
	Calories	Grams	Grams	Grams	Milligrams	Grams	Milligrams	Milligrams	Milligrams	International units	Milligrams	Milligrams	Milligrams	Milligrams
Pork link (16 per 1-lb pkg). cooked[32]............ 1 link............	50	3	4	1.4	11	Tr	4	0.2	168	0	0.10	0.03	0.6	Tr
Salami:														
Cooked type, slice (8 per 8-oz pkg) .... 2 slices............	145	8	11	4.6	37	1	7	1.5	607	0	0.14	0.21	2.0	7[31]

Poultry and Poultry Products

Foods														
Chicken:														
Fried, flesh, with skin.[33]														
Flour coated:														
Breast, ½ breast (4.2 oz with bones) .... 3.5 oz............	220	31	9	2.4	87	2	16	1.2	74	50	0.08	0.13	13.5	0
Drumstick (2.6 oz with bones)............ 1.7 oz............	120	13	7	1.8	44	1	6	0.7	44	40	0.04	0.11	3.0	0
Roasted, flesh only:														
Breast, ½ breast (4.2 oz with bones and skin) .... 3.0 oz............	140	27	3	0.9	73	0	13	0.9	64	20	0.06	0.10	11.8	0
Drumstick, (2.9 oz with bones and skin) .... 1.6 oz............	75	12	2	0.7	41	0	5	0.6	42	30	0.03	0.10	2.7	0
Turkey, roasted, flesh only:														
Dark meat, piece, 2½ by 1⅝ by ¼ in............ 4 pieces............	160	24	6	2.1	72	0	27	2.0	67	0	0.05	0.21	3.1	0
Light meat, piece, 4 by 2 by ¼ in............ 2 pieces............	135	25	3	0.9	59	0	16	1.1	54	0	0.05	0.11	5.8	0
Poultry food products:														
Chicken:														
Frankfurter (10 per 1-lb pkg) .... 1 frankfurter	115	6	9	2.5	45	3	43	0.9	616	60	0.03	0.05	1.4	0

Nutrients in Indicated Quantity

Foods (approximate measures, units, and weight (of edible portion only))	Food energy (Calories)	Protein (Grams)	Fat (Grams)	Saturated fat (Grams)	Cholesterol (Milligrams)	Carbohydrate (Grams)	Calcium (Milligrams)	Iron (Milligrams)	Sodium (Milligrams)	Vitamin A value (International units)	Thiamin (Milligrams)	Riboflavin (Milligrams)	Niacin (Milligrams)	Ascorbic acid (Milligrams)
Soups, Sauces, and Gravies														
Soups:														
Canned, condensed:														
Prepared with equal volume of water:														
Bean with bacon .... 1 cup	170	8	6	1.5	3	23	81	2.0	951	890	0.09	0.03	0.6	2
Beef broth, bouillon, consomme .... 1 cup	15	3	1	0.3	Tr	Tr	14	0.4	782	0	Tr	0.05	1.9	0
Beef noodle .... 1 cup	85	5	3	1.1	5	9	15	1.1	952	630	0.07	0.06	1.1	Tr
Chicken noodle .... 1 cup	75	4	2	0.7	7	9	17	0.8	1,106	710	0.05	0.06	1.4	Tr
Chicken rice .... 1 cup	60	4	2	0.5	7	7	17	0.7	815	660	0.02	0.02	1.1	Tr
Cream of chicken .... 1 cup	115	3	7	2.1	10	9	34	0.6	986	560	0.03	0.06	0.8	Tr
Minestrone .... 1 cup	80	4	3	0.6	2	11	34	0.9	911	2,340	0.05	0.04	0.9	1
Tomato .... 1 cup	85	2	2	0.4	0	17	12	1.8	871	690	0.09	0.05	1.4	66
Vegetable beef .... 1 cup	80	6	2	0.9	5	10	17	1.1	956	1,890	0.04	0.05	1.0	2
Vegetarian .... 1 cup	70	2	2	0.3	0	12	22	1.1	822	3,010	0.05	0.05	0.9	1
Dehydrated:														
Prepared with water:														
Chicken noodle 1 (6-fl-oz)	40	2	1	0.2	2	6	24	0.4	957	50	0.05	0.04	0.7	Tr
Tomato vegetable 1 (6-fl-oz)	40	1	1	0.3	0	8	6	0.5	856	140	0.04	0.03	0.6	5
Sugars and Sweets														
Gelatin dessert prepared with gelatin dessert powder and water. ½ cup	70	2	0	0.0	0	17	2	Tr	55	0	0.00	0.00	0.0	0
Honey, strained or extracted .... 1 tbsp	74	Tr	0	0.0	0	17	1	0.1	1	0	Tr	0.01	0.1	Tr
Jam and preserves .... 1 tbsp	55	Tr	Tr	0.0	0	14	4	0.2	2	Tr	Tr	0.01	Tr	Tr
Jellies .... 1 tbsp	50	Tr	Tr	Tr	0	13	2	0.1	5	Tr	Tr	0.01	Tr	1

Foods approximate measures, units, and weight (of edible portion only)	Nutrients in Indicated Quantity													
	Food energy Calories	Protein Grams	Fat Grams	Saturated fat Grams	Cholesterol Milligrams	Carbohydrate Grams	Calcium Milligrams	Iron Milligrams	Sodium Milligrams	Vitamin A value (IU) International units	Thiamin Milligrams	Riboflavin Milligrams	Niacin Milligrams	Ascorbic acid Milligrams
Popsicle, 3-fl-oz size............1 popsicle.	70	0	0	0.0	0	18	0	Tr	11	0	0.00	0.00	0.0	0
Puddings:														
Canned:														
Chocolate.................5-oz can...	205	3	11	9.5	1	30	74	1.2	285	100	0.04	0.17	0.6	Tr
Tapioca...................5-oz can...	160	3	5	4.8	Tr	28	119	0.3	252	Tr	0.03	0.14	0.4	Tr
Vanilla....................5-oz can...	220	2	10	9.5	1	33	79	0.2	305	Tr	0.03	0.12	0.6	Tr
Dry mix, prepared with whole milk:														
Chocolate:														
Instant................½ cup...	155	4	4	2.3	14	27	130	0.3	440	130	0.04	0.18	0.1	1
Regular (cooked)......½ cup...	150	4	4	2.4	15	25	146	0.2	167	140	0.05	0.20	0.1	1
Rice...................½ cup...	155	4	4	2.3	15	27	133	0.5	140	140	0.10	0.18	0.6	1
Tapioca...............½ cup...	145	4	4	2.3	15	25	131	0.1	152	140	0.04	0.18	0.1	1
Vanilla:														
Instant................½ cup...	150	4	4	2.2	15	27	129	0.1	375	140	0.04	0.17	0.1	1
Regular (cooked)......½ cup...	145	4	4	2.3	15	25	132	0.1	178	140	0.04	0.18	0.1	1
Sugars:														
Brown, pressed down...1 cup...	820	0	0	0.0	0	212	187	4.8	97	0	0.02	0.07	0.2	0
White:														
Granulated.............1 cup...	770	0	0	0.0	0	199	3	0.1	5	0	0.00	0.00	0.0	0
Powdered, sifted, spooned into cup...1 cup...	385	0	0	0.0	0	100	1	Tr	2	0	0.00	0.00	0.0	0
Syrups:														
Chocolate-flavored syrup or topping:														
Thin type.............2 tbsp...	85	1	Tr	0.2	0	22	6	0.8	36	Tr	Tr	0.02	0.1	0
Table syrup (corn and maple)..2 tbsp...	122	0	0	0.0	0	32	1	Tr	19	0	0.00	0.00	0.0	0

Foods

approximate measures, units, and weight (of edible portion only)

Foods	Nutrients in Indicated Quantity													
	Food energy	Protein	Fat	Saturated fat	Cholesterol	Carbohydrate	Calcium	Iron	Sodium	Vitamin A value (IU)	Thiamin	Riboflavin	Niacin	Ascorbic acid
	Calories	Grams	Grams	Grams	Milligrams	Grams	Milligrams	Milligrams	Milligrams	International units	Milligrams	Milligrams	Milligrams	Milligrams
Vegetables and Vegetable Products														
Beans:														
Lima, immature seeds, frozen, cooked, drained:														
Thin-seeded types (baby limas).........1 cup	190	12	1	0.1	0	35	50	3.5	52	300	0.13	0.10	1.4	10
Snap:														
Cooked, drained:														
From raw (cut and French style).........1 cup	45	2	Tr	0.1	0	10	58	1.6	4	830[34]	0.09	0.12	0.8	12
Canned, drained solids (cut).........1 cup	25	2	Tr	Tr	0	6	35	1.2	339[35]	470[36]	0.02	0.08	0.3	6
Beets:														
Cooked, drained:														
Diced or sliced.........1 cup	55	2	Tr	Tr	0	11	19	1.1	83	20	0.05	0.02	0.5	9
Black-eyed peas, immature seeds, cooked and drained:														
From raw.........1 cup	180	13	1	0.3	0	30	46	2.4	7	1,050	0.11	0.18	1.8	3
Broccoli:														
Raw.........1 spear	40	4	1	0.1	0	8	72	1.3	41	2,330	0.10	0.18	1.0	141
Cooked, drained:														
From raw:														
Spear, medium.........1 spear	50	5	1	0.1	0	10	82	2.1	20	2,540	0.15	0.37	1.4	113
Brussels sprouts, cooked, drained:														
From raw, 7–8 sprouts, 1¼ to 1½-in diam.........1 cup	60	4	1	0.2	0	13	56	1.9	33	1,110	0.17	0.12	0.9	96
Cabbage, common varieties:														

Foods — approximate measures, units, and weight (of edible portion only)	Nutrients in Indicated Quantity													
	Food energy Calories	Protein Grams	Fat Grams	Saturated fat Grams	Cholesterol Milligrams	Carbohydrate Grams	Calcium Milligrams	Iron Milligrams	Sodium Milligrams	Vitamin A value (IU) International units	Thiamin Milligrams	Riboflavin Milligrams	Niacin Milligrams	Ascorbic acid Milligrams
Raw, coarsely shredded or sliced ...... 1 cup........	15	1	Tr	Tr	0	4	33	0.4	13	90	0.04	0.02	0.2	33
Carrots:														
Raw:														
Whole, 7½ by 1⅛ in, or strips, 2½ to 3 in long........ 1 carrot or 18 strips........	30	1	Tr	Tr	0	7	19	0.4	25	20,250	0.07	0.04	0.7	7
Cooked, sliced, drained:														
From raw........ 1 cup........	70	2	Tr	0.1	0	16	48	1.0	103	38,300	0.05	0.09	0.8	4
Canned, sliced, drained solids. 1 cup........	35	1	Tr	0.1	0	8	37	0.9	352[37]	20,110	0.03	0.04	0.8	4
Cauliflower:														
Raw, (flowerets) .... 1 cup........	25	2	Tr	Tr	0	5	29	0.6	15	20	0.08	0.06	0.6	72
Cooked, drained:														
From raw (flowerets) .... 1 cup........	30	2	Tr	Tr	0	6	34	0.5	8	20	0.08	0.07	0.7	69
Celery, pascal type, raw:														
Stalk, large outer, 8 by 1½ in (at root end)........ 1 stalk	5	Tr	Tr	Tr	0	1	14	0.2	35	50	0.01	0.01	0.1	3
Pieces, diced........ 1 cup........	20	1	Tr	Tr	0	4	43	0.6	106	150	0.04	0.04	0.4	8
Collards, cooked, drained:														
From raw (leaves without stems) .... 1 cup........	25	2	Tr	0.1	0	5	148	0.8	36	4,220	0.03	0.08	0.4	19
Corn, sweet:														
Cooked, drained:														
From raw, ear 5 by 1¾ in...... 1 ear........	85	3	1	0.2	0	19	2	0.5	13	170[38]	0.17	0.06	1.2	5
Canned:														
Cream style........ 1 cup........	185	4	1	0.2	0	46	8	1.0	730[39]	250[38]	0.06	0.14	2.5	12
Whole kernel, vacuum pack........ 1 cup........	165	5	1	0.2	0	41	11	0.9	571[40]	510[38]	0.09	0.15	2.5	17

Foods — approximate measures, units, and weight (of edible portion only)	Nutrients in Indicated Quantity													
	Food energy	Protein	Fat	Saturated fat	Cholesterol	Carbohydrate	Calcium	Iron	Sodium	Vitamin A value (IU)	Thiamin	Riboflavin	Niacin	Ascorbic acid
	Calories	Grams	Grams	Grams	Milligrams	Grams	Milligrams	Milligrams	Milligrams	International units	Milligrams	Milligrams	Milligrams	Milligrams
Cucumber, with peel, slices, ⅛ in thick (large, 2⅛ in diam.; small, 1¾ in diam.) .....6 large or 8 small......	5	Tr	Tr	Tr	0	1	4	0.1	1	10	0.01	0.01	0.1	1
Lettuce, raw:														
Crisphead, as iceberg: Wedge, ¼ of head...........1 wedge......	20	1	Tr	Tr	0	3	26	0.7	12	450	0.06	0.04	0.3	5
Pieces, chopped or shredded ....1 cup......	5	1	Tr	Tr	0	1	10	0.3	5	180	0.03	0.02	0.1	2
Looseleaf (bunching varieties including romaine or cos), chopped or shredded pieces ....1 cup......	10	1	Tr	Tr	0	2	38	0.8	5	1,060	0.03	0.04	0.2	10
Mushrooms:														
Raw, sliced or chopped ....1 cup......	20	1	Tr	Tr	0	3	4	0.9	3	0	0.07	0.31	2.9	2
Cooked, drained ....1 cup......	40	3	1	0.1	0	8	9	2.7	3	0	0.11	0.47	7.0	6
Canned, drained solids.........1 cup......	35	3	Tr	0.1	0	8	17	1.2	663	0	0.13	0.03	2.5	0
Mustard greens, without stems and midribs, cooked, drained ...1 cup......	20	3	Tr	Tr	0	3	104	1.0	22	4,240	0.06	0.09	0.6	35
Okra pods, 3 by ⅝ in, cooked.................8 pods.....	25	2	Tr	Tr	0	6	54	0.4	4	490	0.11	0.05	0.7	14
Onions Raw: Sliced...............1 cup........	40	1	Tr	0.1	0	8	29	0.4	2	0	0.07	0.01	0.1	10
Cooked (whole or sliced), drained.................1 cup......	60	2	Tr	0.1	0	13	57	0.4	17	0	0.09	0.02	0.2	12
Peas, edible pod, cooked, drained ....1 cup......	65	5	Tr	0.1	0	11	67	3.2	6	210	0.20	0.12	0.9	77
Peas, green: Canned, drained solids.............1 cup......	115	8	1	0.1	0	21	34	1.6	372[41]	1,310	0.21	0.13	1.2	16

Foods	Nutrients in Indicated Quantity													
approximate measures, units, and weight (of edible portion only)	Food energy	Protein	Fat	Saturated fat	Cholesterol	Carbohydrate	Calcium	Iron	Sodium	Vitamin A value (IU)	Thiamin	Riboflavin	Niacin	Ascorbic acid
	Calories	Grams	Grams	Grams	Milligrams	Grams	Milligrams	Milligrams	Milligrams	International units	Milligrams	Milligrams	Milligrams	Milligrams
Potatoes, cooked:														
Baked (about 2 per lb, raw):														
With skin ....1 potato	220	5	Tr	0.1	0	51	20	2.7	16	0	0.22	0.07	3.3	26
Flesh only ....1 potato	145	3	Tr	Tr	0	34	8	0.5	8	0	0.16	0.03	2.2	20
Boiled (about 3 per lb, raw):														
Peeled after boiling ....1 potato	120	3	Tr	Tr	0	27	7	0.4	5	0	0.14	0.03	2.0	18
Peeled before boiling ....1 potato	115	2	Tr	Tr	0	27	11	0.4	7	0	0.13	0.03	1.8	10
French fried, strip, 2 to 3½ in long, frozen:														
Oven heated ....10 strips.......	110	2	4	2.1	0	17	5	0.7	16	0	0.06	0.02	1.2	5
Potato products, prepared:														
Au gratin:														
From home recipe ....1 cup........	325	12	19	11.6	56	28	292	1.6	1,061	650	0.16	0.28	2.4	24
Hashed brown, from frozen ....1 cup........	340	5	18	7.0	0	44	23	2.4	53	0	0.17	0.03	3.8	10
Mashed:														
From home recipe:														
Milk added ....1 cup........	160	4	1	0.7	4	37	55	0.6	636	40	0.18	0.08	2.3	14
Milk and margarine added ....1 cup........	225	4	9	2.2	4	35	55	0.5	620	360	0.18	0.08	2.3	13
Scalloped:														
From home recipe ....1 cup........	210	7	9	5.5	29	26	140	1.4	821	330	0.17	0.23	2.6	26
Pumpkin:														
Canned ....1 cup........	85	3	1	0.4	0	20	64	3.4	12	54,040	0.06	0.13	0.9	10
Spinach:														
Raw, chopped..................1 cup........	10	2	Tr	Tr	0	2	54	1.5	43	3,690	0.04	0.10	0.4	15
Cooked, drained:														
From raw ....1 cup........	40	5	Tr	0.1	0	7	245	6.4	126	14,740	0.17	0.42	0.9	18
Canned, drained solids.....1 cup........	50	6	1	0.2	0	7	272	4.9	683[42]	18,780	0.03	0.30	0.8	31

Nutrients in Indicated Quantity

Foods (approximate measures, units, and weight (of edible portion only))	Food energy (Calories)	Protein (Grams)	Fat (Grams)	Saturated fat (Grams)	Cholesterol (Milligrams)	Carbohydrate (Grams)	Calcium (Milligrams)	Iron (Milligrams)	Sodium (Milligrams)	Vitamin A value (International units)	Thiamin (Milligrams)	Riboflavin (Milligrams)	Niacin (Milligrams)	Ascorbic acid (Milligrams)
Squash, cooked:														
Summer (all varieties), sliced, drained... 1 cup	35	2	1	0.1	0	8	49	0.6	2	520	0.08	0.07	0.9	10
Winter (all varieties), baked, cubes... 1 cup	80	2	1	0.3	0	18	29	0.7	2	7,290	0.17	0.05	1.4	20
Sweet potatoes:														
Cooked (raw, 5 by 2 in; about 2½ per lb):														
Baked in skin, peeled... 1 potato	115	2	Tr	Tr	0	28	32	0.5	11	24,880	0.08	0.14	0.7	28
Boiled, without skin... 1 potato	160	2	Tr	0.1	0	37	32	0.8	20	25,750	0.08	0.21	1.0	26
Canned:														
Solid pack (mashed)... 1 cup	260	5	1	0.1	0	59	77	3.4	191	38,570	0.07	0.23	2.4	13
Vacuum pack, piece 2¾ by 1 in... 1 piece	35	1	Tr	Tr	0	8	9	0.4	21	3,190	0.01	0.02	0.3	11
Tomatoes:														
Raw, 2⅗ in diam. (3 per 12 oz pkg.)... 1 tomato	25	1	Tr	Tr	0	5	9	0.6	10	1,390	0.07	0.06	0.7	22
Canned, solids and liquid... 1 cup	50	2	1	0.1	0	10	62	1.5	391[43]	1,450	0.11	0.07	1.8	36
Tomato juice, canned... 1 cup	40	2	Tr	Tr	0	10	22	1.4	881[44]	1,360	0.11	0.08	1.6	45
Tomato products, canned:														
Paste... 1 cup	220	10	2	0.3	0	49	92	7.8	170[45]	6,470	0.41	0.50	8.4	111
Sauce... 1 cup	75	3	Tr	0.1	0	18	34	1.9	1,482[46]	2,400	0.16	0.14	2.8	32
Turnip greens, cooked, drained:														
From raw (leaves and stems)... 1 cup	30	2	Tr	0.1	0	6	197	1.2	42	7,920	0.06	0.10	0.6	39

Appendix B: continued

[1] Carbohydrate content varies widely because of amount of sugar added and amount and solids content of added flavoring. Consult the label if more precise values for carbohydrate and calories are needed.

[2] For salted butter; unsalted butter contains 12 mg sodium per stick, 2 mg per tbsp, or 1 mg per pat.

[3] Values for vitamin A are year-round average.

[4] For salted margarine.

[5] Based on average vitamin A content of fortified margarine. Federal specifications for fortified margarine require a minimum of 15,000 IU per pound.

[6] Dipped in egg, milk, and breadcrumbs; fried in vegetable shortening.

[7] If bones are discarded, value for calcium will be greatly reduced.

[8] Dipped in egg, breadcrumbs, and flour; fried in vegetable shortening.

[9] Made with drained chunk light tuna, celery, onion, pickle relish, and mayonnaise-type salad dressing.

[10] Also applies to pasteurized apple cider.

[11] Without added ascorbic acid. For value with added ascorbic acid, refer to label.

[12] With added ascorbic acid.

[13] For white grapefruit; pink grapefruit have about 310 IU or 31 RE.

[14] Without added ascorbic acid. For value with added ascorbic acid, refer to label.

[15] With added ascorbic acid.

[16] Egg bagels have 44 mg cholesterol and 22 IU or 7 RE vitamin A per bagel.

[17] Made with vegetable shortening.

[18] Nutrient added.

[19] Value based on label declaration for added nutrients.

[20] For regular and instant cereal. For quick cereal, sodium is 142 mg.

[21] Cooked without salt. If salt is added according to label recommendations, sodium content is 390 mg.

[22] Cooked without salt. If salt is added according to label recommendations, sodium content is 374 mg.

[23] Value based on label declaration for added nutrients.

[24] Excepting angelfood cake, cakes were made from mixes containing vegetable shortening and frostings were made with margarine.

[25] Made with vegetable oil.

[26] Made with vegetable shortening.

[27] Crackers made with enriched flour except for rye wafers and whole-wheat wafers.

[28] Made with lard.

[29] Made with vegetable shortening.

[30] Made with vegetable oil.

[31] Contains added sodium ascorbate. If sodium ascorbate is not added, ascorbic acid content is negligible.

[32] One patty (8 per pound) of bulk sausage is equivalent to 2 links.

[33] Fried in vegetable shortening.

[34] For green varieties; yellow varieties contain 101 IU or 10 RE.

[35] For regular pack; special dietary pack contains 3 mg sodium.

[36] For green varieties; yellow varieties contain 142 IU or 14 RE.

[37] For regular pack; special dietary pack contains 61 mg sodium.

[38] For yellow varieties; white varieties contain only a trace of vitamin A.

[39] For regular pack; special dietary pack contains 8 mg sodium.

[40] For regular pack; special dietary pack contains 6 mg sodium.

[41] For regular pack; special dietary pack contains 3 mg sodium.

[42] With added salt; if none is added, sodium content is 58 mg.

[43] For regular pack; special dietary pack contains 31 mg sodium.

[44] With added salt; if none is added, sodium content is 24 mg.

[45] With no added salt; if salt is added, sodium content is 2,070 mg.

[46] With salt added.

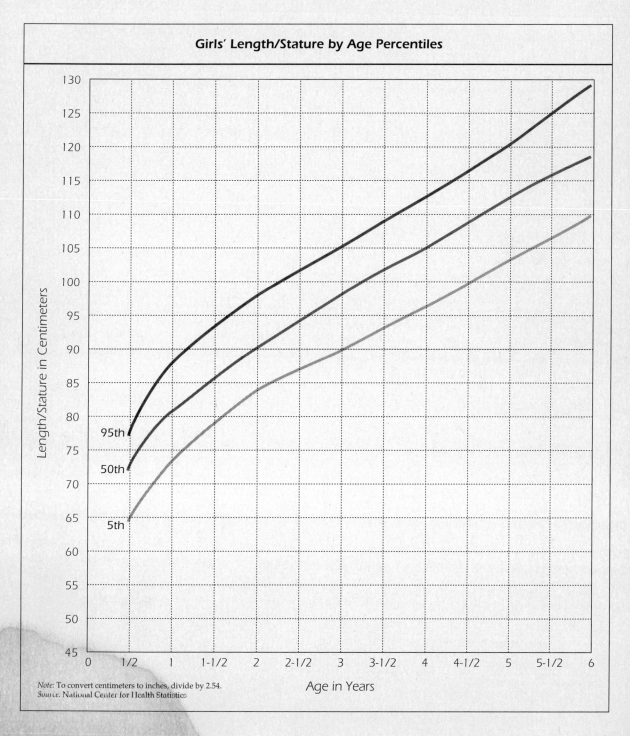

Girls' Length/Stature by Age Percentiles

Length/Stature in Centimeters (y-axis)

Age in Years (x-axis)

95th

50th

5th

Note: To convert centimeters to inches, divide by 2.54.
Source: National Center for Health Statistics

Appendix C: continued

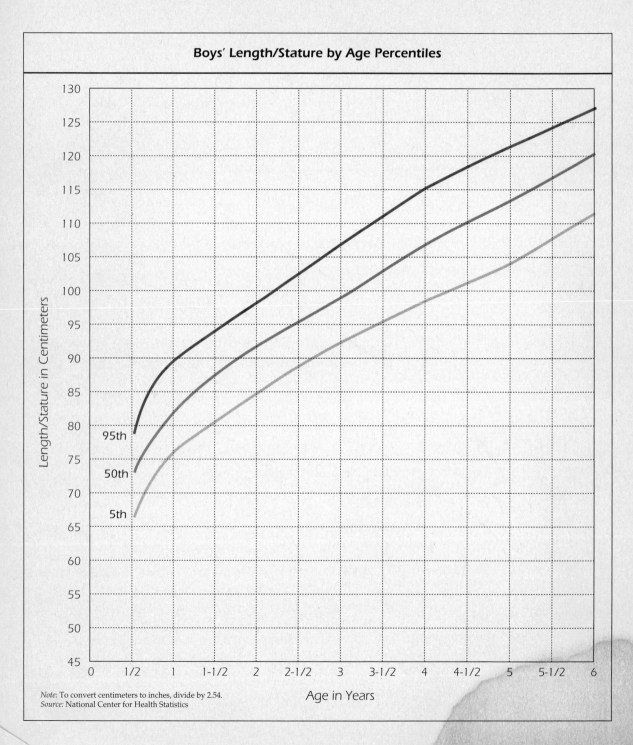

Boys' Length/Stature by Age Percentiles

Length/Stature in Centimeters

95th

50th

5th

Age in Years

Note: To convert centimeters to inches, divide by 2.54.
Source: National Center for Health Statistics

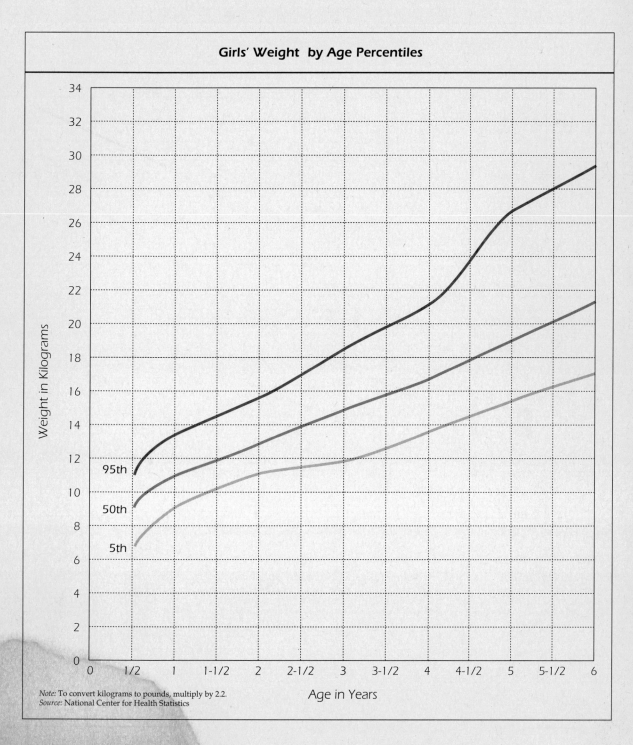

Girls' Weight by Age Percentiles

Note: To convert kilograms to pounds, multiply by 2.2.
Source: National Center for Health Statistics

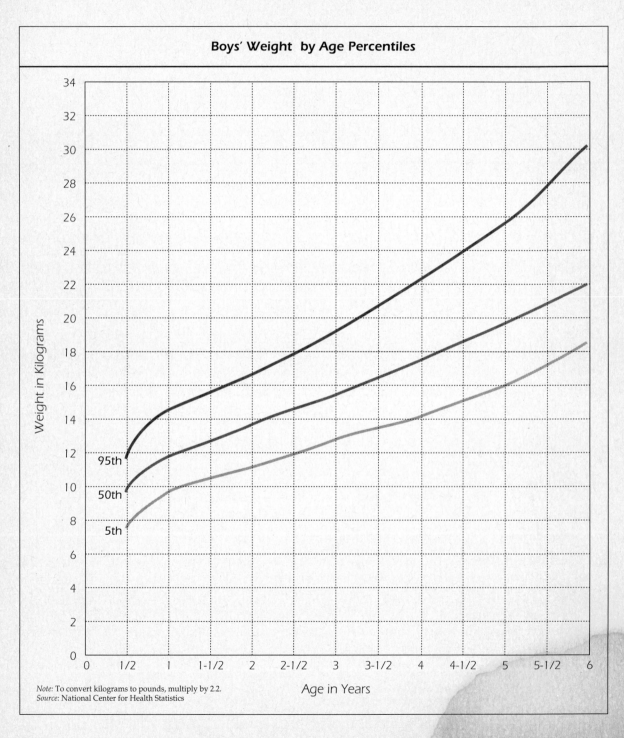

Boys' Weight by Age Percentiles

Weight in Kilograms

95th

50th

5th

Note: To convert kilograms to pounds, multiply by 2.2.
Source: National Center for Health Statistics

Age in Years

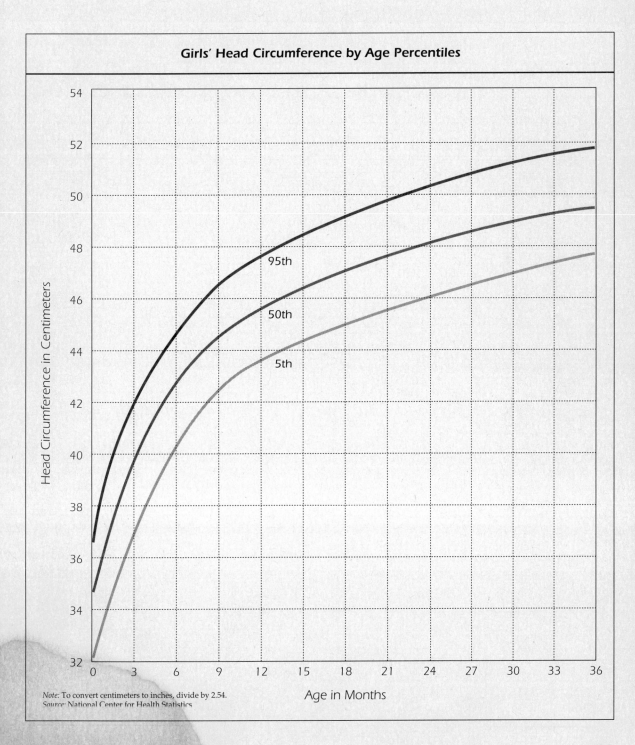

Girls' Head Circumference by Age Percentiles

Head Circumference in Centimeters

95th

50th

5th

Age in Months

Note: To convert centimeters to inches, divide by 2.54.
Source: National Center for Health Statistics

Appendix C: continued

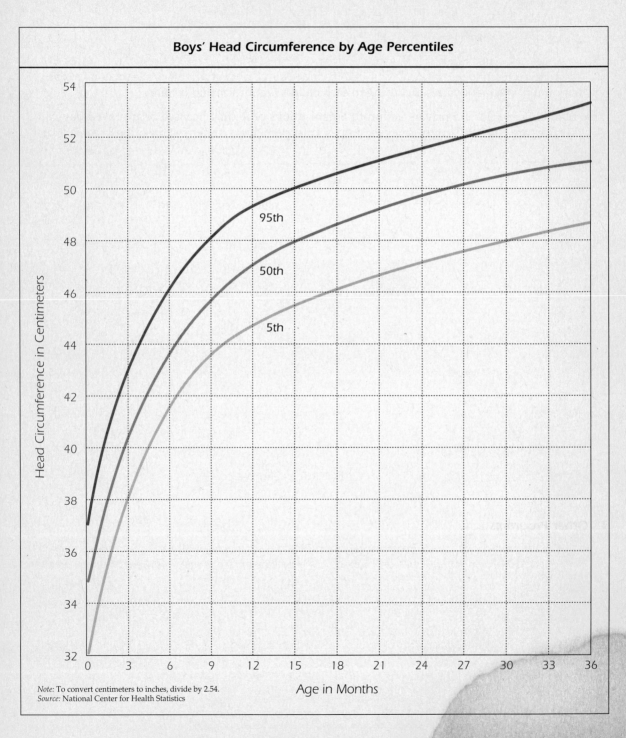

Boys' Head Circumference by Age Percentiles

Note: To convert centimeters to inches, divide by 2.54.
Source: National Center for Health Statistics

Appendix D
Federal Food Programs

1. **The Child Care Food Program**
   - Services: Provides reimbursement for one meal and two snacks or two meals and one snack per day served to children under 12 enrolled in child-care centers or private day-care homes. The amount of payment varies according to each child's family size and income.
   - Eligibility: Public and private nonprofit organizations providing licensed or approved day-care services are eligible. Family day-care homes must participate under a sponsoring organization.
   - Administration: Provided at the state level by the Department of Education.

2. **Special Supplemental Program for Women, Infants, and Children (WIC)**
   - Services: Provides health care referrals, nutrition counseling, and the following foods: iron-fortified infant formula, iron-fortified cereal, fruit/vegetable juices high in vitamin C, fortified milk, cheese, eggs, peanut butter, and dried beans or peas.
   - Eligibility: Pregnant or lactating women, infants, and children up to 5 years of age. Participants must be at nutritional risk and must meet state income standards.
   - Administration: Provided at the state level by the Department of Health.

3. **The Food Stamp Program**
   - Services: Participants buy stamps that are worth more than the purchase price, or they receive them free. Stamps can be exchanged for seeds or *allowed foods,* which do not include soap, cigarettes, paper goods, alcoholic beverages, pet foods, or deli foods that may be eaten on the premises.
   - Eligibility: Low income persons who meet state or local requirements.
   - Administration: Provided by state or local welfare agencies.

4. **Other Programs**
   - The National School Lunch Program reimburses states for nutritionally adequate meals served in schools. Some families may be eligible for free or reduced price meals, based on national poverty guidelines.
   - The School Breakfast Program provides full price, reduced price, and free breakfasts in schools and residential child care facilities.
   - The Summer Food Service Program for Children provides free meals and snacks to children in economically depressed areas during the summer months. School food authorities and state, city, or private summer camps are eligible.

Further information about any of the above programs may be obtained by calling the Federal Information Center at 1-800-347-1997.

Glossary

A

acute stage Time period in the course of an infectious illness during which a person displays definite symptoms typical of a specific infection. [Ch. 11]

allergen Any substance that causes an allergic reaction. [Ch. 9]

amino acids The building blocks of proteins. [Ch. 3]

anemia Condition in which insufficient hemoglobin or red blood cells are present to carry oxygen from the lungs to all parts of the body. [Ch. 9]

antioxidant A substance that removes free radicals, by-products of metabolism that can damage cells and their genetic material. [Ch. 3]

appetite A psychological desire to eat, usually influenced by food habits and a pleasant association with food. [Ch. 2]

aspiration The inhaling of a foreign object into the airway; it is the leading cause of accidental death in infants. [Ch. 6]

asthma A condition in which swelling of lung tissues interferes with breathing. [Ch. 10]

attitudes A person's feelings, beliefs, or opinions about a person, object, or event. [Ch. 14]

attractive nuisance An object that entices people to a restricted area or private property and may also pose a danger. [Ch. 12]

B

bottle-feeding Using a bottle to provide nourishment to a baby. [Ch. 6]

breast-feeding Providing nourishment to a baby directly from the mother's breast. [Ch. 6]

C

calories A measure of energy applied to the energy content of food and the amount of energy the body uses for physiological processes. [Ch. 3]

carrier Person whose body contains a disease organism and who spreads it to other people without showing symptoms of the disease himself. [Ch. 11]

child abuse According to Kendrick, Kaufmann, and Messenger, a nonaccidental injury or pattern of injuries to a child for which there is no 'reasonable' explanation (Kendrick, et al., 1991). [Ch. 13]

child-initiated Approach to curriculum in which children are given opportunities to choose their own activities and decide for themselves how to explore new materials and pursue new experiences. [Ch. 14]

child neglect The failure of a parent to provide for the physical care, safety, education, and emotional well-being of a child. [Ch. 13]

cholesterol A fatlike substance important in human metabolism and found only in animals. [Ch. 3]

chronic Persisting for a long time; chronic disorders are not generally communicable. [Ch. 10]

communicable diseases Infections that can be passed from one person to another. [Ch. 11]

communication The exchange of messages between people. [Ch. 15]

complete proteins Dietary proteins that contain all nine essential amino acids. [Ch. 3]

complex carbohydrates Chains of chemically linked glucose units that may serve as a fuel source for the body (dietary fiber is the exception). [Ch. 3]

cooperative Type of preschool in which parent governing boards make policy decisions and hire staff members, act as assistants for teachers, and generally participate in the operations of the school. [Ch. 15]

critical periods Time frames during which children should have appropriate experiences if they are to continue to develop normally. [Ch. 6]

cross-contamination The spread of bacteria from one food to another. [Ch. 4]

culture The beliefs, customs, knowledge, and habits that people share. [Ch. 2]

curriculum The process of identifying goals and making plans to provide educational experiences for young children. [Ch. 14]

cystic fibrosis An inherited disease that affects the mucus-producing glands of both the lungs and the digestive system. [Ch. 9]

D

deficiency disease A condition that may result from a diet lacking in a particular nutrient or group of nutrients. [Ch. 5]

dehydration Serious loss of water from the body. [Ch. 5]

dental caries Tooth decay. [Ch. 4]

development A change in function from simple to more complex. [Ch. 5]

diabetes mellitus Condition in which the body produces an inadequate amount of the hormone insulin. [Ch. 9]

dietary fiber The parts of plants that cannot be fully broken down in the human digestive tract. [Ch. 3]

drowning To suffocate by submersion in water or another liquid. [Ch. 12]

E

eczema A condition characterized by skin inflammation; it may be a symptom of a food allergy. [Ch. 9]

electrolytes Substances that maintain the proper water balance within the body by regulating fluids that move into and out of every cell; they are also needed for sending nerve impulses throughout the body. [Ch. 3]

emotional abuse Verbally threatening, rejecting, ignoring, belittling, isolating, or placing unreasonable demands on a child. [Ch. 13]

enriched A governmentally regulated descriptor used on grain products. An enriched product must include such vitamins and minerals as niacin, thiamin, riboflavin, folic acid, and iron. [Ch. 4]

entrapment Situation in which a child enters an appliance, shuts the door, and is unable to open it from inside. [Ch. 12]

enzymes Proteins that speed up chemical reactions in the body. [Ch. 5]

ethnic foods Foods common to a specific ethnic group. A preference for these foods is often passed on from parents to children generation after generation. [Ch. 2]

F

failure to thrive Failure to grow at the expected rate over time. [Ch. 5]

fatty acids The building blocks of fats. [Ch. 3]

fetal alcohol syndrome Abnormal development of a fetus caused by the mother's use of alcohol during pregnancy. [Ch. 10]

fine motor skills Abilities that require control of the small muscles of the body. [Ch. 5]

flame-retardant Difficult to set on fire; often used to describe specially prepared fabrics. [Ch. 12]

food allergy Condition in which the body's immune system reacts to a food substance as if it were an attacking organism. [Ch. 9]

food-borne illness Food poisoning; results from eating food that has been contaminated by bacteria or the poisons some bacteria produce. [Ch. 4]

food environment The sum total of a child's encounters with food, including such elements as furniture, utensils, cleanliness, atmosphere, eating companions, and meal scheduling. [Ch. 2]

Food Guide Pyramid A visual aid, designed by the U. S. Department of Agriculture, that translates commonly accepted dietary guidelines into daily food selection advice. [Ch. 4]

food intolerances Conditions in which the body lacks an enzyme or enzymes needed to make use of a particular food. [Ch. 9]

food jags Periods of days or weeks during which toddlers become obsessive about certain foods. [Ch. 7]

food patterns How, when, where, and how much food people eat. [Ch. 2]

food preferences Propensities toward certain types of food preparation or certain groups of foods; characteristic of most preschoolers. [Ch. 8]

frostbite   Freezing of body tissues from exposure to cold temperatures. [Ch. 13]

G

glycogen   A form of carbohydrate, made by the body from glucose, that is stored in the muscles, liver, and other body cells. [Ch. 3]

gross motor skills   Abilities that involve the use of large muscle groups. [Ch. 5]

growth   Process that occurs when cells increase in number and/or size. [Ch. 5]

H

HDL cholesterol   High-density lipoprotein cholesterol; sometimes called "good cholesterol," it is associated with a lower risk of cholesterol deposits on artery walls. [Ch. 3]

health   The state of a person's overall physical, mental, and emotional well-being. [Ch. 1]

heat exhaustion   Condition resulting from dehydration and/or the loss of salts from the body due to excessive exposure to high temperatures. [Ch. 13]

hemophilia   A condition in which blood does not clot properly. [Ch. 10]

heredity   The sum of the traits, characteristics, and defects that are passed from parents to their children through genetic mechanisms. [Ch. 1]

hormones   Substances formed in one organ and carried, usually by the bloodstream, to another organ whose function they regulate. [Ch. 5]

host   Person or animal on which parasites live and from which they draw their nourishment. [Ch. 11]

hunger   A physical sensation signaling that it is time to eat. [Ch. 2]

hyperlipidemia   The presence of excess lipids, including cholesterol, in the blood. [Ch. 9]

hypertension   High blood pressure. [Ch. 4]

I

immunization   A process that stimulates the immune system to make substances that protect the body from specific infectious diseases. [Ch. 10]

incest   Sexual activity among members of a family who are not married to one another. [Ch. 13]

incubation period   Length of time between the contraction and the onset of an infectious illness during which a pathogen multiplies inside the body without giving signs that the person is infected. [Ch. 11]

infant botulism   A disease caused when spores of the *Clostridium botulinum* bacterium grow in an infant's intestines and release a poison. The spores are sometimes found in honey. [Ch. 6]

infectious diseases   Conditions caused by organisms capable of entering the body and damaging tissue. [Ch. 11]

instructional objective   An expression of the intended outcome of a lesson. It states the specific skill, behavior, knowledge, or attitude that the teacher wants the children to acquire, accomplish, or understand. [Ch. 14]

iron-deficiency anemia   Anemia caused by a lack of iron. Symptoms may include weakness, fatigue, headaches, and irritability. [Ch. 5]

L

lactose intolerance   An inability to digest lactose, the sugar found in milk. [Ch. 9]

LDL cholesterol   Low-density lipoprotein cholesterol; often called "bad cholesterol," at high levels it tends to deposit cholesterol on artery walls. [Ch. 3]

legumes   Edible seeds found in the pods of certain plants; they include beans, peas, lentils, peanuts, and soybeans and are a source of high-quality protein. [Ch. 3]

listening skills   Abilities to concentrate on what is being said and to participate actively in the communication process. [Ch. 15]

M

malabsorption   Poor assimilation into the body; with iron, it can cause iron-deficiency anemia. [Ch. 9]

malnutrition   A condition that results when a person is poorly nourished for an extended period of time. [Ch. 1]

mechanical suffocation Fatal condition that occurs when oxygen cannot get to the lungs because an object is covering the mouth or nose, pressure is being placed upon the throat or chest, or a person is trapped in an airtight enclosed space. [Ch. 12]

metabolism The whole range of physical and chemical processes that sustain life. [Ch. 3]

minerals Substances that help regulate body processes. Minerals, unlike many vitamins, are not destroyed by heat. [Ch. 3]

molars The broad-surfaced teeth at the back of the mouth that are used for grinding food. [Ch. 7]

mouth patterns Ways that babies manipulate food in their mouths, including rooting and suckling reflexes, sucking, and chewing. [Ch. 6]

N

noncommunicable diseases Infections that do not pass from person to person. [Ch. 11]

nursing bottle syndrome Tooth decay that results when babies are repeatedly permitted to fall asleep while drinking from their bottles. [Ch. 6]

nutrient density A measure of the ratio of the amount of nutrients to the number of calories supplied by a food. [Ch. 4]

nutrients Substances in food that provide nourishment and help the body to function. [Ch. 1]

nutrition The study and science of the foods people consume as well as the physical processes involved in taking in and using food. [Ch. 1]

nutritional status A comparison of ingested nutrients with those required for growth and health. [Ch. 5]

O

obesity The excessive storing of fat in the body. [Ch. 9]

observation Watching and listening to classroom activities, usually without direct participation. [Ch. 15]

otitis media Infection of the middle ear; it is a common complication of colds and throat infections in young children. [Ch. 10]

overnutrition A condition caused by consuming too much of one or more nutrients. [Ch. 1]

P

palmar grasp Type of grip in which the four fingers hold an object against the palm of the hand. [Ch. 6]

pathogens Disease-causing organisms. [Ch. 11]

Percent Daily Value Unit of nutritional information included on a packaged food label. Provided for various nutrients in the product, it is expressed as a percentage of the amount of the nutrient that an average person needs for a 2,000- or 2,500-calorie-a-day diet. [Ch. 4]

phenylketonuria Often called PKU; condition caused by the inability to metabolize properly the essential amino acid phenylalanine. [Ch. 9]

physical abuse Injuring a child by shaking, hitting, beating, burning, or performing other violent acts. [Ch. 13]

pincer grasp Type of grip in which an object is held between the thumb and forefinger. [Ch. 6]

prodromal stage Time period in the course of an infectious illness during which a person begins to show nonspecific signs of sickness such as restlessness, discomfort, mild fever, or headaches. [Ch. 11]

R

Recommended Dietary Allowances Amounts of key nutrients, suggested by the Food and Nutrition Board of the National Research Council, that an average healthy person needs each day for optimum health. [Ch. 4]

recovery stage Time period in the course of an infectious illness during which the symptoms begin to disappear and health gradually returns. [Ch. 11]

reflective statement A restatement of another person's feelings or concerns made to show that the feelings are understood and valued. [Ch. 15]

reportable disease   Illness whose occurrence must, by law, be reported to local or state public health agencies. [Ch. 11]

rickets   A deficiency disease caused by a lack of vitamin D and characterized by improper formation of the bones. [Ch. 5]

rituals   A characteristic of toddler behavior involving rigidly specific circumstances or requirements—often relating to food. [Ch. 7]

S

safety   Freedom from risk, harm, and injury. [Ch. 1]

satiety   A feeling of fullness or satisfaction that comes with eating. [Ch. 2]

saturated fats   Fats that contain mostly saturated fatty acids; they are usually solid at room temperature. [Ch. 3]

screenings   Tests performed on apparently healthy people, designed to detect disorders at an early stage. [Ch. 10]

seizure disorder   Commonly known as epilepsy, this condition is caused by unusually strong discharges of electricity in the brain. [Ch. 10]

sexual abuse   Exploiting a child for the sexual gratification of an adult. [Ch. 13]

shock   Condition in which insufficient blood reaches important parts of the body. [Ch. 13]

sickle-cell disease   A condition in which the red blood cells are misshapen and unable to carry necessary oxygen to the body's tissues. [Ch. 10]

skinfold measurement   Test that uses a caliper (a measuring instrument) to determine the amount of fat under the skin at specific locations on the body. [Ch. 8]

sudden infant death syndrome   Commonly called SIDS, it refers to instances in which a child suddenly and unexpectedly dies in her crib. [Ch. 10]

sunburn   Inflammation of the skin, ranging from mild reddening to extensive blistering, caused by prolonged exposure to the sun. [Ch. 13]

T

teacher-directed   Approach to curriculum in which the teacher determines and leads the lesson or activity. [Ch. 14]

teething   The process whereby an infant's teeth erupt through the gums into the mouth. [Ch. 6]

tissue differentiation   The separation and specialization of groups of cells by function. Occurs in the development of an embryo. [Ch. 5]

toxic   Harmful or poisonous, especially to people. [Ch. 12]

transition times   Periods when one activity is ending and another is about to begin. [Ch. 14]

U

undernutrition   A condition caused by not eating enough foods containing essential nutrients. [Ch. 1]

unintentional injuries   Accidents; injuries that could have been foreseen and possibly prevented. [Ch. 12]

universal precautions   Preventive measures people should take in order to avoid infection; they are used whenever it is necessary to handle body fluids, which may contain infectious organisms. [Ch. 11]

usable space   Total area in a child care center that is free of furniture and equipment and is available for play. [Ch. 12]

V

vegetarian   Term that encompasses a variety of eating styles in which plant sources of foods are central. [Ch. 4]

vitamins   Substances that help regulate body processes. Unlike minerals, many vitamins can be destroyed by heat. [Ch. 3]

W

weaning   The process of changing a child's food pattern from obtaining nourishment from the breast or bottle to drinking from a cup and eating table food. [Ch. 6]

References

ABOUD, F. (1988). *Children and prejudice.* New York: Basil Blackwell.

AINSWORTH, M. D. S., & WITTIG, B. A. (1969). Attachment and the exploratory behavior of one-year-olds in a strange situation. In B. M. Foss (Ed.), *Determinants of infant behavior* (Vol. 4, pp. 113–136). London: Methuen.

ALFORD, B. B., & BOGLE, M. L. (1982). *Nutrition during the life cycle.* Englewood Cliffs, NJ: Prentice-Hall.

ALTMAN, L. K. (1993, August 10). Sleeping face down seems to put babies at risk, studies say. *The New York Times*, C11.

AMERICAN ACADEMY OF PEDIATRICS, COMMITTEE ON NUTRITION. (1989). Iron fortified infant formulas, *Pediatrics, 84*, 114–115.

AMERICAN PUBLIC HEALTH ASSOCIATION & THE AMERICAN ACADEMY OF PEDIATRICS. (1992). *Caring for our children, national health and safety performance standards: Guidelines for out-of-home child care programs.* Elk Grove Village, IL, and Washington, DC: Author.

ANDERSEN, R. D., BALE JR., J., BLACKMAN, J., & MURPH, J. (1986). *Infections in children.* Rockville, MD: Aspen Publishers.

BARER-STEIN, T. (1991). *You eat what you are: A study of ethnic food traditions.* Toronto: Culture Concepts.

BASSUK, E. L., & ROSENBERG, L. (1990). Psychosocial characteristics of homeless children and children with homes. *Pediatrics, 85* (3), 257–261.

BJORKLUND, G., & BERGER, C. (1987). Making conferences work for parents, teachers, and children. *Young children, 41* (2), 26–31.

BRODY, J. (1993, August 11). Skipping vaccinations puts children at risk. *The New York Times*, C11.

BROWN, J. D., & SIEGEL, J. M. (1988). Exercise as a buffer of life stress: A prospective study of adolescent health. *Health Psychology, 7* (4), 341–353.

BURT, J. V., & HERTZLER, A. A. (1978). Parental influence on the child's food preference. *Journal of Nutrition Education, 10*, 127–128.

CARLSSON-PAIGE, N., & LEVIN, D. E. (1992). Making peace in violent times: A constructivist approach to conflict resolution. *Young Child.* Washington, DC: National Association for the Education of Young Children.

CENTERS FOR DISEASE CONTROL, Chicken Pox (Varicella) Statistics, Document #248006, July 8, 1992.

CHILD HEALTH ALERT. (1993, January). Reader's mailbag, p. 3.

CHILDREN'S DEFENSE FUND. (1992). *The state of America's children 1991.* Washington, DC: Author.

CHIRA, S. (1993, September 22). Census data show rise in child care by fathers. *The New York Times*, A20.

CORNACCHIA, H. J., OLSEN, L., & NICKERSON, C. J. (1991). *Health in elementary schools* (8th ed.). St. Louis: Mosby–Year Book.

CRANWELL, P. D. (1984). Blood pressure teaching and screening programs for school children in grades 5–8. *Home Healthcare Nurse, 2* (3), 42–46.

CRESSWELL, W. H., & NEWMAN, I. M. (1993). *School health practice* (10th ed.). St. Louis: Mosby–Year Book.

DIETZ, W. H., & GORTMAKER, S. L. (1985). Do we fatten our children at the television set? Obesity and television viewing in children and adolescents. *Pediatrics, 75*, 807–812.

DIVISION OF INJURY CONTROL, CENTER FOR ENVIRONMENTAL HEALTH AND INJURY CONTROL, CENTERS FOR DISEASE CONTROL. (1990). Childhood injuries in the United States. *American Journal of Diseases of Children, 144* (6), 627–646.

DRAKE, M. A. (1992, May-June). The nutritional status and dietary adequacy of single homeless women and their children in shelters. *Public Health Reports, 107,* 312+.

EDELSTEIN, S. (1992). *Nutrition and meal planning in child-care programs: A practical guide.* Chicago: The American Dietetic Association.

EIGER, M. S., & OLDS, S. W. (1987). *The complete book of breastfeeding.* New York: Workman.

FARLEY, D. (1992, May). Vegetarian diets: The pluses and the pitfalls. *FDA Consumer,* pp. 21–22.

FARRELL, K. A. (1985). *Reach out and teach.* New York: American Foundation for the Blind.

FENWICK, K. (1993, September). Diffusing conflict with parents: A model for communication. *Exchange,* pp. 59–60.

FETAL ALCOHOL SYNDROME—UNITED STATES, 1979–1992. (1993). *Morbidity and Mortality Weekly Reports (MMWR), 42* (17), 339–341.

GALLER, J. R. (1984). Behavioral consequences of malnutrition in early life. In J. R. Galler (Ed.), *Nutrition and behavior* (pp. 63–117). New York: Plenum.

GREER, F., & MARSHALL, S. (1989). Bone mineral content, serum vitamin D metabolite concentrations, and ultraviolet B light exposure in infants fed human milk with and without vitamin D_2 supplements. *Journal of Pediatrics, 114* (2), 203–212.

HENDRICK, J. (1990). *Total learning: Developmental curriculum for the young child* (3rd ed.). Columbus, OH: Merrill.

HENDRICK, J. (1992). *The whole child: Developmental education for the early years* (5th ed.). New York: Merrill/Macmillan.

HILDEBRAND, V. (1990). *Guiding young children* (4th ed.). New York: Macmillan.

Implications for day-care: Epidemic of food poisoning on the west coast . . . , (1993, February). *Child Health Alert, 11,* 1–2.

INSTITUTE OF MEDICINE. (1991). *Improving America's diet and health.* Report of the Committee on Dietary Guidelines Implementation, Food and Nutrition Board. Washington, DC: National Academy Press.

JEWELL, D. S. (1988). The psychology of stress: Run silent, run deep. *Advances in Experimental Medicine and Biology, 245,* 341–352.

KATZ, P. (1982). Development of children's racial awareness and intergroup attitudes. In L. Katz (Ed.), *Current topics in early childhood education* (Vol. 4, pp. 17–54). Norwood, NJ: Ablex.

KENDRICK, A. S., KAUFMANN, R., & MESSENGER, K. P. (Eds.). (1991). *Healthy young children: A manual for programs.* Washington, DC: National Association for the Education of Young Children.

KITTLER, P. G., & SUCHER, K. (1989). *Food and culture in America.* New York: Van Nostrand Reinhold.

LANZKOWSKY, P. (1985). Problems in diagnosis of iron deficiency anemia. *Pediatric Annuls, 14* (9), 618–636.

LOWENBERG, M., TODHUNTER, E. N., WILSON, E. D., SAVAGE, J. R., & LUBAWSKI, J. L. (1979). *Food and people.* New York: Macmillan.

LOWRY, R., & SAMUELSON, R. (1993, April 12). How many battered children? *National Review,* p. 46.

MATAS, L., AREND, R., & SROUFE, L. A. (1978). Continuity of adaptation in the second year: The relationship between quality of attachment and later competence. *Child Development, 49,* 547–556.

McBEAN, L. (1993, March/April). Breakfast: Its effects on health and behavior. *Dairy Council Digest, 64,* 2.

MCBEAN, L. (1993, September/October). Calcium: Newly emerging roles in disease prevention. *Dairy Council Digest, 64,* 5.

MILUNSKY, A. (1987). *How to have the healthiest baby you can.* New York: Simon & Schuster.

MITCHELL, A. (Ed.). (1993, March). Diet and Nutrition. *Child Health Alert, 11,* 4–6.

MOTT, S. R., JAMES, S. R., & SPERHAC, A. M. (1990). *Nursing care of children and families* (2nd ed.). Redwood City, CA: Addison-Wesley Nursing.

NATIONAL CENTER FOR THE PREVENTION OF CHILD ABUSE. (1988). *Basic facts about child sexual abuse* (3rd ed.). Chicago: Author.

NATIONAL RESEARCH COUNCIL. (1989). *Diet and health: Implications for reducing chronic disease risk.* Report of the Committee on Diet and Health, Food and Nutrition Board. Washington, DC: National Academy Press.

NATIONAL RESEARCH COUNCIL. (1989). *Recommended dietary allowances* (10th ed.). Washington, DC: National Academy Press.

NEWBURGER, J. (1990). Management of dyslipidemia in childhood and adolescence. In D. F. Fyler (Ed.), *Nadas's pediatric cardiology.* Philadelphia: Hanly & Belfus.

NORA, J. J., & FRASER, F. C. (1989). *Medical genetics* (3rd ed.). Philadelphia: Lea & Febiger.

PARCEL, G. S. (1989). *Basic emergency care of the sick and injured* (4th ed.). St. Louis: Mosby–Year Book.

PILLITTERI, A. P. (1992). *Maternal and child health nursing: Care of the childbearing and childrearing family.* Philadelphia: J. B. Lippincott.

PIPES, P. L., & TRAHMS, C. M. (1993). *Nutrition in infancy and childhood.* St. Louis: Mosby–Year Book.

PLESS, I. (1987). Morbidity and mortality among the young. In Hoekelman, R. A., Friedman, S. B., Nelson, N. M., & Seidel, H. M., (Eds.), *Primary pediatric care.* St. Louis: Mosby–Year Book.

PUBLIC HEALTH SERVICE. (1991). *Healthy people 2000: National health promotion and disease prevention objectives.* DHHS Publication No. (PHS) 91-50213. U. S. Department of Health & Human Services.

RALLISON, M. L. (1986). *Growth disorders in infants, children, and adolescents.* New York: Churchill Livingstone.

RIVARA, F. P., & BARBER, M. (1985). Demographic analysis of childhood pedestrian injuries. *Pediatrics, 76,* 375–381.

ROBERTS, J. (1993, February/March). Otitis media: Implications for early intervention. *Zero to Three.*

ROTHENBERG, M. B. (1983). The role of television in shaping attitudes of children. *Journal of the American Academy of Child Psychiatry, 22,* 86.

SATTER, E. (1986). *Child of mine.* Menlo Park, CA: Bull Publishing.

Stronger data link smoking to asthma in young. (1993, June 15). *The New York Times.*

STRUNKARD, A. J., HARRIS, J., PEDERSEN, N., & MCCLEARN, G. (1990). The body-mass index of twins who have been reared apart. *New England Journal of Medicine, 322* (21), 1483–1487.

STRUNKARD, A. J., SORENSEN, T., HANIS, C., TEASDALE, T., CHAKRABORTY, R., SCHULL, W., & SCHULSINGER, F. (1986). An adoption study of human obesity. *New England Journal of Medicine, 314* (4), 193–198.

TAYLOR, J. M., & TAYLOR, W. S. (1989). *Communicable disease and young children in group settings.* Boston: Little, Brown.

TUCHASCHERER, P. (1988). *TV interactive toys: The new high tech threat to children.* Bend, OR: Pinnaroo Publishing.

University of California at Berkeley Wellness Newsletter, 9. (1993, April).

U. S. DEPARTMENT OF AGRICULTURE. (1988). *Feeding infants: A guide for use in the child care food program.* Publication FNS-258. Washington, DC: Author, Food and Nutrition Service.

U. S. Department of Agriculture. (1989). *A planning guide for food service in child care centers.* Publication FNS-64. Washington, DC: Author, Food and Nutrition Service.

U. S. Department of Agriculture. (1990). *Preventing foodborne illness.* Home and Garden Bulletin Number 247. Washington, DC: Author, Food Safety and Inspection Service.

U. S. Department of Agriculture and U. S. Department of Health and Human Services. (1990). *Nutrition and your health: Dietary guidelines for Americans* (3rd ed.). Home and Garden Bulletin Number 232. Washington, DC: Author.

Whaley, L. F., & Wong, D. L. (1991). *Nursing care of infants and children* (4th ed.). St. Louis: Mosby–Year Book.

Whitener, C. B., & Keeling, M. H. (1984). *Nutrition education for young children: Strategies and activities.* Englewood Cliffs, NJ: Prentice-Hall.

Wotecki, C. E., & Thomas, P. R. (1992). *Eat for life.* Washington, DC: National Academy Press.

Wrecha, J. L., Dwyer, J. T., & Dunn-Strohecker, M. (1991, July-August). Nutrition and health services needs among the homeless. *Public Health Report, 106,* 364 + .

York, S. (1991). *Roots & wings: Affirming culture in early childhood programs.* St. Paul, MN: Toys 'n Things Press.

Index